Essentials of Toxicology for Health Protection

A handbook for field professionals

SECOND EDITION

Edited by

David Baker

Lakshman Karalliedde

Virginia Murray

Robert L. Maynard

Norman H.T. Parkinson

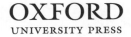

OXFORD
UNIVERSITY PRESS

OXFORD

UNIVERSITY PRESS

Great Clarendon Street, Oxford, OX2 6DP,
United Kingdom

Oxford University Press is a department of the University of Oxford.
It furthers the University's objective of excellence in research, scholarship,
and education by publishing worldwide. Oxford is a registered trade mark of
Oxford University Press in the UK and in certain other countries

© Health Protection Agency, 2008

© Oxford University Press, 2012

The moral rights of the authors have been asserted

First Edition published by Health Protection Agency in 2008
Second Edition published in 2012

Impression: 1

British Library Cataloguing in Publication Data
Data available

Library of Congress Cataloging in Publication Data
Data available

ISBN 978–0–19–965254–9

Printed in Great Britain on acid-free paper by
Ashford Colour Press Ltd, Gosport, Hampshire

Preface

David Baker
Virginia Murray
Norman H.T. Parkinson

The establishment of the United Kingdom Health Protection Agency (HPA) in 2003 created a new focus for skills development and training in environmental public health. At that time HPA found that most existing postgraduate courses in public health were generic in nature, and did not necessarily provide the depth of specialist health protection knowledge, skills, and competencies needed to enable HPA staff to fulfill their roles in advising and supporting local authorities, the UK National Health Service, the emergency services, and other agencies.

It was also recognized that there was a continuing need for specialist training of environmental public health personnel in other agencies, such as local authority environmental health practitioners and emergency planning officers.

Overall there was a requirement for a comprehensive and structured national approach to the provision of such education and training, within the framework of continuing professional development and a national scheme of accredited masters level modules and programmes in health protection.

Spiby (2006) developed a model of core competencies required of those working in environmental public health that reflected the need for a 'coming together of the knowledge and skills base of environmental science, public health, clinical toxicology and environmental epidemiology'.

Two main domains of competency were recognized:

1. Specialist environmental public health knowledge and skills, and

2. Generic organizational skills.

The first domain contains five areas of competency:

A. Toxicology

B. Environmental Science

C. Environmental Epidemiology

D. Risk Assessment and Risk Management

E. Environmental Public Health.

The second identified the following areas:

A. Teaching

B. Research

C. Management and Leadership.

The need for this book

In developing the *Essentials of Toxicology for Health Protection* module it became clear that there was no suitable text for students coming from a variety of specialist backgrounds. In a study of London health protection professionals by Paddock (2006), it was found that 89% (33/37) of respondents did not feel confident about their knowledge of toxicology, and most had had limited experience of chemical incidents.

The first edition of this book was therefore produced to meet the need for a single text that covered not only the basics of toxicology, but also its application to issues of topical concern such as contaminated land, food additives, water and air pollution, and emerging issues such as 'traditional' medicines.

The book was intended as both a course reader and a handbook for all health protection field professionals. Feedback from the students of the courses indicated that it was fulfilling a genuine need.

The current second edition of this book is a complete revision of the original material based upon input from readers and students of the King's College *Essentials of Toxicology for Health Protection* course. It contains new chapters on products of combustion and the increasingly important field of nanotoxicology. Also, having found during the course that some students from non-medical backgrounds lacked sufficient understanding of basic human sciences, an appendix covering basic medical concepts was included in the first edition. This was found to be very useful by many students and has been retained and revised in this edition. There is also a glossary of technical and medical terms.

Readership

This new edition is aimed at a wide range of professionals working in environmental public health, including health protection consultants, specialists and trainees, public health practitioners, environmental health practitioners, environmental scientists, and staff of the emergency services, the water and waste industries, and other industrial and regulatory bodies.

Most readers will be graduates with a good knowledge of public health sciences but the editors have tried to make the book accessible and readily understood by all field practitioners who require a basic understanding of the essentials of toxicology.

The scope of the book

As before, each chapter of the book has been written by an invited expert in specific topics covering a broad spectrum of toxicology.

Section 1. *Fundamentals of Toxicology* provides a general introduction to the subject and explains how toxicological information is derived.

Section 2. *Applications of Toxicology* addresses exposure assessment, susceptible populations, and the medical management of chemical incidents. It also provides valuable pointers to sources of toxicological data. The section on occupational toxicology considers the problems of toxic exposures in the workplace.

Section 3. *Environmental Toxicology* considers pollutants in air, water, and land, and food contaminants and additives.

Section 4. *A Review of Some Toxic Agents* addresses in detail a selection of important toxic agents: carbon monoxide; pesticides; heavy metals and trace elements as well as the emerging issues of traditional medicines and the deliberate release of toxic agents in warfare and terrorism. There are new chapters covering the toxic products of combustion and the increasingly important area of nanotoxicology.

We hope that this new edition of *Essentials of Toxicology for Health Protection* will prove useful not only to those requiring an understanding of toxicology as part of their work as health professionals but to all who seek a greater understanding of the impact of toxic substances on our society.

References

Paddock R. (2006) Chemical Incident Training Assessment Via a Health Professional Questionnaire. Chemical Hazards and Poisons Report (6):56–57. Health Protection Agency, UK.

Spiby J. (2006) Developing Competencies in Environmental Public Health. Chemical Hazards and Poisons Report (6):57–59. Health Protection Agency.

Acknowledgements

The editors wish to acknowledge the helpful comments and input from all the participants of the *Essentials of Toxicology for Health Protection* course held at King's College London over the past few years which have guided us in presenting the new edition of this book in a form most appropriate, relevant, and useful for future participants and other health professionals from different educational backgrounds.

The editors also thank Dr Jill Meara for reading through the text and making many helpful suggestions and also Karen Hogan and Anita Cooper for their invaluable secretarial help.

Contents

Section 4 **A Review of Some Toxic Agents**

Contributors

Editors

Professor David Baker
Emeritus Consultant Anaesthesiologist,
SAMU de Paris
Hôpital Necker – Enfants Malades, Paris,
France
Consultant Medical Toxicologist
Centre for Radiation, Chemical and
Environmental Hazards (London)
Health Protection Agency, United
Kingdom

Professor Lakshman Karalliedde
Visiting Senior Lecturer
Department of Public Health Sciences
School of Medicine, King's College
London, United Kingdom
Honorary Professor in Toxicology and
Clinical Pharmacology
Faculty of Medicine, Peradeniya
University, Sri Lanka

Professor Robert L. Maynard CBE
Honorary Professor of Environmental
Medicine
University of Birmingham, United
Kingdom
Honorary Principal Fellow
Department of Occupational and
Environmental Medicine
National Heart and Lung Institute,
London, United Kingdom

Professor Virginia Murray
Visiting Professor in Health Protection
Department of Public Health Sciences

School of Medicine, King's College,
London, United Kingdom
Consultant Toxicologist and Head of
Extreme Events Health Protection Section
Centre Radiation, Chemical and
Environmental Hazards (London)
Health Protection Agency,
United Kingdom

Norman H.T. Parkinson
Senior Fellow
Department of Public Health Sciences
King's College, London, United Kingdom

Assistant Editors

Anita Cooper
Section Administrator
Centre for Radiation, Chemical and
Environmental Hazards (London)
Health Protection Agency, United
Kingdom

Catherine Keshishian
Environmental Public Health Scientist
Centre for Radiation, Chemical and
Environmental Hazards (London)
Health Protection Agency, United
Kingdom

Karen Hogan
Training Administrator
Centre for Radiation, Chemical and
Environmental Hazards (London)
Health Protection Agency, United
Kingdom

Contributors

Dr Diane Benford
Senior Consultant Toxicologist
Food Standards Agency, United Kingdom

Nicholas Brooke
Environmental Public Health Scientist
Centre for Radiation, Chemical and
Environmental Hazards (London)
Health Protection Agency, United Kingdom

Dr Simon F.J. Clarke
Consultant Emergency Physician
Frimley Park NHS Foundation Trust,
United Kingdom
Honorary Consultant in Emergency
Response and Medical Toxicology
Centre for Radiation, Chemical and
Environmental Hazards (London)
Health Protection Agency, United Kingdom

Nicholas Castle
Consultant Nurse
Resuscitation & Emergency Care
Frimley Park NHS Foundation Trust,
United Kingdom
Department of Emergency Medical Care
and Rescue
Durban Institute of Technology, South
Africa

Professor James Kevin Chipman
Professor of Cell Toxicology
School of Biosciences
University of Birmingham,
United Kingdom

Dr Robin Fielder
Formerly Head of General Toxicology Unit
Centre for Radiation, Chemical and
Environmental Hazards (Chilton)
Health Protection Agency, United Kingdom

Dr John Gray
Consultant in Water Safety and Security
Formerly Deputy Chief Inspector
(Operations) with the Drink Water
Inspectorate, United Kingdom

Robie Kamanyire
Head of Environmental Hazards and
Emergencies London Unit
Centre for Radiation, Chemical and
Environmental Hazards (London)
Health Protection Agency, United Kingdom

Dr Ishani Kar-Purkayastha
Specialist Registrar in Public Health and
Clinical Toxicology
Centre for Radiation, Chemical and
Environmental Hazards (London)
Health Protection Agency, United Kingdom

Dr Gary Lau
Environmental Public Health Scientist
Centre for Radiation, Chemical and
Environmental Hazards (London)
Health Protection Agency, United Kingdom

Dr Timothy C. Marrs
Edentox Associates,
University of Central Lancashire,
National Poisons Information Service,
Birmingham Centre, UK

Dr Ovnair Sepai
Principal Toxicologist, Lead for Human
Biomonitoring
Centre for Radiation, Chemical and
Environmental Hazards (Chilton)
Health Protection Agency, United Kingdom

Dr Sohel Saikat
Environmental Public Health Scientist
Centre for Radiation, Chemical and
Environmental Hazards (London)
Health Protection Agency, United Kingdom

Professor Vicki Stone
Professor of Toxicology
School of Life Sciences
Heriot-Watt University, Edinburgh

Dr James C. Wakefield
Research Scientist
Centre for Radiation, Chemical and
Environmental Hazards (Chilton)
Health Protection Agency, United Kingdom

Dr James Wilson
Formerly Senior Environmental Scientist
Centre for Radiation, Chemical and
Environmental Hazards (London)
Health Protection Agency, United Kingdom

Section 1

Fundamentals of Toxicology

Chapter 1

Introduction to toxicology

Lakshman Karalliedde, David Baker,
and Virginia Murray

Learning outcomes

At the end of this chapter and any recommended reading the student should be able to:

1. explain the commonly used terms and definitions in toxicology;
2. explain the role of toxicology in health protection;
3. classify toxicological agents and toxins,
   a) based on physico-chemical properties, and
   b) based on types of toxic effects;
4. discuss and describe the routes of exposure;
5. describe the fate of toxins in the body;
6. describe the principles of risk assessment, and
7. apply acquired knowledge in the analysis and management of hazardous situations.

1.1 Introducing toxicology as a speciality

Simply and concisely, toxicology is the study of the nature and mechanism(s) of toxic effects of substances on living organisms and other biological systems. Toxic substances, commonly known as poisons, have the ability to cause harm or damage (toxicity) to living organisms. Poisons vary in their origin, chemical structure, and physical properties, and most importantly in the manner in which they cause toxicity.

Toxicology is thus essentially the science of poisons. It is also a speciality in medicine which studies the manner in which poisons cause harmful effects to living organisms, the amounts (doses) that cause such harm, the consequences of harm (e.g. disordered function, disease, death), the manner in which such harm can be prevented, and the methods by which the harmful effects can be treated.

It is necessary to be aware that harmful effects may not be immediately visible or detectable, for example the ability to cause cancers or abnormalities in the development or function of organs. These effects may only occur months or years after the poison has entered the living organism. The time lag before such effects are manifest is known as the lead time.

The discipline of toxicology has several essential components:

- Scientific and experimental toxicology: the study of basic toxic effects using animal and other models.

- Medical toxicology: the application of medical knowledge (diagnosis, treatment, and prevention) to patients who have had toxic exposures and to chemical population exposure assessments.

- Clinical toxicology: the direct provision of clinical care to poisoned patients.

- Occupational toxicology: the study of toxic effects as a direct consequence of an occupation.

- Environmental toxicology: the study of toxic effects on humans as a result of the release of toxic substances into the biosphere.

All of these approaches to toxicology are linked by the common pathway of the effects of chemical substances on the systems/organs within the human body, which enables an individual to maintain good health.

The dose is the critical factor in the consideration of the potential toxicity of a substance. This means the amount (e.g. weight or volume—milligrams, micrograms, litres, or millilitres—or the concentration in air in units such as milligrams per cubic metre (mg/m^3)) taken at a particular time (with a single exposure) or the amounts in total taken over a specified period of time. Thus the quantity of the substance and the duration during which the toxic exposure has taken place (orally, by skin contact (dermally), or by inhalation) are critical in the assessment of the harmful effects a substance would produce in the human body (Box 1.1).

1.1.1 History

The development of toxicology has a colourful history. Early cave dwellers knew through personal experience of the dangers that some plants could cause to humans. As early as 1500 BC there were written records of the effects of hemlock, opium, and animal poisons, which were used to smear arrows to kill or immobilize animals for food and clothing. The harmful effects of some heavy metals have also been recorded in ancient crypts associated with traditional medicines.

Poisons were used from the times of the origin of man to kill fellow human beings—be they enemies or relatives—or as punishment for crimes by the state or governing authorities. Historical figures who have been fatally poisoned include Socrates, Cleopatra, and Claudius. During the Renaissance, the study of poisons began to emerge as a science. Paracelsus (*c.* AD 1500) is considered by many to be the father of toxicology. In his writings he noted '*Sola dosis facit venenum*' (the dose of a substance determines its toxicity.)

Box 1.1 Toxicity is the association between dose and exposure

Dose (single or repeated) × exposure (single or repeated) = toxic effect

In other words, no substance is a poison by itself: it is the dose that makes a substance a poison. This observation laid the foundations for the concept of dose-response.

Alcohol (ethanol) provides a good example of the fundamental concept of Paracelsus. The non-toxic or beneficial dose of alcohol (social drinking) occurs at a blood level of 0.05%. In the short term a blood level of 0.1% is a toxic dose and a blood level of 0.5% is lethal. However, repeated short-term elevations of lower doses can lead to serious health effects that can have a range of long-term effects affecting a wide range of target organs, particularly the liver.

A Spanish physician, Matteo Orfila (1787–1853), considered by many to be the founder of toxicology, developed a description of the relationship between chemicals and the effects each of these chemicals produced in the human body. He studied the harmful changes a poison had on the organs of the human body and demonstrated the nature of damage caused by that particular poison.

1.2 The role of toxicology in health protection

Ill-health due to chemicals present in the environment has become a matter of concern in medical practice, particularly in industrialized countries but also in developing countries that may be using cheaper substances that are potentially more toxic and where regulations for the disposal of toxic waste are often lax.

Industrialization has greatly increased the manufacture and use of chemicals beneficial to humans in diverse ways and in diverse situations. However, they all have the potential to cause harm to human health. There are over 34 million chemicals which have been allocated Chemical Abstract Service (CAS) numbers. These are chemicals which are in existence in stable form (not intermediates). However, there is scant information on the potential toxicity or toxicology of the majority of these compounds (see Table 1.1).

Manufactured chemicals have specific uses and are intended to be used in a safe manner but there is always the potential for misuse, overuse, or inappropriate use. As most of these chemicals have the ability to cause toxicity or harm to human health, it is necessary to ensure that theys are properly manufactured, stored, and used, with appropriate safeguards at each stage. Some of the chemicals that have been introduced to destroy lower organisms (e.g. pesticides) are not selective in their toxicity and can adversely affect humans. It is necessary to ensure that workers involved in their production or manufacture

Table 1.1 Details of toxic chemical agents

Numbers of chemicals	Information source
Over 60,000,000 chemicals assigned CAS numbers	Chemical Abstract Service (March 2008)
160,014 commercially available chemicals	Chemfinder (Cambridge Soft Corporation)
About 70,000 chemicals routinely transported in UK	National Chemical Emergency Centre (UK)
About 500 new chemicals introduced to UK market each year	Health and Safety Executive (UK)
About 5000 chemicals have reliable medical toxicology information for acute and chronic exposure	Baxter (1991)

and those using them (e.g. those that spray insecticides or use them in sheep dipping) are supplied with clear practical guidance in the safe handling of the particular chemical or chemical mixtures. This may include the use of personal protective equipment (PPE), health and safety actions to take in the event of an accident, and occupational health and hygiene guidance to reduce possible exposure.

There are many scenarios where the potential of chemical substances to cause ill-health to exposed populations is a matter of public health protection concern. These include:

(1) The entry of chemicals to water supplies.

(2) The effects of toxic vapours contaminating the environment of public places and housing complexes.

(3) The presence of chemicals in land where buildings or recreational activities are planned—land contamination.

(4) Instances where there would be deliberate release of toxic chemicals, either during warfare or as an act of terrorism.

Toxicology is concerned with the study of the potential of these chemicals to cause harm to the various systems/organs of the human body, depending on the concentration, duration, and route of exposure. Thus the role of toxicology is to reduce or prevent ill-health due to exposure to chemicals. A related role is the research of, investigation into, and treatment of exposures, documenting them for other medical disciplines, public health, and government. Another aspect is to advise or provide governments or regulatory bodies with the appropriate information to facilitate policy formation and regulation in relation to the import, export, manufacture, and use of potentially harmful chemicals.

1.3 Types of toxic agents

Toxic agents can be classified according to their properties (Box 1.2) and their effects on human health (Box 1.3).

Box 1.2 Chemical classification based on physico-chemical properties

Physical agents	Chemical agents	Biological agents
Ionizing radiation	Human medicines	Vaccines
Non-ionizing radiation	Veterinary medicines	Allergens
Noise	Consumer products	Endotoxins
Vibration	Industrial chemicals	
Synthetic pesticides		
Food additives		
Chemicals of natural origin		
Chemical warfare agents		

Source: Data from Illing P. (2001) Toxicity and Risk; Context, Principles & Practice. Taylor & Francis.

Box 1.3 Chemical classification of toxic agents based on toxic effects

Class of substance	Toxic effects
Irritant	Causes inflammation of the skin and mucous membranes (skin, eyes, nose, or respiratory system). Skin (dermal) irritants cause irritant contact dermatitis (acute inflammation of the skin), symptoms of which include itching and skin changes ranging from reddening to blistering or ulceration. Examples: dilute solutions of acids, alkalis, and some organic solvents.
	Respiratory irritants cause injury to the nose, mouth, throat, and lungs. Materials that are very water soluble affect mainly the nose and throat. Less water-soluble materials act deeper in the lungs.
Corrosive	A material that can destroy human tissue. Includes both acids and alkalis and may be a solid, liquid, or gas.
Asphyxiant	A material that deprives tissues of oxygen and causes suffocation by displacing oxygen or interfering chemically with oxygen absorption, transport, or utilization.
	Simple: A simple asphyxiant displaces oxygen from the atmosphere, which prevents its absorption. Examples: carbon dioxide, methane, and nitrogen.
	Chemical: A chemical asphyxiant prevents the uptake of oxygen by cells. Examples: carbon monoxide combines with haemoglobin and prevents it transporting oxygen to the cells; cyanides prevent uptake of oxygen by cells by inhibiting the action of the cytochromes in the mitochondria that are necessary for this process.
Sensitizer	A chemical that causes an allergic reaction, such as urticaria or breathing problems. Examples: nickel, toluene di - isocyanate.
Systemic effect	A response to chemical exposure that affects the whole body. Systemic illnesses may cause symptoms in one or two areas, but the whole body is affected.
Anaesthetic	Depresses the central nervous system. Examples: ether, halogenated hydrocarbons.
Pulmonary toxin	Irritates or damages the lungs. Examples: asbestos, silica, chlorine, phosgene.
Neurotoxin	Affects the nervous system. Examples: mercury, lead, carbon disulphide.
Cardiotoxin	Affects the heart. Example: Atropa Belladonna (Deadly Nightshade), volatile anaesthetics.
Hepatotoxin	Causes liver damage. Example: ethyl alcohol, carbon tetrachloride, chloroform.
Haematopoietic toxin	Affects the function of the cellular components of blood. Examples: benzene, 2,4,6-trinitrotoluene, mustard gas.
Nephrotoxin	Causes kidney damage. Examples: chloroform, mercury, lead.
Carcinogen	A material that can cause cancer. Examples: asbestos, benzene, acrylonitrile, 1,2 napthphylamine, vinyl chloride monomer.
Mutagen	Anything that causes a change in the genetic material of a living cell. Many mutagens are also carcinogens.
Reproductive toxins	Causes impotence or sterility in men and women. Examples: lead, dibromodichloropropane.
Teratogen	A material that interferes with the developing embryo when a pregnant female is exposed to that substance. Examples: lead, thalidomide.

1.4 **Routes of exposure to toxic substances**

Figure 1.1 summarizes routes of exposure and pathways of absorption, distribution, and excretion of toxic chemicals in humans.

A potentially harmful substance may enter a living organism by the following routes:

A. **Ingestion (orally)**: This is entry by mouth, when absorption of the administered dose usually occurs in the gastrointestinal tract (i.e. stomach, intestines). On occasions, absorption may occur through the mucous membrane of the mouth, particularly

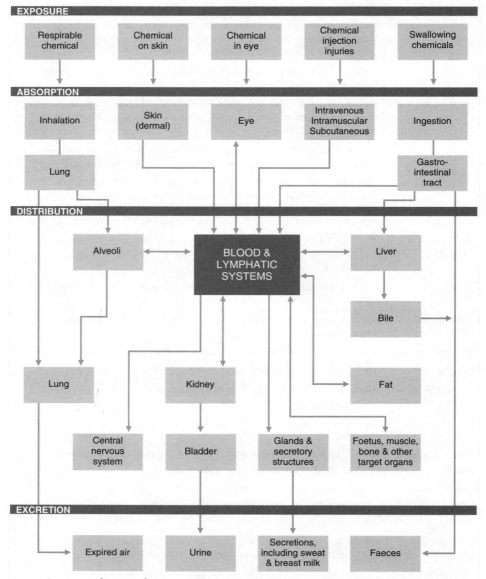

Fig. 1.1 Summary of routes of exposure, absorption, distribution, and excretion of toxins in the body.

under the tongue (sublingual). Some drugs, such as glyceryl trinitrate tablets, are prescribed for use sublingually.

B. **Injection**: This is direct administration into the bloodstream, usually into a vein (intravenous injection), but sometimes (rarely) into an artery. Injections can also be given into a muscle (intramuscular). The substance is distributed more slowly around the body after an intramuscular injection than after an intravenous injection, and the rate depends on the blood flow to the muscle. Substances are also injected into the skin (intradermally or subcutaneously), into joints (intra-articularly), or into the fluids and spaces surrounding certain structures or organs within the body (e.g. intrathecally, when a substance is injected into the space between the layers covering the spinal cord, which contains cerebrospinal fluid).

C. **Dermal**: One of the most common routes of exposure is where the potentially harmful substance is absorbed through the layers of the skin. In such instances, the rate of absorption into the body depends on the vehicle or substances in which the toxic substance is dissolved.

D. **Inhalation**: This is also a common route of exposure, particularly in occupational settings. The harmful substances are inhaled via the nose and breathing tubes (trachea, bronchi, and bronchioles) into the lung and finally into the thinly lined air cells (alveoli), which are surrounded by blood vessels. The harmful substances diffuse easily, depending on their chemical properties, across the thin lining of the alveoli into the bloodstream.

E. **Through mucous membranes**: Substances may enter the body following absorption through the mucous membrane of the rectum (through suppositories) or the vagina.

1.5 Fate of a toxic substance in the body

When a toxic substance enters the human body, it is subjected to a number of processes which result either in the total elimination of the toxic substance, with no ill-health, or in toxic ill-effects on the body, leading to the death of cells and failure of body systems. The fate of a toxic substance in a human body, including the metabolism, excretion, or binding to tissues, cells, or protein blood components, is referred to as **toxicokinetics**. This may be regarded as the way in which the body deals with the toxin. Similarly, when drugs used in the treatment of disease are considered, the term used is pharmacokinetics. How a toxic substance affects the cells and organs of the human body is known as **toxicodynamics**. The parallel term in drug therapy is pharmacodynamics.

For most toxic substances it is their chemical and physical properties which determine the manner in which they are handled by the human body and the nature of the harmful effects they produce. For example, if a substance is volatile (i.e. has a strong tendency to evaporate), it will usually be absorbed by inhalation. Substances which are lipophilic (dissolve easily in fat) will enter cells more easily than those that are essentially water soluble because cell membranes have high lipid (fat) contents and allow lipophilic molecules to pass through them easily. The size of a molecule (usually described in terms of molecular weight) influences both its absorption and excretion; large molecules are absorbed less readily than small molecules, and large molecules are poorly excreted by the kidneys. Equally the shape of a molecule is important in determining whether or not it will bind to specific controlling sites on the surface of body cells, known as receptors.

When a toxic substance enters the body by mouth (orally), it is usually absorbed from the gut (gastrointestinal system) and this may occur in the stomach or in the small or large intestines. Once absorbed, the toxic substance is taken by the portal veins from the intestine to the liver, where cellular enzymes can either make it non-toxic (inactivated) or more toxic. Detoxification is the more common occurrence. Amongst the enzymes present in the liver, the most important group is referred to as the cytochrome enzymes— notably the cytochrome P 450 enzymes. There are many components to this enzyme complex and each of the components has a specific affinity or ability to change the toxicity of the absorbed toxic agent. Amongst the cytochrome enzymes are CYP2C8 and CYP2C9. These enzymes are best known as metabolizers or inactivators of drugs used in the treatment of disease. What is important is that these enzymes can either increase or decrease their intrinsic activity, independently of the toxic substance. These changes to enzyme activity are predominantly brought about by other agents, usually drugs, but also by alcohol and cigarette smoking. Agents that increase the activity of the metabolizing enzymes are called inducers and those that decrease the activity of the enzymes are called inhibitors. It is important to know whether the metabolizing enzymes of the liver and other parts of the body are induced or inhibited by a toxic substance since this information will influence the potential adverse effects.

It is now established that there are agents that facilitate the absorption of substances by the gut (intestine) and also the excretion of substances from the gut, kidney, and bile. These are P-glycoproteins (P-gp) and organic anion transporting polypeptides (OATPs). These active transport systems play an important role in the elimination of drugs and also of toxins. These systems are affected by genetic factors and also by foods and drugs. The importance of these transport systems is that they influence the amount or concentration of a drug or toxic substance absorbed in the blood by altering absorption or loss (excretion) from the intestine, loss through the kidney (proximal renal tubular excretion), and loss through bile. The net result is that the amount of a substance that is available to produce effects in the human body by acting at various sites or target organs will be affected by the relative contributions of the transport agents that promote removal or exit/efflux (P-gp) and entry/influx (OATP mechanisms). What makes toxicity a complex process is that most agents that influence efflux and influx also affect the metabolizing enzymes in the liver, intestine, and kidney.

How chemicals may enter, be absorbed, become metabolized and are excreted from the body is illustrated in Figure 1.2 which illustrates the essentials of toxicodynamics and toxicokinetics.

As stated earlier, the toxic or harmful effect of a toxic substance on an organ is determined primarily by the dose of the toxic substance that reaches the susceptible organ (also known as the target organ—see Chapter 2). The dose of the toxic substance that reaches the target organ is known as the target dose.

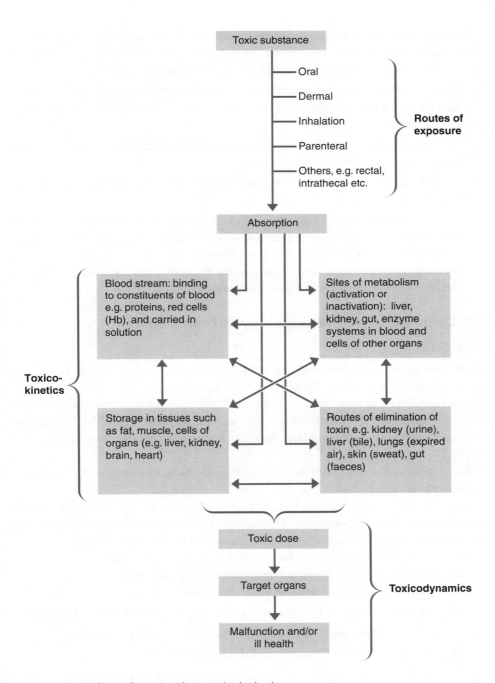

Fig. 1.2 Possible fates of a toxic substance in the body.

The target dose is determined not only by the dose which reaches the body by inhalation, ingestion, through the skin or by any other exposure route, but also by the processes that take place once the toxic substance is within the body. These processes include:

- the rate of absorption: this includes the rate of absorption from the gut if intake is oral, rate of breathing if intake is inhalational and blood flow if intake is by intramuscular or intravenous injection;

- binding to proteins (especially in the blood), to fat, and to other tissue, which may prevent the toxin from reaching the target organ;

- metabolism by processes usually in the liver, kidney, or intestine that turn the toxin into a less harmful chemical;

- excretion, that is, removal of the potentially toxic substance from the body through the urine, the faeces, in the bile or breath, or through the skin. It should be noted that there is a double excretion through the faeces. Through this route the bile from the liver containing detoxified metabolites is excreted and faeces will also contain toxic substances that have been ingested but not absorbed through the gut.

1.6 Commonly used terminology in toxicology

1.6.1 Dose

Dose: The amount of the potentially harmful substance that is administered at one time, i.e. the amount that enters the living organism at a given time.

Exposure dose: The amount of the potentially harmful substance that is present in the environment or the source from which the harmful substance enters the living organism, i.e. the amount of contaminated air, water, and liquids that come into contact with the body.

Absorbed dose: The exact amount of the potentially harmful substance that enters the living organism and is absorbed by it.

Administered dose: The amount of the potentially harmful substance that is given (administered) to a living organism. A harmful substance may be administered by mouth or injected or applied to the skin or given by inhalation as an aerosol or spray.

Target dose: The dose of a toxic substance that reaches a target organ.

Total dose: The sum of all individual doses, from all exposure routes.

Toxic dose (TD): The dose that causes adverse or harmful effects:

- TD_0 is the maximum dose that would cause harmful effects to 0% of the population
- TD_{10} is the dose that would cause harmful effects to 10% of the population
- TD_{50} is the dose that would cause harmful effects to 50% of the population
- TD_{90} is the dose that would cause harmful effects to 90% of the population.

Threshold dose: The dose at which a toxic effect is first observed or detected.

LD_{50}: The statistically derived dose at which 50% of individuals will be expected to die (based on experimental observations, mostly in animals). This is the most frequently used estimate of the toxicity of substances.

LC_{50}: The calculated concentration of a gas lethal to 50% of a group when exposure is inhalational. Occasionally LC_0 and LC_{10} are also used.

Effective dose (ED): This term indicates the effectiveness of a therapeutic substance. In most instances, the effective dose refers to a beneficial effect, for example relief of pain. For certain drugs, such as muscle-relaxing drugs, which are used in anaesthesia to facilitate surgery, the effective dose of a substance would cause an effect that would be harmful in an uncontrolled setting (i.e. would cause muscle paralysis and respiratory failure). Thus, depending on the nature of the use of a substance, the effective dose could either indicate a beneficial effect or a harmful effect. A dose effective for 0% of the population would be indicated as ED_0, a dose effective for 10% of the population would be ED_{10}, analogous to the toxic doses defined above.

The importance of knowing the toxic doses and the effective doses is that an indication of the safety of an agent may be expressed. If the effective dose and the toxic dose for 50% of the population are similar the margin of safety within which the agent can be used is very small. In contrast, if there is a relatively large difference between the effective dose and the toxic dose for 50% of the population, then the agent would be regarded as being safe, having a high safety margin.

1.6.2 Dose–response curve

This is a fundamental concept in the discipline of toxicology and has evolved from the speciality of pharmacology (the study of the effects, actions, and adverse effects of therapeutic agents and drugs used in the treatment or prevention of disease).

The dose–response curve describes graphically the size of the effect or response to a particular dose of a drug used in the treatment of disease or a chemical that has the potential to cause beneficial as well as harmful effects. It provides an indication of the doses at which a particular harmful effect is likely to occur, as well as information about when a maximal beneficial effect would occur.

A dose–response curve is calculated experimentally by using the lowest possible dose and noting the response, then increasing the dose at consistent increments and determining the response. These data are then plotted on a graph, as in Figure 1.3. On most dose–response curves the dose is plotted logarithmically along the *x*-axis, which gives the curve its characteristic sigmoidal shape.

The dose–response curve is a very valuable tool in understanding the health effects of toxins. If lethality is plotted against dose LD_{50} can be determined. This is the dose of a toxic substance that would cause death in 50% of the subjects exposed. In the case of a therapeutic drug the dose–response curve also provides information on what an effective dose or ED_{50} of a substance would be, that is the dose at which an effective response would be obtained in 50% of the subjects exposed In the case of a drug the comparison of the toxic and effective dose–response curves provides a valuable indication of safety, known as the therapeutic index. This is defined as the ratio LD_{50}/ED_{50}.

The dose–response curve also provides an indication of the potency of a drug, as shown in Figure 1.3. If the curve is shifted to the right, the drug has less potency than a drug with

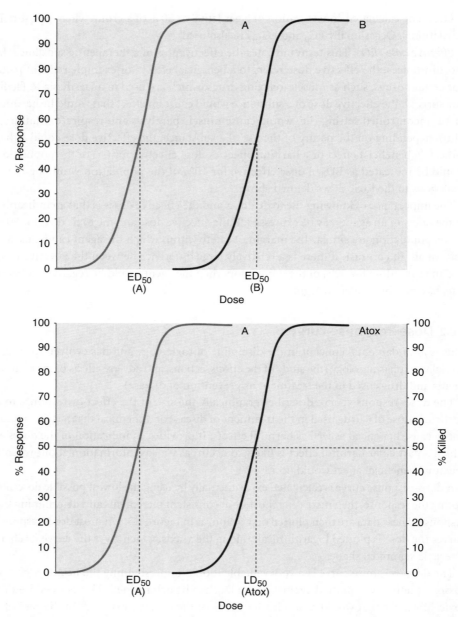

Fig. 1.3 Typical dose–response and toxicity curves. In the upper figure both curves show variation in response to increasing doses of two substances A and B. Substance A is more potent than substance B because the ED_{50} (the dose that is effective in 50% of the population) is lower. In the lower figure the right-hand curve shows the toxic effects of A and the ED_{50} becomes LD_{50} (the dose causing death in 50% of the population). The ratio LD_{50}/ED_{50} is known as the therapeutic index and indicates the margin of safety.

a curve shifted to the left. The other parameter indicated by the curve is efficacy, which may be defined as a measure of the ability of a drug to produce a specific effect.

1.6.3 Other toxicology terms

1.6.3.1 NOAEL/LOAEL

Following human and animal studies on substances that have the potential to cause harm, it is possible to obtain values or doses at which no harm would be expected. The highest level or dose at which there was no observed harmful or adverse effect is referred to as the **no o**bserved **a**dverse **e**ffect **l**evel (NOAEL). The lowest dose at which a harmful or adverse effect was observed is referred to as LOAEL, the **l**owest **o**bserved **a**dverse **e**ffect level. As with effective doses, the terms NOAEL and LOAEL are applicable for harmful or adverse effects as well as for desired therapeutic or clinical effects. In order to be more conservative, the terms no observed effect level (NOEL) or lowest observed effect level (LOEL) are sometimes used to reassure the public of actual toxicity with regard to substances that are frequently encountered in food or domestic use (e.g. pesticides).

1.6.3.2 Half-life

The elimination half-life of any toxin refers to the time taken for the quantity of a toxin in the body (or plasma concentration) to be reduced to half its original level through various elimination processes. Half-life may vary between individuals (and species) depending on genetic make-up, state of health, age, and several other factors.

Half-life is an important concept as it provides a timescale during which toxic effects may decrease due to the fall in concentration in the body, and also indicates how long a toxin is likely to remain within the body. The half-life is also dependent on the site in which the toxin is found. For example, with cadmium, the half-life in the blood is measured in days (approximately 5–7 days), whilst in the liver it is measured in months (7 months or so) and in the kidney it is measured in years (15 years or so). It should be noted, however, that certain toxic effects, such as the capacity to cause mutations in cells, may persist long after the original toxin has been eliminated from the body. An example of this is poisoning from mustard gas (see Chapter 17).

1.7 An introduction to risk assessment

A **hazard** is something (in the context of this book, a chemical) with the potential to cause an adverse, or 'harmful', effect. **Harm** may be physiological or psychological. While psychological harm is a controversial issue, it should not be underestimated when potential risks are communicated to the public by the media.

Risk is usually defined as a measure of the likelihood of the occurrence of a particular adverse effect. It is therefore a probability, a number between 0 and 1, such as 10^{-6}. This might sometimes be expressed as a ratio, e.g. one in a million. Risk may also be defined as the product of the probability of the adverse effect and the magnitude of the effect.

The public usually seeks an assurance of zero risk, but this is rarely, if ever, possible. A lifetime risk of 10^{-6} (about the same as the risk of being struck by lightning) is often considered to be 'acceptable', but public acceptability depends on whether the risk arises from a hazard that is perceived as elective/pleasurable or beneficial, such as alcohol consumption or antibiotic medication, or imposed/involuntary, such as emissions from factory chimneys. The public more readily accept risk when it is a matter of personal choice (such as smoking) rather than an imposition (food additives, water treatment chemicals). There are also more concerns about the exposure of perceived at-risk groups in the population such as children.

'Safe' and 'dangerous' are imprecise and subjective terms that are best avoided because they are likely to be interpreted very differently by different people. There is no substance that can be considered completely 'safe' In lay terms safe/dangerous risks could be defined as 'risks which are acceptable/unacceptable to a particular individual or population'.

Relative risk is the ratio of the risk of a particular adverse effect in the population exposed to the hazard to the risk of this effect to the population not exposed to the hazard.

1.7.1 Risk management

In managing risk, setting standards, and communicating with the public about hazards, public health agencies and regulatory bodies must balance the risks of a hazardous agent with its benefits to society. To do this effectively, they need sound **risk assessment** procedures, and these must be based on good toxicological data. Unfortunately, there are many uncertainties and gaps in scientific knowledge and these have to be taken into account. Some of the methods and models used involve multiple assumptions, approximations and scientific judgements. Somewhat arbitrary 'safety factors' and 'uncertainty factors' may have been used in the extrapolation from animal studies to humans, in allowing for variations in animal and human populations, and in extrapolating risk estimates calculated on small samples. These factors are all open to challenge. Risk assessment is certainly *not* an exact science (Cooper et al. 2007)!

Most models for risk assessment are based on the following four steps:

(1) hazard identification;

(2) dose–response assessment;

(3) exposure assessment;

(4) risk characterization.

Hazard identification, in the context of chemicals, involves the extensive search of the published scientific evidence of adverse effects associated with exposure to the particular chemical and similar substances. More than one hazard may result from exposure to a single substance.

The **dose–response assessment** involves detailed study of the available toxicological data with an understanding of the dose–response curve, threshold effects, elimination half-lives, LD_{50}s, NOAEL, and LOEL. There may also be other relevant data, such as epidemiological studies and incident reports.

Exposure assessment includes a study of the frequency, duration, magnitude, concentrations, and doses of chemicals to which humans will be exposed. This includes the possible pathways and routes of entry, noting that an individual may be exposed to more than one source of the chemical, or more than one chemical. Exposures may be both acute and chronic.

Risk characterization brings together the other three steps to estimate risk and make recommendations for **risk management**, including the setting of exposure standards and industrial codes of practice. It will include a detailed consideration and analysis of the robustness of the toxicological data, the appropriateness of analytical procedures and modelling techniques, and the reasonableness of assumptions, including the magnitude of uncertainty and safety factors. With so many assumptions, uncertainties, and subjectivity outcomes are generally very conservative.

1.8 Conclusions

This chapter has given a general introduction to toxicology and its terminology. In the following sections the applications of toxicology in specific situations are considered in terms of the situations where exposure to toxins may occur, the damage toxins cause to the systems of the body, and the medical management required.

1.9 References

Baxter PJ. (1991) Major chemical disasters. *BMJ* **302**(6768):61–62.

Cooper R, Fielder R, Jefferson R, Meara J R, Smith K R, Stather J W. (2007) Comparison of Processes and Procedures for Deriving Exposure Criteria for the Protection of Human Health: Chemicals, Ionising Radiation and Non-ionising Radiation (RCE-3). Health Protection Agency: **ISBN**: 978-0-85951-599-3 Available at http://www.hpa.org.uk/Publications/Radiation/DocumentsOfTheHPA/RCE03ComparisonofProcessesandProceduresRCE3/.

Illing P. (2001) *Toxicity and Risk; Context, Principles & Practice*. Taylor & Francis, London & New York.

1.10 Further reading

Ballantyne B, Marrs T, Syversen T. (eds) (1999) *General and Applied Toxicology*. 2nd edition. MacMillan, London.

Gilbert SG. (2004) *A Small Dose of Toxicology: The Health Effects of Common Chemicals*. CRC Press, New York.

Klaassen C. (ed.) (1996) *Casarett & Doull's Toxicology: The Basic Science of Poisons*. 5th edition. McGraw Hill, New York.

National Research Council (1983) *Risk Assessment in the Federal Government: Managing the Process*. National Academy Press, Washington DC, USA.

NRPB (2004) In Terms of Risk: Report of a Seminar to Help Define Important Terms Used in Communicating about Risk to the Public 2004. Available at http://www.hpa.org.uk/Publications/Radiation/NPRBArchive/DocumentsOfTheNRPB/Absd1504/.

http://www.hpa.org.uk/Publications/Radiation/DocumentsOfTheHPA/RCE03ComparisonofProcesses-andProceduresRCE3/.

Rodricks JV. (2007) *Calculated Risks*. Cambridge University Press, Cambridge.

Timbrell JA. (2002) *Introduction to Toxicology*. 3rd edition, Taylor and Francis, London.

1.11 Useful internet links

Chemical Abstract Service: www.cas.org.
Chemfinder: http://chemfinder.cambridgesoft.com/.
Health and Safety Executive: www.hse.gov.uk.
National Chemical Emergency Centre: www.the-ncec.com.

Chapter 2

Target organs

David Baker

Learning outcomes

At the end of this chapter and any recommended reading the student should be able to:

1. explain the normal structure and function of the human body systems, and the concept of target organs and systems;

2. explain, with the use of examples, how dysfunction in each of the important body systems may occur following exposure to toxic agents;

3. describe and discuss the manifestations of dysfunction in each of the important systems of the human body;

4. demonstrate awareness of the common chemicals causing ill-health and the associated symptoms and signs, and

5. apply acquired knowledge in the analysis and management of hazardous situations.

2.1 Body systems and target organs

The human body can be regarded as a number of systems operating in parallel with each other to maintain normal life. The nervous, cardiovascular (heart and circulation), digestive and urinary systems are examples. Each system contains a number of key structures which are essential for its function. These are vulnerable to injury by foreign substances and in this context are termed target organs, since they are the clinical target of the toxic assault. Toxic substances do not affect all target organs equally. Differences can be explained generally in terms of different susceptibilities or higher concentrations of the toxic substance or its metabolites at the site of action.

Target organs and systems will be discussed in this chapter using a standardized approach. This is:

1. the definition of the system in terms of its anatomy and physiology;

2. a brief description of normal function;

3. the medical expressions of abnormal function.

Note that medical signs and symptoms (Box 2.1) are the final pathway of many biochemical processes that are covered by the science of biochemical toxicology. Some examples are provided in Table 2.1.

Box 2.1 Definition of signs and symptoms

A symptom is an indication of disease, illness, injury, or that something is not right in the body. Symptoms are felt or noticed by a person, but may not easily be noticed by anyone else. For example chills, weakness, aching, shortness of breath, and a cough may be symptoms of pneumonia.

A sign is also an indication that something is not right in the body. But signs are defined as things that can be seen by a doctor, nurse, or other healthcare professional. Fever, rapid breathing rate, and abnormal breathing sounds heard through a stethoscope may be signs of pneumonia.

Our analysis will include key chemical changes (for example in the disturbance of chemical transmitters in the body) but will emphasize the overall somatic disturbances produced by toxic exposure. This is the role of medical toxicology.

The normal function of each target organ and system will only be presented in outline. The non-medical reader is advised to read this chapter in conjunction with the basic medical concepts appendix, where the normal function of the body is described in more detail.

2.2 The nervous system

The nervous system controls all aspects of body function. It consists of the central nervous system, which includes the brain and spinal cord, and the peripheral nervous system, which transmits messages from the brain to all the organs of the body and also receives messages about the body and the environment from the sensory system. The nervous system is made up of nerve cells and fibres, which carry electrical impulses from the brain, and also chemical transmitters, which amplify these electrical impulses at relay stations called synapses. The peripheral nervous system is subdivided into the voluntary system, which controls all muscular movements, and the autonomic system, which is not under voluntary control and ensures the function of all organs except the muscular system. There are many chemical transmitters involved in both the central and peripheral nervous systems. One of the most important is acetylcholine, which is the chemical transmitter between the end of the motor nerves and muscle fibres, and also in the end synapses of the parasympathetic nervous system.

2.2.1 The central nervous system

Key target: brain (including cerebrum, cerebellum hindbrain)

2.2.1.1 Normal function

The brain is a complex array of neurons grouped to control motor, sensory, posture and higher cognitive function. The brainstem controls much of the essential physiological activity, such as breathing. See section A4.1 of the appendix for more information on the normal functioning of the central nervous system.

Table 2.1 Some signs and symptoms, and possible chemical causes

Signs and symptoms	Substance
Alopecia (loss of hair on the head)	Arsenic, barium, bismuth, borates, carbon monoxide, gold compounds, lead, thallium
Amnesia (forgetfulness)	Bromides, ethanol, hydrogen sulphide, methyl bromide
Aplastic anaemia (lack of blood cells due to failure of production by the bone marrow)	Arsine, benzene, carbon tetrachloride, lindane, nitrous oxide
Chest pain (heart-attack like)	Cocaine, carbon disulphide
Convulsions (fits)	Carbon monoxide, cyanide, lindane, opiates, arsenic, lead
Diplopia (double vision)	Bromide, carbomates, carbon dioxide, carbon disulphide, carbon monoxide, ethanol, ethylene glycol, lead, mercury, methanol, methyl bromide, methyl chloride, organophosphate, trichloroethylene, triethyl tin
Eye irritation or redness	Chlorine, ammonia, crowd control agents (e.g. CS gas)
Fasciculations (visible involuntary twitching of muscles)	Organophosphates, carbamates
Hallucinations	Methyl chloride, some solvents, thiocyanates
Hearing loss	Bromates, carbon monoxide aminoglycosides such as kanyamycin, toluene
Haematemesis (vomiting of blood)	Acetone, acids, alkalis fluoride, formaldehyde, hypochlorites, phosphorus
Miosis (small or pinpoint pupils)	Acetone, carbamates, organophosphates, opiates
Mydriasis (large or dilated pupils)	Atropine, carbon dioxide, chloroform, cyanide, ethyl bromide, ethylene glycol, fluoride, methyl bromide, thallium, toluene
Nystagmus (jerky movements of the eyeball)	Arsenic, carbon disulphide, carbon monoxide, ethanol, ethyl bromide, ethylene glycol, gold compounds, manganese, methyl bromide, methyl chloride, organophosphates, toluene, xylene
Photophobia (intolerance of or hypersensitivity to light by the eyes)	Bromide, carbon dioxide, methanol, mercury
Skin irritation with defatting of skin and/or rashes	Acids, alkalis, alcohols, chlorinated compounds, ketones, nickel, phenol, trichloroethylene
Tinnitus (ringing in the ears)	Arsenic, ethanol, trimethyltin, toluene
Upper respiratory tract irritation	Oxides of nitrogen, oxides of sulphur, crowd control agents (e.g. CS gas)
Wheezing	Chlorine, phosgene, oxides of nitrogen or sulphur, organophosphates (inhalation), acrolein, asbestos, chromium, hydrogen sulphide, nickel, nitrogen dioxide, ozone, silica

2.2.1.2 Abnormal function

The cells of the central nervous system are very vulnerable to both direct and indirect actions of toxic substances, in particular lack of oxygen. Toxic effects on the central nervous system have profound effects on both higher cerebral functions, including consciousness, and the movements of the body and their control. Examples of manifestations of toxic damage or injury to the brain are coma, convulsions, impairment of memory, and disturbances in gait.

2.2.2 The peripheral nervous system

Key targets: sensory, autonomic, and motor nerves

2.2.2.1 Normal function

Sensory nerves. These are of varying sizes and transmit information about the body, such as pain and temperature, from special receptors.

Acetylcholine. Acetylcholine (ACh) is a major chemical neurotransmitter. It is released in small packets or vesicles from the nerve terminal and creates an amplified electrical response on the other side of the synapse. When this has happened the transmitter is very rapidly broken down by an enzyme called acetyl cholinesterase, which is present throughout the cholinergic nervous system.

The cholinergic nervous system. The control of the concentration of ACh is essential to the functioning of the cholinergic nervous system. This includes:

- Voluntary motor nerves: acetylcholine transmission at the neuromuscular junction.

- The autonomic nervous system: this comprises the parasympathetic and sympathetic systems. The parasympathetic system uses ACh as a transmitter whereas the sympathetic system uses noradrenaline. In general, the sympathetic system causes stimulation of body systems whereas the parasympathetic has the reverse effect. A good example is found in the nervous control of the heart.

Cholinergic effects are divided into muscarinic and nicotinic effects. These terms were derived from the actions of the compounds muscarine and nicotine during the early research into the cholinergic system. Muscarinic ACh receptors are found in the gut, heart (vagus), and pupil and accommodation muscles of the eye. The actions are blocked by atropine. Nicotinic ACh receptors control the voluntary nerve endings to muscle.

See section A4.2 of the appendix for more information on the normal functioning of the peripheral nervous system.

2.2.2.2 Abnormal function

Failure of the peripheral nervous system affects both the sensory and motor systems. The autonomic nervous system can also be affected. A direct toxic effect on nerves is called toxic neuropathy. This causes failure of nerve transmission due to the dysfunction of motor and large sensory fibres.

Failure of nerve conduction Toxic neuropathy affects nerve conduction by toxic effects on the myelin sheath of the nerve, which is essential for normal function. Many chemical substances cause damage to nerve conduction, a condition called toxic peripheral neuropathy. Examples include some organophosphate pesticides (no longer used in the UK) and industrial substances such as lead, thallium, triorthocresyl phosphate, carbon disulphide, n-hexane, and acrylamide. Nerve conduction can also be affected by toxins. These are naturally occurring compounds that are produced by plant, animal, and aquatic organisms and bacteria. Examples are tetrodotoxin and saxitoxin, which interrupt nerve conduction by blocking essential sodium ion channels in the nerve.

Finally, nerve conduction can also be interrupted by an inappropriate immune reaction from the body. An example is the Guillain Barré syndrome (acute idiopathic inflammatory polyneuropathy), which may be caused by a cell-mediated hypersensitivity (see section 2.8.2 in this chapter).

Failure of chemical transmission If the acetyl cholinesterase at the cholinergic synapses is reduced, this causes an **increase** in ACh at cholinergic synapses, causing poisoning by over-stimulation of the voluntary and autonomic cholinergic nervous systems. This is the case in organophosphate (OP) and carbamate pesticide poisoning. Increases in the ACh concentrations cause effects at all cholinergic synapses, both peripheral and in the central nervous system (Box 2.2). Further information on OP poisoning is found in Chapter 15 on pesticides.

Cholinergic synaptic transmission can also be affected by a **reduction** in the release of ACh from the nerve terminal. This is the case following intoxication by botulinum toxin as a result of food poisoning. In botulism there is muscle weakness, but the clinical picture is one of failure of cholinergic transmission rather than overstimulation, as in the case of pesticide poisoning. The muscles of the shoulder girdle, respiration and swallowing are particularly affected, creating the classic syndrome of botulism. The onset of paralysis is much slower than with anticholinesterase poisoning and the weakness can be overcome to an extent in the early stages by extra voluntary effort.

Alterations in transmission of impulses at cholinergic synapses have far-reaching effects on other body systems and target organs which are considered below.

2.3 The cardiovascular system (the heart and circulatory system)

Blood is transported through the body via a continuous system of blood vessels. This comprises arteries, capillaries, and veins. Arteries carry oxygenated blood away from the

Box 2.2 Classic signs and symptoms of organophosphate anticholinesterase poisoning

- Pinpoint pupils
- Excess salivation
- Lachrymation
- Urination
- Involuntary defecation
- Muscle fasciculation and paralysis
- Central nervous stimulation and fitting
- Failure of respiratory control in the brain stem

heart into capillaries supplying tissue cells. Veins collect the blood from the capillary bed and carry it back to the heart. The main purpose of blood flow through body tissues is to deliver oxygen and nutrients to cells and to remove waste products. Circulation outside the heart and pulmonary circulation is known as the systemic circulation.

The cardiovascular system forms the transport system of the body. As such it carries:

1. oxygen from the lungs to the tissues;
2. carbon dioxide from the tissues to the lungs so that it may be eliminated during the expiration phase of breathing;
3. food components from the digestive tract to cells to provide nutrition for growth and energy;
4. waste products from cells to the kidneys to be removed in the urine;
5. hormones from the glands that produce them (endocrine glands) to other organs;
6. heat produced in other parts of the body to the skin so that the surplus heat can be given off.

2.3.1 The heart

Key target: heart (including nerve control, conducting system, heart muscle)

2.3.1.1 Normal function

See section A5.1 of the appendix for information on the normal functioning of the heart.

2.3.1.2 Abnormal function

Direct toxic effects The heart beats by contraction of its individual muscle fibres or myocytes. The heart muscle itself can be a target for toxic attack. Toxic effects may occur on:

- the **conducting system**. The conducting system carries impulses from the sino atrial node in the atria through to the ventricles and controls the timing and synchronization of the heart. Interference with this system may be either direct or indirect and lead to irregular heart beats or dysrhythmias.
- **myocytes** (the heart muscle fibres). Many toxic substances, such as inhaled hydrocarbons, including volatile anaesthetics, produce atrial and ventricular ectopic beats. These compounds can also affect conduction at the junction between the atria and the ventricles.

Indirect toxic effects These are mediated via the autonomic nervous system. The heart is controlled by the vagus nerve, which is cholinergic, and also by sympathetic nerves. Stimulation of these nerves causes:

- slowing of the heart via stimulation of the vagus nerve muscarinic receptors. This is most commonly seen in pesticide poisoning. The effect can be blocked by atropine, which causes block of the vagal impulses. In poisoning by *Atropa belladonna* (deadly nightshade), tachycardia is a key sign.
- acceleration of the heart via stimulation of the sympathetic nervous system and noradrenaline receptors. This is seen in cases of adrenaline overdose.

2.3.2 The arterial system

Key targets: veins, arteries

2.3.2.1 Normal function

See section A5.2 of the appendix for information on the normal functioning of the arterial system.

2.3.2.2 Abnormal function

In addition to the heart, the arterial system can be a target organ. Both constriction and dilation of vessels can occur, as with ergotamine poisoning (from the fungus *Claviceps purpurea*) and vasodilators such as nitrites and alcohol. Vasodilation is also a beneficial effect in the coronary arteries when drugs such as glyceryl trinitrate are used. Overdose with vasodilators can lead to a major fall in blood pressure.

2.4 The gastrointestinal system

Key targets: small intestine, large intestine, stomach, mouth, oesophagus

2.4.1 Normal function

See section A7 of the appendix for information on the normal functioning of the gastrointestinal system.

2.4.2 Abnormal function

Toxic actions on the gut mediated by nervous control The gut is controlled by the parasympathetic autonomic nervous system. Toxic effects begin at the mouth, where there may be hyper- and hypo-salivation caused by OP and atropine, respectively. Intestinal motility may be increased by OP or carbamate pesticides, leading to colic and diarrhoea, or decreased by morphine and related compounds.

Direct effects
Direct effects on the gut may occur through:

+ corrosive effects on the stomach (e.g. by acids);
+ acute toxic effects on gut absorption (e.g. by enterotoxins), and
+ chronic effects such as neoplasia and carcinoma of the mouth, tongue, and oesophagus (e.g. by chillies, betel nuts, tobacco).

2.5 The liver

Key target: liver

2.5.1 Normal function

The liver is a major target organ which is associated with the alimentary system. It has an essential role in the body in nutrition and in the removal of a number of toxic substances. Normal biochemical detoxification functions are part of balanced excretion and detoxification.

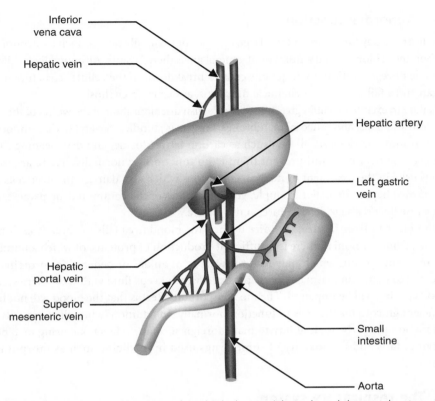

Inferior
vena cava

Hepatic vein

Hepatic artery

Left gastric
vein

Hepatic
portal vein

Superior
mesenteric vein

Small
intestine

Aorta

Fig. 2.1 Blood supply to the liver comes from both the arterial supply and the portal system from the gut. Courtesy of Timbrell (2002).

The liver is a key target organ for many toxic substances because:

- it receives a rich blood supply from the gut, where toxic substances may be absorbed (Figure 2.1);
- it has a unique structure based upon hepatocytes which are metabolically very active, and
- it has a major metabolic and excretory role.

The liver receives 25% of the blood supply from the heart. Toxic substances absorbed from the gut are transported directly to the liver which is therefore the first target organ exposed after the gut itself. Hepatocytes are cells that make up most of the structure of the liver and are very metabolically active. Normally they are involved in many essential biochemical processes, such as removal of nitrogen as urea, synthesis of glycogen as a glucose store, and lipid metabolism. Many toxic substances inhibit protein synthesis because of their action in the liver. Apart from metabolizing the body's own waste products, the liver also has a key role in removing external poisons (xenobiotics) such as carbon tetrachloride and alcohol. Carbon tetrachloride blocks protein synthesis through a free radical mechanism.

See section A8 of the appendix for more information on the normal functioning of the liver, including the excretion of bilirubin.

2.5.2 Abnormal function

The liver is a key target organ for a large number of toxic substances, such as alcohol and carbon tetrachloride, and a number of general anaesthetic agents. Although liver cells are capable of regeneration, toxic actions cause a breakdown in the cellular structure of the organ and a failure of its biochemical functions, as occurs in cirrhosis.

Failure to excrete bilirubin gives rise to a yellowish discolouration of the whites of the eyes, the skin and nails, and mucosal membranes, known as jaundice. Several toxic compounds such as some pesticides, solvents such as carbon tetrachloride, and dry-cleaning fluids damage the liver cells and prevent them from functioning normally. There are many drugs used in the treatment of medical conditions which also damage the liver cells and are termed hepatotoxic. For example, very high doses of the common drug paracetamol can cause liver damage, liver failure, and jaundice.

Therefore in **liver failure**, jaundice occurs, the blood urea falls (as urea is no longer formed from ammonia), there is insufficient production of proteins, of which albumin is the most important, which may lead to swelling of ankles or oedema (as proteins are essential to maintain plasma osmotic pressure, which keeps fluid within capillaries), and blood clotting will be impaired. The most important effect is that the blood will not have sufficient glucose for the cells to function normally. In addition, when the liver cells fail to function properly, their ability to make foreign substances less toxic using metabolic enzymes fails and the toxicity of some drugs used in medicine such as morphine is increased.

2.6 The respiratory system

Respiration involves the transport of oxygen from the atmosphere to the cells of the body and carbon dioxide in the opposite direction. It is divided into external respiration, which describes the passage of oxygen to the red blood cells in the lung sacs (alveoli), and internal respiration, which describes the carriage of oxygen from the lungs to the cells and carbon dioxide back to the lungs.

2.6.1 External respiration

Key targets: brainstem (respiratory control), lungs (airways and alveoli)

2.6.1.1 Normal function

The respiratory centres in the mid brain and brain stem control cyclical active inflation and passive deflation of the lungs, commonly called breathing. Breathing ensures the passage of oxygen to alveoli and removal of carbon dioxide to the atmosphere via upper and lower airways. The exchange of gases to and from the blood in the alveoli takes place at the alveolar membrane (where internal respiration starts). Normal external respiration is designed to maintain the oxygen and carbon dioxide levels in the blood at levels that allow the body cells to operate normally. The thin membrane between the alveolar sac and the pulmonary capillary is highly vulnerable to direct attack by inhaled toxic compounds.

In addition to its role in exchanging gases, the pulmonary capillary bed acts as an active filtration and detoxification system. This makes it very vulnerable to a number of toxic substances.

See section A6 of the appendix for more information on the normal functioning of the external respiratory system.

2.6.1.2 Abnormal function

Depression of central control of respiration Many toxic substances act on the brain and depress breathing, for example opioids and organophosphates. This leads to a build up of carbon dioxide in the lung sacs and in the blood, causing hypoxia and respiratory acidosis. If breathing depression is not reversed or artificial ventilation started, the hypoxia will worsen followed by cardiac arrest (stoppage of the heart beat due to lack of oxygen to the heart muscle).

Effects on lung parenchymal tissue The air sacs of the lung (the alveoli) have many functions apart from exchange of gases. They are very fragile and susceptible to toxic attack either directly by inhaled toxic substances, for example phosgene, causing toxic pulmonary oedema, or indirectly as a result of filtering out toxic substances such as paraquat (a weedicide), which attacks the pulmonary capillaries.

The outcome of toxic effects on the lung and airways may be divided into:

◆ acute respiratory failure. Failure of breathing and ventilation of the lungs leads to increasing carbon dioxide levels and hypoxia in the alveoli. Hypoxic myocardium leads to secondary cardiac arrest.

◆ chronic respiratory failure where there is fibrosis and adult respiratory distress syndrome;

◆ neoplastic effects, including carcinoma of the bronchus from tobacco smoke and mesothelioma from the inhalation of asbestos particles.

2.6.2 Blood and internal respiration

Key targets: red blood cells, mitochondria

2.6.2.1 Normal function

The red cells of the blood contain haemoglobin, which carries oxygen from the lungs to the cells of the body. In the cells, oxygen is delivered to the mitochondria—intracellular structures that are the 'powerhouses' of the cells. Mitochondria have cytochromes, which generate energy in the form of adenosine triphosphate (ATP) and ensure normal life function.

2.6.2.2 Abnormal function

Red cells Haemoglobin can be a target if the oxygen-carrying capacity is blocked by toxic gases. This is the case in carbon monoxide (CO) poisoning, where CO combines with haemoglobin more easily than oxygen (see Chapter 13 on carbon monoxide for more information).

Mitochondria The other key targets in the internal respiratory system are the mitochondria in the cells. The interaction of oxygen with the cytochrome system in the mitochondria can be blocked, leading to a failure of internal respiration. This is the case in cyanide poisoning and is also thought to follow exposure to carbon monoxide.

2.7 The haemopoietic system

Key targets: bone marrow, white blood cells

2.7.1 Normal function

The bone marrow is the source of both white and red blood cells. White cells have an essential role in inflammatory, coagulation, and immune function. Red cells, as noted above, have an essential role in the carriage of oxygen.

See section A5.3 of the appendix for more information on the normal functioning of the haemopoietic system.

2.7.2 Abnormal function

The bone marrow is a major target for many toxic substances. As a result of failure of generation of new cells, there may be failure of the red cell system (aplastic anaemia) and failure of the white cell system, causing both overwhelming infection due to absence of granulocytes (agranulocytosis) and failure of the immune system from a total reduction on the white cell count, including lymphocytes (pancytopaenia).

Failure of cellular development can be caused by a number of toxic agents, including drugs, mustard gas, and heavy metals. Toxic effects on the bone marrow may cause generation of a type of cancer called leukaemia.

2.8 The immune system

Key targets: immune reactions are mediated by a number of cell types in the body, each of which may be regarded as a system in its own right

2.8.1 Normal function

See section A11 of the appendix for information on the normal functioning of the immune system.

2.8.2 Abnormal function

Toxic reactions involving the immune systems may involve direct or indirect immunotoxicity.

Direct immunotoxicity Direct effects are caused by immunosuppression or immunostimulation. In immunosuppression, the toxic agent reduces the activity of the immune system, causing malfunction. This may be due to an effect on a target organ of the system such as the thymus, which produces B lymphocytes, or the bone marrow, which produces blood cells. Examples of substances causing immunosuppression include dioxin and polonium 210.

In immunostimulation, the immune system is stimulated by a challenge from an administered protein that is similar to that found in humans but is treated by the body as an antigen. Examples include drugs derived from recombinant DNA.

Indirect immunotoxicity Indirect effects include hypersensitivity, allergic reactions, and autoimmunity. These are caused by a toxic substance presenting a challenge to the immune system as an antigen. Most toxic chemicals are too small to do this and have to combine with a larger molecule such as a protein (called a hapten) to be able to create an effective foreign antigen.

Immune reactions which result from indirect immunotoxicity are classified as type 1–type 4.

Type 1 reactions
In these reactions, free antigen fixes to IgE antibody, which then attacks mast cells, releasing vasodilator mediators (e.g. 5-hydroxytryptamine). This type of reaction causes acute collapse following a priori sensitization (anaphylaxis) or pulmonary sensitization/asthma-like effects. Examples include drugs such as penicillins or industrial compounds such as toluene di-isocyanate.

Type 2 reactions
In these reactions there is a break-up of the cell (cytolysis). Antigen bound to cell membranes associates with free antibodies (IgG, IgM, IgA) to produce agglutination with complement fixation and cell lysis. Examples include drugs such as aminopyrine.

Type 3 reactions
In these reactions there is free soluble antigen in excess of antibody, which combines with free antibody. This then causes a complex known as precipitin to be deposited in the inner lining of blood vessels (the vascular endothelium). An example is the drug hydralazine, sometimes used for the emergency reduction of high blood pressure.

Type 4 reactions
These are cell-mediated hypersensitivity reactions in which part of the cell membrane becomes an antigen. This then combines with killer T lymphocytes, causing death of cells. An example is the familiar nickel contact dermatitis.

2.9 The urinary system

Key targets: kidney, bladder

2.9.1 Normal function

See section A9 of the appendix for information on the normal functioning of the kidney.

2.9.2 Abnormal function

The kidney, like the liver, has a high blood supply and metabolic activity, but its major role is in excretion of urea and maintenance of the somatic acid–base balance, rather than metabolic activity. Substances that cause kidney damage are those which are concentrated in the organ. This accumulation may produce acute and chronic toxic effects on the tubule system, which can lead to acute and chronic renal failure. Examples include heavy metals such as ionized mercury, lead, and the antibiotic gentamycin.

In addition to the kidney, other parts of the urinary tract may be the target of toxic attack, such as the neoplastic effects on the bladder of aniline dyes.

2.10 The reproductive system

Key targets: ovaries, testes, oocytes, spermatozonia

2.10.1 Normal function

The reproductive system comprises the ovaries in the female, which release oocytes, and spermatozonia in the male, which are involved in fertilization of the oocyte.

2.10.2 Abnormal function

Toxic effects on the reproductive system may be manifest as effects on fertility or on development of offspring. Impaired fertility has been noted with chemicals but only following prolonged exposure, whereas developmental toxicity may occur following a single exposure. Teratogenicity, the production of congenital malformations following exposure during pregnancy, is a particular concern. The actions of certain drugs as teratogens have been well known since the problem was first highlighted by thalidomide in the 1960s. The foetus is very vulnerable to teratogenic effects during the first trimester of pregnancy, and during the second and third trimesters drugs may affect growth and functional development. Since the 1960s, detailed rules for prescribing have been published (see British National Formulary 2011), which underline the fact that drugs should only be prescribed in pregnancy if the expected benefit to the mother is thought to be greater than the risk to the foetus. All drugs should be avoided if possible during the first trimester except those for life-threatening conditions.

2.11 The epithelial system

Key targets: eyes, skin and mucous membranes

2.11.1 Normal function

The epithelial system includes the skin, the mucous membranes, which line the mouth, and the eyes. The system has an important role in the body's defences. The skin is not usually regarded as an organ (some consider the skin to be the largest organ in the body) but it should nevertheless be included as a toxic target organ. The skin, like the liver and the alimentary tract, is constantly under renewal, with new cells being created in the dermis and migrating outwards to the epidermis. This process of cellular renewal is a target for a number of toxic pathways.

2.11.2 Abnormal function

The eye The pupil is a good indicator of toxic effects. The constrictor muscle is cholinergic (muscarinic) and is affected by toxic agents with an action on this system. Pupils may be small (pinpoint pupils) as a result of OP pesticide poisoning. Morphine also causes the same result but by a different central mechanism.

The pupil may also be dilated following a blocking of the constrictor muscle, as is the case following atropine (deadly nightshade) poisoning. The cornea of the eye is very vulnerable to attack by corrosive and vesicant agents such as mustard gas (see Chapter 17 on chemical warfare agents).

The skin A number of toxins have a direct effect on the skin. Ricin acts due to a generalized inhibition of protein synthesis and leads to a multiple breakdown of body organ systems prior to death (multiple organ dysfunction syndrome). *Clostridium welchii*, the organism causing gas gangrene, produces dramatic clinical effects on the skin with widespread necrosis due to its action on phospholipase C. There are possibilities that this toxin may have been considered for development as an agent of chemical warfare.

There may be direct toxic effects on the DNA structure of the dermis, leading to DNA cross-linking, which is thought to be behind the vesicant effects of mustard gas. Mustard gas causes damage presenting as severe blistering and ulceration. Equally, corrosive substances such as strong acids cause chemical burning by direct chemical disruption of the cells.

The skin may also be affected by allergic reactions, leading to eczema–dermatitis (as in the case of nickel contact—see type 4 immune reactions above) and also urticaria produced as a result of a generalized allergic reaction.

2.12 Conclusions

A wide variety of toxic substances produce a medical expression through target organs and systems in the body. Effects may be considered in terms of normal and abnormal function of organs and systems. Expression of toxicity may be acute and chronic through pharmacological, physiological, immune, teratogenic and carcinogenic mechanisms. Target organ toxicology provides the link between biochemical toxicology and overall signs and symptoms which are the end stage of toxic exposure.

2.13 References

British National Formulary. (2011) www.bnf.org.
Timbrell J. (2002) *Introduction to Toxicology*. 3rd edition. CRC Press, London.

2.14 Further reading

Lu FC, Kacew S. (2002) *Lu's Basic Toxicology*. 4th edition. Taylor and Francis, London.

Chapter 3

Experimental methods for investigating the safety of chemicals

James Kevin Chipman

Learning outcomes

At the end of this chapter and any recommended reading the student should be able to:

1. explain how toxicological data are produced and be able to describe some of the methods used;

2. understand the limitations of data obtained *in vitro* and *in vivo* and understand how toxicological data can be used in the setting of standards;

3. take a critical and analytical approach to the application of standards set by advisory and regulatory bodies;

4. apply acquired knowledge in the analysis and management of hazardous chemicals, and

5. have awareness of new directions and strategies for chemical safety assessment.

3.1 Introduction

For most chemicals there are little, if any, sound human data from experience in use on which to base an assessment of their effects on health. Thus such assessments must be based largely on results of toxicological studies *in vitro* and in animals.

In order to draw up a toxicological profile of a chemical, information from the following studies would generally be expected:

+ acute toxicity;
+ skin and eye irritancy and skin sensitization;
+ repeated dose toxicity (28 or 90 days);
+ mutagenicity (and hence potential carcinogenicity);
+ toxicity to the reproductive system;
+ additional specific studies such as on the immune and neurological systems;
+ chronic toxicity and carcinogenicity bioassays (as required), and
+ absorption, distribution, metabolism and excretion (ADME).

In addition, an understanding of the mechanisms of toxicity is always valuable in helping to determine modes of action and in the extrapolation process so as to determine the
relevance of *in vitro* and animal studies to humans and also to understand the shape of the
dose–response curve.

3.1.1 *In vitro* alternatives to the use of animals

Every effort is made to ensure that tests are carried out using the minimum number of
animals and with minimal distress to the test animals. EU member states have a legal
requirement in this respect, often referred to in the animal welfare context as the 3Rs
(Reduction, Refinement and Replacement when practical and validated alternatives are
available) (Council Directive 1986). However, despite considerable research into alternatives to animals, there are only a few specific areas of toxicology where reliable predictive
toxicity may be obtained *in vitro*, although these systems can aid compound prioritiza-
tion. Assessing mutagenic potential or local effects such as skin and eye irritation represent particular areas in which *in vitro* prediction is valuable. *In vitro* systems based largely
on cell culture have limitations for prediction of whole organism toxicity, particularly
because of the lack of inter-tissue interactions and difficulties in mimicking repeat exposures over long periods of time. Nevertheless there has been successful application of such
systems in two major ways. The first is in the context of helping to understand the mechanisms of toxicity and the relevance of toxic mechanisms to humans. In the case of various non-genotoxic carcinogens that appear to have a specific effect in rodent liver at
relatively high dose levels, this has been particularly successful (Roberts et al. 2003).
The second way is the initial screening of potential toxicity. This can rank-order toxic
potential in early drug development, for example, and thereby prioritize chemicals for
further analyses. This method has had benefit in relation to the 3Rs in toxicity testing.
Early screening can also be aided by *in silico* analysis of quantitative structure activity
relationships (QSARs), but these 'expert systems' are only as good as the databases that
describe them.

3.1.2 Integration of new technologies and the move to a greater investigative approach

New technologies relating to, for example, imaging, genomics, and stem cell biology are
increasingly being integrated into toxicological assessments both *in vitro* and *in vivo*, with
an emphasis on understanding the mechanisms of toxic responses and the dose–response
relationships. Mechanistic toxicology has been strongly aided by the 'omic' technologies
that allow unbiased analysis of the changes in the levels of many thousands of mRNA,
protein, and metabolite levels in cells or tissues in response to chemical agents. Thus the
field of toxicogenomics is now well established (Blomme et al. 2009; Van Hummelen and
Sasaki 2010). Although not regularly integrated into safety assessment and utilized for
regulatory decisions, such information can be useful as a supplement in the interpretation
of biological responses and bioinformatic approaches, such as reverse engineering, and
recognition of adverse effect pathways from molecular networks has great potential for
the detection of toxicity and the development of molecular biomarkers. It is emerging

that characteristic profiles of gene expression changes, for example, arise from different classes of chemicals, thus providing the potential to detect *in vitro* pathways that lead to, for example, hepatoxicity or cancer through non-genotoxic versus genotoxic mechanisms (e.g. Ellinger-Ziegelbauer et al. 2005; Blomme et al. 2009). Extensive interactions between toxicologists, mathematicians, and computer scientists are needed to enhance this field further. Overall, there is a move towards a greater emphasis on an investigative and comprehensive approach to chemical safety in which toxicological responses can be defined mechanistically whilst optimizing the use of *in vitro* systems (Li 2004; Andersen and Krewski 2010; Kimber et al. 2011).

3.1.3 Integration of information on absorption, distribution, metabolism, and excretion

An important part of the safety assessment of chemicals is the analysis of metabolism and pharmacokinetics. This allows predictions of the levels of a chemical or its derivatives that may be achieved in the body and assist in the extrapolation of toxicity data from animals to humans. Although metabolism of chemicals generally results in detoxication and greater water solubility to aid excretion, some chemicals can be metabolically activated into more toxic intermediates. It is essential in toxicity assessment to be able to determine the relative ability of animal models and humans to produce such toxic metabolites. This is aided by the ability to express different human and animal enzymes in cell culture through heterologous gene expression systems. This approach is also highly valuable in determining which human enzymes are responsible for the metabolism of foreign compounds since this information is needed to determine the likelihood of inter-individual differences in toxicity that may result from there being polymorphic forms of various drug-metabolizing enzymes (Johansson and Ingelman-Sundberg 2011; Pinto and Dolan 2011).

3.1.4 Animal general toxicity

For assessing general toxicological effects of single and repeated exposure to chemicals, animals have to be used in laboratory studies.

General toxicology aims to survey any possible effects of chemicals predominantly in rodent (e.g. rat) and non-rodent (e.g. dog) animal models, and is conducted in conjunction with assessment of ADME studies. A short single-dose acute study aims to detect severe general toxicity. Originally this was in the form of an LD_{50} test but these were not very informative and did not comply with the principles of the 3Rs. Clinical observations and animal growth and food consumption are particularly informative in studies of general toxicity, although there are more specific functional analyses that can test, for example, for neurotoxicity. Indirect information on target organ toxicity can come from analysis of blood and urine for indicators of toxicity. The elevation of transaminases in the blood, for example, can be useful in the detection of liver toxicity. A further example is the detection of effects on the bone marrow through the haematological analysis of quantitative and qualitative changes in erythrocytes and leucocytes in the peripheral blood. Detailed histopathology is then completed on tissues from organs at the end of the study in addition to assessment of the weight and macroscopic appearance of organs. Additional analyses are also completed to assess for effects on specific organs or systems such as the immune, reproductive, and neurological systems. In some cases, depending on the routes of anticipated exposure, dermal and respiratory toxicity analyses are also needed.

The key guidelines for methods for investigating the toxic effects of chemicals are those produced under the auspices of the Chemicals Programme of the Organisation of Economic Cooperation and Development (see OECD Guidelines). These are internationally recognized and have done much to reduce the needless duplication of studies to satisfy specific requirements of different countries and regulatory agencies. They are updated with regard to both advances in science and animal welfare considerations. Figure 3.1 gives a summary of the general strategy of drug identification and development through preclinical safety assessment into clinical trials and Figure 3.2 gives a more focused summary of the specific strategy for preclinical safety assessment. The methodology of the latter is given in more detail throughout this chapter.

3.2 Methodology within preclinical safety assessment

3.2.1 Acute toxicity

The aim of an acute toxicity study is to investigate effects following a single exposure for a period of up to 24 hours using the oral, dermal, or inhalation route as appropriate. Normally three dose levels are used except for relatively non-toxic compounds, when a single limit dose is acceptable (2000 mg/kg bodyweight/day by the oral route). Current methods place emphasis on noting signs of toxicity (onset and duration) rather than calculating an LD_{50} value, as used in the past. One approach, first proposed by a working group of the British Toxicology Society and now recognized as an OECD guideline, does not use death as an endpoint, the maximum dose level used being designed to produce less severe signs of toxicity. In all acute toxicity studies animals are observed carefully during the first 4 hours post dosing, and then on a daily basis for at least 14 days (van den Heuval et al. 1990). Animals are subject to autopsy at termination, when all gross pathological changes are recorded together with microscopic examination of organs showing gross pathology.

Results from these studies are used for hazard assessment and for classification of chemicals on the basis of acute toxicity.

3.2.2 Repeated dose toxicity study (28- or 90-day)

Assessment of the possible health hazards arising from repeated exposure is usually determined by either a 28-day or a 90-day study in rodents. There are OECD guidelines for such studies by the oral, dermal, and inhalation routes. The 28-day study is designed for use with chemicals for which a 90-day study would not be warranted, for example because of low production volume and limited potential for human exposure. Many aspects of the 28-day and 90-day studies are common. At least three dose levels are used, together with a control group, using 5 males and 5 females per group in the 28-day study, and double these numbers in the 90-day study.

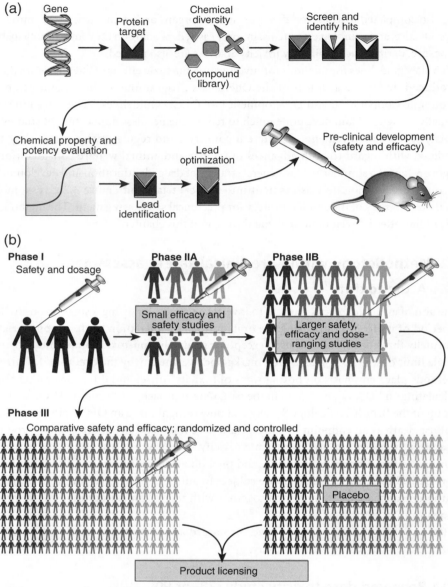

Fig. 3.1 The overall strategy of drug identification and safety assessment. Reprinted with permission from Macmillan Publishers Ltd: Allen D. Roses, Pharmacogenetics and drug development: the path to safer and more effective drugs, Nature Reviews Genetics, 5(9), 645–656 ©2004, Nature Publishing Group.

In addition to the general clinical observations daily (with observations for morbidity and mortality twice daily), haematology and clinical chemistry studies are carried out at the end of the test period, with interim samples being taken in the 90-day study during the course of the experiment. Full gross autopsies are carried out on all animals at the end

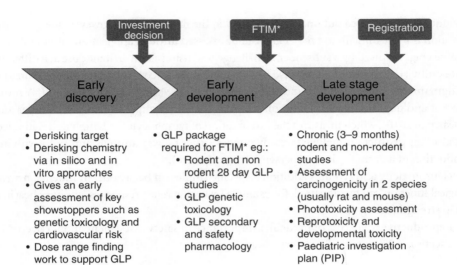

Fig. 3.2 The stages of preclinical drug safety evaluation. The investment decision refers to the decision that a candidate drug has the right properties for development. FTIM, first time in man. Courtesy of Professor Ruth Roberts.

of the exposure period, with a wide range of organs/tissues being observed (slightly more in the 90-day study than in the 28-day). Full histopathology is carried out on all the preserved organs/tissues from animals in the high-dose group, together with tissue/organs from any group showing gross lesions.

For most chemicals information will not be available from studies of longer than 90 days, and for risk assessment purposes there will be a need to extrapolate the findings to more prolonged exposure. It is recognized that the 'No Observable Adverse Effect Level' (NOAEL) in a 90-day study in the rat may be higher than the NOAEL for the same endpoint in a chronic or essentially lifetime study (2 years in the rat), although this is not always the case and the variability is often in the range two- to fourfold (Doe et al. 2006). Account for this is made in extrapolation to essentially lifetime exposure by dividing the NOAEL by an additional uncertainty factor.

There are a number of specific studies that are required beyond the tests described above to provide a more complete assessment of compound safety. Immunotoxicity as expressed by, for example, hypersensitivity is one particular area in which general pathology is not sufficient as an assessment due to the complex interaction of a range of tissues such as the thymus, bone marrow, spleen, and other lymphoid tissues. Although relevant information is obtained from analysis of lymphoid tissues and peripheral blood, additional assessment of any changes in, for example, cytokine release and antibody production enhances the confidence in safety assessment. Allergic sensitization is a feature of dermal toxicity carried out in addition to tests of irritancy. Both skin and eye irritancy can be assessed *in vitro* with good prediction. It is now possible by consideration of various factors (physico-chemical properties and results from validated *in vitro* tests for skin corrosivity or irritation of eyes) to predict severe effects without using live animals. The animal tests are used to confirm lack of irritancy or to grade mild to moderate irritation. If there is any doubt, tests are carried out on a single animal in the first instance. However, allergic sensitization is more difficult to predict and can be assessed through application into the skin of guinea pigs followed by a subsequent 'challenge test' using a non-irritant dose at a different site and visualization of a response in skin compared to controls. The Magnusson and Kligmann maximization test and the Buehler test are variants of this method. A more recent and quantitative test commonly used is the local lymph node assay (Kimber and Dearman 2010), which measures the proliferation of lymphocytes in lymph nodes in mice. It also has distinct animal welfare advantages (use of fewer animals and not involving induction of a dermal (skin) hypersensitivity response).

Neurotoxicity also requires additional specific studies on behaviour. In rodents, neurological function can be measured, for example by testing reflex responses, auditory hearing, grip strength, and gait.

Reproductive toxicity is of particular importance in safety assessment and is covered in the section 3.2.3.

3.2.3 Toxicity to the reproductive system

Considerable research is ongoing into the development of *in vitro* methods to investigate aspects of reproductive toxicology (Bremer et al. 2005). Clearly, in view of the complexities of mammalian reproduction, it is most unlikely that complete replacement of animal tests will be possible. *In vitro* tests are likely, however, to play an important role in identifying priority compounds for investigating reproductive toxicology in animal studies and also for studies on the mechanism of action. One particularly promising area such as that originally developed by Scholz et al. (1999) is the development of *in vitro* assays for embryotoxicity. This embryonic stem cell test (EST) can measure differentiation of stem cells into cardiac myocytes (heart muscle cells), neuronal cells (nerve cells or neurones), and chondrocytes (bone forming cells). Although some indication of potential impact on development can be obtained *in vitro*, such as in the use of whole embryo cultures, these are sufficiently reliable only as pre-screens. Reproductive toxicity is often assessed in rabbits as well as in rodents. These tests include assessment of fertility, organogenesis, teratogenicity, and perinatal and postnatal development. Measurements in reproductive toxicity studies will include assessment of food intake, bodyweight, litter size, and weight. Fertility studies include measurement of the time for successful mating, and sperm counts and mobility are measured coupled with histological analyses of testis. Embryonic toxicity can be detected to some extent by measurement of foetal weight but more sophisticated analyses include examination for skeletal or visceral abnormalities. For later stages of development, the survival and gain of weight of pups is assessed and features of subsequent development are monitored, including physical development (e.g opening of eyes), sensory development (e.g. reflex reactions and learning ability), and sexual organ development (e.g. vaginal opening). These tests can be multigenerational.

There are two different endpoints on which reproductive toxicity data are necessary: (i) developmental toxicity, namely the effects on developing offspring following *in utero* (inside the uterus) or neonatal exposure, and (ii) effects on reproduction over one or more generations, including effects on male and female fertility. There are established animal studies (see Woolley 2003) to provide information on these endpoints which are described below.

3.2.3.1 Developmental toxicity

An OECD guideline is available for measuring prenatal developmental toxicity. Pregnant animals (rodents or rabbits) are exposed from implantation to one day prior to the day of scheduled sacrifice, which is as close as possible to the normal day of delivery. Shortly before caesarean section, the animals are killed and uteri and contents are evaluated for soft tissue and skeletal effects. Key endpoints noted are death of offspring, resorptions, embryonic development, foetal growth, morphological variations, and malformations. This study does not detect functional deficiencies in the offspring, but these are covered in the studies considered later. At least three dose levels and a concurrent control group are used. The top dose is chosen to produce some evidence of toxicity in the maternal animal, the intermediate dose to have minimal observable toxic effects, and the lowest dose no maternal or developmental toxicity.

3.2.3.2 One- and two-generation reproductive toxicity studies

These studies are designed to provide general information on the effect of the test substance on the integrity and performance of the male and female reproductive systems, including gonadal function, the oestrous cycle, mating behaviour, conception, gestation, parturition, lactation and weaning, and growth and development of offspring. The test substance is given in graduated doses to several groups of male and female animals. Males of the parent generation are dosed for at least one complete spermatogenic cycle (c. 70 days in rats, the preferred species) prior to mating. Females are dosed for several oestrogenic cycles before mating. The test substance is then administered to the parental animals throughout the mating period and the resultant pregnancies, and through weaning of first generation (F1) offspring. In the second generation study the administration of substance is continued during their growth into adulthood, mating, and production of the F2 generation, until the F2 is weaned. Clinical observations and pathology and histopathology examinations at autopsy are carried out with emphasis on the integrity and performance of reproduction and growth, and development of offspring.

3.2.4 Mutagenicity and non-genotoxic carcinogens

Mutagenicity is the ability to induce a permanent change in the amount or structure of the genetic material (DNA) in an organism or cell. Data on the mutagenicity of a chemical are important both because of concerns about heritable effects due to mutations in germ cells and also as a screen for potential carcinogenicity that may arise as a result of mutations in somatic cells.

The crucial role of mutagenesis in carcinogenicity is well established. It is known that certain dominant inherited conditions predispose to cancer, for example mutation of the Rb gene (a tumour suppressor gene) can predispose to retinoblastoma (a malignant tumour within the eye). Furthermore, a large proportion of cancers contain mutated oncogenes such as the Ras gene or mutated or deleted tumour suppressor genes such as Rb or p53. Indeed, there is a good correlation between chemicals shown to be *in vivo* mutagens and those that are carcinogenic in animal bioassays. This evidence was suffi- cient for the Committee on Mutagenicity of Chemicals in Food, Consumer Products and the Environment (COM) and its sister committee on carcinogenicity (COC) in the UK to conclude that it is prudent to assume that a chemical capable of producing *in vivo* somatic mutations in mammals has carcinogenic potential (Department of Health 1991). There are some chemicals, however, that have been shown to cause tumours in animal models despite a lack of mutagenicity. These non-genotoxic carcinogens are often species- and tissue- specific (e.g. rodent liver) and appear in many cases to exhibit a threshold dose for effect since their mechanisms often involve a disruption of the balance between cell proliferation and cell death through apoptosis (Roberts et al. 2003). In some cases these are mediated through hormonal effects. Thus many non-genotoxic animal carcinogens appear not to have relevance for humans at achievable exposure levels. This is a particularly good example of where an understanding of the mechanisms of toxicity is important in safety assessment and extrapolation from animals to humans.

3.2.5 Strategy for investigating mutagenicity of chemicals

There are well-established strategies for the investigation of the mutagenicity of chemicals (Department of Health 2000). The overall strategy involves initial testing *in vitro* to assess the mutagenic potential of a chemical, followed by *in vivo* testing of compounds with positive *in vitro* responses to assess whether the activity can be expressed in somatic cells in the whole animal, and finally, and if appropriate, testing in germ cells *in vivo* for potential heritable effects.

Before any testing is carried out, some idea as to whether a chemical would be expected to have any mutagenic potential can be provided by considering whether it has any structural alerts for DNA reactivity (Ashby and Paton 1993) and this can be aided by QSARs.

3.2.5.1 Stage 1: *In vitro* testing

The initial testing *in vitro* needs to cover all three types of mutation, namely gene muta- tion (alterations in DNA involving a single gene), clastogenicity (structural chromosome aberrations), and aneuploidy (numerical chromosome aberrations). These tests are lim- ited in number and are well validated and informative. Three tests are recommended and for each there are OECD test guidelines. Testing is carried out in the presence and absence of an appropriate exogenous metabolic activation system (a liver subcellular fraction) since it is known that many chemical mutagens are only able to react with DNA following metabolic activation by enzymes present in the liver and other tissues of mammals. At least three to five concentrations are generally used, the highest producing evidence of cytotoxicity. Negative and appropriate positive controls are used and all results con- firmed in an independent experiment.

Bacterial reverse mutation test The bacterial assay for gene mutation uses *Salmonella typhimurium* (this test was developed by Bruce Ames and is often referred to as the Ames test).

The strains of Salmonella used all require an essential amino acid, histidine, for growth due to a pre-existing mutation. A reverse mutation to the wild type caused by the chemical being tested removes this dependency and the revertant bacteria may be detected by growth on medium deficient in histidine. A range of bacterial strains are available that measure different types of point mutation (both base-pair or frame-shift, resulting in addition or deletion of one or a few DNA base pairs).

Test for clastogenicity and indications of aneuploidy in mammalian cells The second *in vitro* test is for clastogenicity and indications of aneugenicity. The most widely used approach is metaphase analysis for chromosome damage. Either cell lines, for example, Chinese hamster ovary (CHO) or primary cultures of human lymphocytes (stimulated by addition of a mitogen) are used. At least three concentrations of test compound are investigated at levels up to those causing marked cytotoxicity (effects on mitotic index) and cells are harvested for metaphase analysis to detect chromosome damage after treatment. Some information on aneugenicity is obtained from the incidence of hyperdiploidy, polyploidy, or modification of the mitotic index.

An alternative approach commonly used is the *in vitro* micronucleus test. This assay measures micronuclei in interphase cells rather than chromosome aberrations in metaphase cells. Micronuclei may arise either from acentric fragments (chromosome fragments lacking a centromere) or whole chromosomes that are unable to migrate with the rest of the chromosomes during the anaphase of cell division. The assay thus detects both clastogenic and aneugenic chemicals.

Mammalian cell gene mutation test A third *in vitro* test commonly used is the mouse lymphoma assay. This has the advantage of detecting both gene mutations and chromosome aberrations. The assay uses L5178Y mouse lymphoma cells and measures mutations at the thymidine kinase (TK) locus. Cells deficient in TK due to the mutation are resistant to the cytotoxic effects of the pyrimidine analogue trifluorothymidine (TFT). TK proficient cells are sensitive to TFT. Thus mutant cells are able to proliferate in the presence of TFT whereas normal cells are not.

Implication of results from the three *in vitro* tests In the event of evidence of mutagenicity in any of the above tests, assessment *in vivo* is required to determine if the mutagenic potential can be manifested in the body. Sometimes mutagenicity of *in vitro* mutagens is not evident in the body, for example due to lack of absorption or differences in metabolism. In addition, for compounds where there is likely to be high, or moderate and prolonged levels of direct exposure to humans (e.g. most medicines), then an *in vivo* assay is also recommended even in the absence of effects *in vitro*.

3.2.5.2 Stage 2: *In vivo* studies in somatic cells

For compounds that have shown mutagenic potential *in vitro*, negative results from *in vivo* studies from at least two different tissues will be needed before adequate reassurance is provided that activity cannot be expressed *in vivo*. Generally, three dose levels are used up to the maximum tolerated dose (i.e. one that produces signs of toxicity such that higher dose levels would be expected to produce lethality) together with a negative and positive control group. In most cases the first test will involve the bone marrow as this tissue is readily exposed to chemicals present in the blood.

Most data are available from the bone marrow micronucleus test and there is an OECD guideline outlining the methodology. The micronucleus test indirectly detects clastogens by measuring micronuclei in newly formed cells in the bone marrow. It can identify the induction of both structural and numerical aberrations by appropriate staining techniques. The mouse is usually used for this assay since in this species (unlike the rat) the spleen does not remove micronucleated erythrocytes. Alternatively, chromosome damage in bone marrow may be measured by metaphase analysis. The rat is usually used for these studies and bone marrow is harvested at two different time intervals.

A negative result in these *in vivo* tests will not be sufficient to conclude that the compound is not an *in vivo* mutagen and further testing in at least one additional tissue *in vivo* will be required. The appropriate additional test needs to be considered on a case-by-case basis, taking into account the structure of the compound, its toxicokinetic properties, the results from earlier studies, and the available expertise. There are a number of possible approaches that the COM document (Department of Health 2000) recommends be considered. One useful assay is one that detects unscheduled DNA synthesis (UDS) in liver cells obtained from treated animals. This is important as the liver is often the most appropriate second tissue in which to investigate *in vivo* activity, largely because this organ maximizes the opportunity for metabolic activation. The endpoint UDS is indicative of DNA damage and subsequent repair. Studies are usually in the rat. UDS is measured by determining the uptake of labelled nucleotides, usually tritiated thymidine by autoradiography, in liver cells that are not undergoing scheduled (S phase) DNA synthesis. Additional assays often employed include the Comet assay (single-cell gel electrophoresis), which measures DNA strand breaks via microscopy imaging following electrophoresis of nucleoids. The breaks can be produced directly by the chemical or arise as a result of the DNA excision repair process and thus the assay is sensitive and non-specific. A particular advantage of this assay is that it can be applied to most nucleated cells in the body, enabling different potential target cells to be assessed. DNA–chemical adducts can also be measured, usually through the use of a radiolabelled chemical, use of accelerator mass spectrometry or by an indirect ^{32}P post-labelling assay for DNA adducts. There are also commercially available transgenic animal models that have the potential for measuring gene mutations in any tissue but often the sensitivity can be low (e.g. Muta[TM] Mouse and Big Blue[TM]).

If a positive effect is observed in any of the above *in vivo* tests it can be concluded that the compound is an *in vivo* somatic cell mutagen and hence a potential carcinogen and possible germ cell mutagen.

3.2.5.3 Stage 3: *In vivo* germ cell assays

In vivo data on mutagenic effects in germ cell DNA are also needed before drawing definite conclusions regarding heritable effects. However, in most cases such testing will not be justified since once established as an *in vivo* somatic cell mutagen, the compound will be assumed to be a potential genotoxic carcinogen and appropriate risk management procedures adopted. In some cases germ cell studies may be undertaken for the specific purpose of demonstrating whether an *in vivo* somatic cell mutagen is, or is not, a germ cell mutagen. There are two possible approaches for which there are methods in the OECD guidelines. A dominant lethal mutation is one occurring in a germ cell that does not cause dysfunction of the gamete but is lethal to the fertilized egg or developing embryo. The assay measures embryo-lethal genetic changes (mainly chromosomal) expressed as death of the conceptus as a blastoma or soon afterwards. Alternatively, there is an assay for structural chromosome aberrations in rodent spermatogonia and spermatocytes.

3.2.6 Carcinogenicity

As noted above, almost all *in vivo* somatic cell mutagens are also animal carcinogens when adequately tested and it is thus prudent to assume that they are also potential human carcinogens. However, mutagenicity tests do not detect non-genotoxic carcinogens whose mechanism is not primarily related to mutagenicity. For example, some carcinogens appear to act by sustained cell proliferation, for instance due to hormonal effects on certain tissues or to compensatory hyperplasia following cytotoxicity. Many of these agents have also been shown to inhibit cell death by apoptosis, to interfere with gap junctional intercellular communication, and to alter DNA methylation, and all of these effects may contribute to non-genotoxic mechanisms of action.

There are well-established methods for investigating the carcinogenicity of chemicals. Because of the long latent period it is essential to expose the animals to the chemical for a high proportion of their life span, namely 2 years in the rat or 18 months for mice. Also, because of the need, as far as practical, to detect low incidence effects, large numbers of animals have to be used. Hence the carcinogenicity bioassay requires a major commitment in animal resources, time, and expense, and should only be carried out when justified by the very real need to ascertain whether or not a chemical is a carcinogen.

The general principles governing these assays have not changed over several decades. In addition to carcinogenicity, information may also be obtained on chronic (essentially lifetime) toxicity. There are OECD guidelines for both the carcinogenicity bioassay and a combined chronic toxicity/carcinogenicity bioassay. In the latter case satellite groups are used for investigating clinical chemistry and haematology.

The objective of the carcinogenicity bioassay is to dose and observe animals for a major proportion of their lifespan for the development of tumours. Full autopsies are carried out on all animals that die or are killed during the test or at termination, with detailed histopathology. For pragmatic reasons testing is generally limited to rats and mice. Three dose levels are used, the highest being the maximum tolerated dose. This is described as being sufficient to elicit signs of minimal toxicity (e.g. slight depression of body weight gain, less than 10%) without substantially altering lifespan. For pragmatic reasons, group size is usually 50 males and 50 females, with higher numbers in the control groups. Exposure is from shortly after weanling for at least 2 years in the rat and 18 months in the mouse. It is important to have good knowledge of the spontaneous incidence of tumours at specific sites in test animals (i.e. good historic control data) for comparative purposes.

There are several transgenic and gene-knock-out mouse models that have been developed as potentially sensitive models for carcinogenicity testing. For example, a mouse line with a knock-out of the p53 tumour suppressor gene (used as a heterozygote) has been used as a sensitive model in which many carcinogens can be detected within a much smaller timescale than 18 months.

3.3 How are toxicological studies used in the risk assessment process and in setting standards?

The concept of risk assessment was introduced in Chapter 1, section 1.7.

It is recognized that there are uncertainties in extrapolating from animal data to humans. This is taken into account by dividing the critical NOAEL in animal studies by uncertainty factors (or assessment factors). A value of 100 is commonly used, comprising 10 to account for inter-species differences and 10 for intra-individual variability that may arise from, for example, genetic polymorphisms in genes such as those coding for enzymes involved in xenobiotic metabolism and which can influence susceptibility (IGHRC 2003). This value may be modified. For example, the uncertainty factor might be increased in the event of there being an incomplete data set or if the severity of effects in toxicity studies is high. Several reviews give more details of the use of uncertainty factors and their possible replacement by chemical specific factors if sufficient data are available, but this is rarely the case (IPCS 2005).

The approach described above of estimating a safe exposure level is appropriate for toxicological effects that have a threshold dose required for toxicity. This is true for most toxic effects but there is one important exception. Compounds that are mutagenic, namely those that damage DNA, which may be expressed as carcinogenicity or induction of heritable mutations, may not have a threshold dose. This is because one 'hit' on DNA may, in theory, result in a mutation in a single cell that can, after clonal expansion, contribute to tumour formation. Although in practice there may be a threshold, due for example to effective detoxification of the chemical or DNA repair, this is difficult to demonstrate convincingly. For these compounds a risk management approach of reducing exposure to **As L**ow **A**s **R**easonably **P**racticable (ALARP) is generally adopted.

Guidance on general principles for assessing chemical carcinogens is provided in an IGHRC document (IGHRC 2002).

3.4 References

Andersen ME, Krewski D. (2010) The vision of toxicity testing in the 21st century: moving from discussion to action. *Toxicol Sci* **117**:17–24.

Ashby J, Paton D. (1993) The influence of chemical structure on the extent and sites of carcinogenesis for 522 rodent carcinogens and 55 different human carcinogen exposures. *Mutat Res* **286**(1):3–74.

Blomme EA, Yang Y, Waring JF. (2009) Use of toxicogenomics to understand mechanisms of drug-induced hepatotoxicity during drug discovery and development. *Toxicol Lett* **186**:22–31.

Bremer S, Cortvrindt R, Daston G, Eletti B, Mantovani A, Maranghi F, Pelkonen O, Ruhdel I, Spielmann H. (2005) Reproductive and development toxicity. *Altern Lab Anim.* **33** Suppl 1: 183–209.

Council Directive. (1986) On the approximation of laws, regulations and administrative provisions of the Member States regarding the protection of animals used for experimental and other scientific purposes (86/609/EEC). *Official Journal of the European Communities* **L358**:1–29.

Department of Health. (1991) Guidelines for the evaluation of chemicals for carcinogenicity. Committee on Carcinogenicity of Chemicals on Food, Consumer Products and the Environment (COC). Report on Health and Social Security Subjects No 42. London, HMSO.

Department of Health. (2000) Guidance on a strategy for testing of chemicals for mutagenicity. Committee on Mutagenicity of Chemicals in Food, Consumer Products and the Environment (COM). Available at: http://www.advisorybodies.doh.gov.uk/com/publications.htm.

Doe JE, Boobis AR, Blacker A, et al. (2006) A tiered approach to systemic toxicity testing for agricultural chemical safety assessment. *Crit Rev Toxicol* **36**(1):37–68.

Ellinger-Ziegelbauer H, Stuart R, Wahle B, Bomann W, Ahr HJ. (2005) Comparison of the expression profiles induced by genotoxic and nongenotoxic carcinogens in rat liver. *Mutat Res* **575**:61–84.

IGHRC. (2002) Assessment of chemical carcinogens: Background to general principles of a weight of evidence approach. Interdepartmental Group on Health Risks from Chemicals. Institute for Environment and Health, University of Leicester. (IEH is now based at Cranfield University, Silsoe.) Available at: http://www.silsoe.cranfield.ac.uk/ieh/publications/publications.html.

IGHRC. (2003) Uncertainty factors: their use in human health risk assessment by UK Government. Interdepartmental Group on Health Risks from Chemicals. Institute for Environment and Health, University of Leicester. (IEH is now based at Cranfield University, Silsoe.) Available at: http://www.silsoe.cranfield.ac.uk/ieh/publications/publications.html.

IPCS. (2005) Chemical-specific adjustment factors for interspecies differences and human variability: Guidance document for use of data in dose/concentration- response assessment. International Programme on Chemical Safety. World Health Organization, Geneva. Available at: http://whqlibdoc.who.int/publications/2005/9241546786_eng.pdf.

Johansson I, Ingelman-Sundberg M. (2011) Genetic polymorphism and toxicology-with emphasis on cytochrome P450. *Toxicol Sci* **120**:1–13.

Kimber I, Dearman RJ. (2010) The local lymph node assay and skin sensitization testing. *Methods Mol Biol* **598**:221–231.

Kimber I, Humphris C, Westmoreland C, Alepee N, Negro GD, Manou I. (2011) Computational chemistry, systems biology and toxicology. Harnessing the chemistry of life: revolutionaizing toxicology, a commentary. *J Appl Toxicol* **31**:206–209.

Li AP. (2004) An integrated, multidisciplinary approach for drug safety assessment. *Drug Discov Today* **9**:687–693.

OECD Guidelines for the Testing of Chemicals. Organisation for Economic Co-operation and Development. Available at: http://www.oecd.org/department/0,2688,en_2649_34377_1_1_1_1_1, 00.html.

Pinto N, Dolan ME (2011) Clinically relevant genetic variations in drug metabolising enzymes. *Curr Drug Metab* **12**:487–497.

Roberts RA, Goodman JI, Shertzer HG, Dalton TP, Farland WH. (2003) Rodent toxicity and nongenotoxic carcinogenesis: knowledge-based human risk assessment based on molecular mechanisms. *Toxicol Mech Methods* **13**:21–29.

Scholz G, Genschow E, Pohl I, Bremer S, Paparella M, Raabe H, Southee J, Spielmann H. (1999) Prevalidation of the Embryonic Stem Cell Test (EST) – A new *in vitro* embryotoxicity test. *Toxicol in vitro* **13**(4–5):675–681.

van den Heuval MJ, Clark DG, Fielder RJ, Koundakjian PP, Oliver GJ, Pelling D, Tomlinson NJ, Walker AP. (1990). The international validation of a fixed dose procedure as an alternative to the classical LD_{50} test. *Food Chem Toxicol* **28**(7):469–482.

Van Hummelen P, Sasaki J. (2010) State of the art genomics approaches in toxicology. *Mutat Res* **705**:165–171.

Woolley A. (2003) Reproductive toxicology. In: *A Guide to Practical Toxicology*. Taylor and Francis, London and New York, pp 95–106.

Chapter 4

Introduction to human biomonitoring for public health

Ovnair Sepai

Learning outcomes

At the end of this chapter and any recommended reading the student should be able to:

1. discuss the application of human biomonitoring in the evaluation of human exposure, uptake, and effect of exposure to environmental chemicals;

2. describe the different classes of biomarkers;

3. explain the need for an understanding of the toxicokinetics and toxicodynamics when designing a biomonitoring study;

4. discuss the current knowledge base for the appropriate application of human biomonitoring in the management of both acute and chronic environmental chemical exposures;

5. explain the stages of a biomonitoring study;

6. evaluate the interpretation and utility of human biomonitoring data, and

7. apply acquired knowledge in the analysis and management of hazardous situations.

4.1 Introduction

Human biomonitoring (HBM) is a powerful tool used extensively to assess human exposure and uptake of chemicals, particularly following occupational exposures. However, human biomarkers of environmental exposure are increasingly being used to determine the presence of a chemical(s). There are several national human biomonitoring programmes, the most extensive being that of the Centers for Disease Control and Prevention (CDC) in the USA. CDC began their National Health and Nutrition Examination Survey (NHANES) in 1971 and published a third extensive report in 2005 (CDC 2005). The German Environmental Health Survey started in 1985 and since 1995 has focused on childhood exposure (Becker et al. 2006). These surveys are two good examples of the application of human biomonitoring to public health. A Pan-European HBM project, funded by Directorate Generals for Environment and Research was launched in 2010 (www.eu-hbm.info). This pilot study will be competed in 2012.

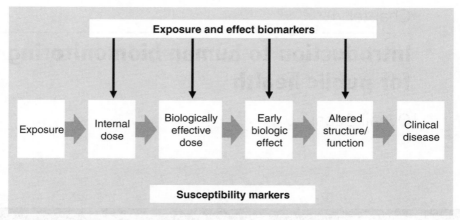

Fig. 4.1 Human biomonitoring continuum.

The use of biomarkers to assess human exposure and uptake or the effect of the uptake of environmental chemicals is not a simple analytical exercise. There are wider considerations such as the appropriate use and interpretation of the data as well as due consideration of the ethical issues and communication of the results. Advances in analytical technology in the 1980s reduced detection limits and extended the utility of biomarkers from high-level occupational exposure to low-level environmental exposures. With the more recent advancements in technology, including but not exclusively genomics-based approaches, the field of biomarker development and application has assumed an even greater importance. The advances in technology have overtaken our ability to understand and interpret much of the data that are being produced, thus there is a need for the development of a framework for appropriate application and interpretation of human biomarkers in public health.

Back in 1987 the National Research Council (NRC) in the USA recognized that biomarkers of exposure/uptake and effect may potentially be developed for any of the stages between exposure to the chemical and development of clinical disease (NRC 1987). This is outlined in Figure 4.1.

The NRC report established three classes of biomarker, namely, exposure/uptake, effect, and susceptibility. It is clear that the application of biomarkers to public health monitoring is a complicated undertaking but one which represents clear advantages over exposure estimates by measuring uptake and in some cases early effects. This chapter is a primer to human biomonitoring as a tool in public health surveillance and research.

4.2 Defining biomarkers and biomonitoring

4.2.1 Classification

A biomarker can be defined for the purposes of environmental exposure as:

> A chemical, biochemical, or functional indicator of exposure to and uptake of (or the effect of exposure to) an environmental chemical, physical, or biological agent.

Biomarkers can be divided into four broad categories (WHO 2001).

4.2.1.1 Biomarkers of exposure (and uptake)

A biomarker of exposure and uptake can be defined as the chemical or its metabolite or the product of an interaction between a chemical and some target molecule or cell that is measured in a biological fluid. Examples include lead in blood, cadmium in urine, buta-diene adducts to haemoglobin, and dioxin levels in human breast milk.

Biomarkers of exposure and uptake are measures of internal dose and in some cases biologically effective doses. The internal dose is that which has been absorbed or taken up via all three routes of exposure (see Chapter 1, Section 1.6.1). The advantage of such a biomarker is that it reflects individual exposure from ingestion, skin absorption, and inhalation, and can be a proxy for population exposure. Biomarkers of exposure are by definition relatively simple to interpret as a measure of exposure and uptake. The challenge here is determining what the health risks, if any, from the internal dose are and, where environmental exposure limits are available, how the internal dose relates to external exposure.

4.2.1.2 Biomarkers of effect

A biomarker of effect is a measurable biochemical, physiological, or behavioural change resulting from exposure to the chemical, which can be recognized as associated with an established or possible adverse health effect. Examples include 8-hydroxyldeoxyguanine in urine as a marker of oxidative damage, acetyl cholinesterase activity as a marker of exposure to an acetyl cholinesterase inhibitor, such as an organophosphate pesticide, and chromosomal aberrations or DNA adducts as a marker of exposure to genotoxic agents.

Biomarkers of effect are often not specific for a given chemical exposure and thus are often difficult to interpret. However, markers of effect are potentially important in the determination of mechanisms of action. Biomarkers of effect are often used in epidemiological studies to relate the occurrence of adverse health effects to exposure to a substance in a study. A full review of effect markers is beyond the scope of this chapter but it should be noted that there are significant advances in this area that may in the future lead to valuable tools for health protection.

4.2.1.3 Biomarkers of susceptibility

A biomarker of susceptibility is an indicator of an inherent or acquired ability of an organism to respond to the challenge of exposure to a specific chemical. Examples include genetic polymorphisms in metabolic enzymes, cytochrome P450s, glutathione transferases, N-acetyl transferases, DNA repair genes, and excision repair cross-complementing 1 and 2. All these polymorphisms have the potential to affect individual susceptibility, but analysis is often complex and interpretation is difficult.

Variations in absorption, distribution, metabolism, DNA repair, and cell turnover processes can modify the risk for adverse effects and the levels of biomarkers after exposure to toxic agents. Some of these differences are due to heritable variation, individual susceptibility (genetic polymorphisms), and gene-environment interactions. Biomarkers of susceptibility are by their nature complex and although they may have a role to play in modulating individual responses to exposure, the interpretation from a health risk point of view is difficult. There are many environmental epidemiological studies that include the measurement of genetic polymorphisms, and metabolic variations could affect the level of biomarkers detected.

In the public health context biomarkers—or markers of susceptibility—can also be expanded to socio-economic susceptibility, where lifestyle and many other factors may affect population exposure patterns. These aspects are discussed in some detail in Chapter 7, section 7.2 on individual susceptibility. Examples include smoking status and household income.

4.2.1.4 Biomarkers of clinical disease

A fourth category, biomarkers of clinical disease, is to the right of the continuum in Figure 4.1. These biomarkers include liver function enzymes, kidney function enzymes and even ECG and lung function tests. Again, although these biomarkers indicate a disease state they are non specific and the contribution of environmental toxicants to the disease state is hard to determine. Biomarkers of disease will not be considered further in this chapter.

4.2.2 Biomonitoring

As applied in this text, biomonitoring is a scientific technique used to sample blood, urine, breast milk, and other tissue to assess human exposure uptake of or effect on natural and synthetic chemicals.

The use of human biomarkers in environmental epidemiology enables the epidemiologist to determine more accurately population exposure and to associate exposure with adverse health effects.

4.3 Biomarker utility

Our ability to interpret the health significance of any human biomonitoring data lags behind the analytical technology that allows us to measure ever decreasing concentrations of organic and inorganic pollutants. There is an increasing number of studies, subjects, and substances determined in human biomonitoring and a parallel increasing in awareness of the general public of those chemicals in our bodies. Statements to the effect that the presence of an environmental pollutant in a biological sample is not a reflection of risk to health or a cause of disease will not fully address public anxiety (CDC 2005). There have to be clear guidelines for the appropriate interpretation and use of biomarkers. There have been attempts to develop frameworks for the interpretation and utility of biomarkers (Boogart 2007).

Four broad categories of activity where biomarkers can be used are (i) scoping, (ii) trend analysis, (iii) exposure and health research, and (iv) risk assessment (Burke et al. 1992). These are considered in turn. Scoping studies are exploratory studies to determine the level of a pollutant in human tissue and compare this to 'normal' values or background levels if they exist. However, if background levels are not available these preliminary scoping studies can be used to develop reference ranges. Trend analyses assess the concentration of the chemical and whether there are any temporal or spatial trends. Such studies provide valuable information on the effectiveness of control measures aimed at reducing or eliminating exposure. This information also assists in population studies. Biomonitoring studies in health research investigate correlations between health effects in population.

Biological data can be used in risk-based assessments and clinical evaluation to assess individual risks or exposure. Here data are available on the correlation with internal dose (marker of exposure) and effect. Health-risk assessment can only be determined with dose–response relationships, ideally in humans (or using animal data with the appropriate uncertainty factors). The classic example of this is blood lead levels and effect.

The interpretation of the significance of biomarker concentration will ultimately depend on the quantum of knowledge about the biomarker. This includes the toxicity, toxicokinetics, and individual and population-based variability (genetic susceptibility).

4.4 Study design, conduct and communication

When designing a biomonitoring study it is important to consider in the first instance what the purpose of the study is. Only with this in mind can the appropriate biomarker in the appropriate population be selected. The ethical and communication issues must be considered at the planning or design stage of the project. Biomonitoring study design should also consider in particular the toxicokinetics of the substance under investigation (see Chapter 1) in the selection of appropriate biomarkers.

4.4.1 Selection of the appropriate study population: criteria for taking a human sample

The study population is dependent on the hypothesis to be tested. As a basis for developing a hypothesis it is necessary to use the four categories: (i) scoping, (ii) trend analysis, (iii) exposure and health research, and (iv) risk assessment. These have been described briefly above. In addition there should be knowledge of the potential exposure to investigate as well as a knowledge of epidemiology. It may be possible to select a population, a sampling strategy, and where necessary, appropriate controls. An understanding of the intra- and interindividual sources of variation in exposure is vital when developing a sampling strategy.

Of particular interest to health protection is the place of biomonitoring in investigations of acute incidents and chronic exposure to environmental chemicals.

The ideal situation is where the health professional has the luxury of developing a hypothesis and sound study design and is able to include the appropriate biomonitoring protocol following the acute incident. However, there are great pitfalls in taking human samples following an acute incident. Thus there is a need for a set of criteria or an algorithm that will aid the decision as to when and where to take biological samples or when biological samples should not be taken. These criteria are listed in Box 4.1.

4.4.2 Selection of the appropriate biomarker

Environmental chemical exposure levels generally are much lower than occupational exposures and therefore there is a need to develop sensitive analytical methods. The analytical procedure must be validated at the exposure levels in question. The exposure may be intermittent and hence the integrated exposure measured at a point in time needs to reflect a known exposure period.

Box 4.1 Criteria for the use of biological samples to investigate a chemical incident

1) *Exposure assessment to guide clinical interventions*
Testing may be of direct patient benefit where there is the option to use a therapeutic intervention (e.g. antidotes or other medical treatment).

2) *Exposure assessment to monitor clinical effects*
Testing may be appropriate even where there is no specific treatment to counteract the effect of the chemical (e.g. monitoring the levels of a chemical and/or the specific clinical effects of exposure).

3) *Confirmation of exposure to a known or unknown agent*
Where there is no specific antidote or other clinical intervention option, testing may still be appropriate in order to confirm exposure to an agent and to quantify the degree of exposure, for a number of reasons:

A) identification of an unknown chemical agent

B) epidemiological follow up

C) reassurance monitoring

D) clinical research

E) medico-legal reasons.

An understanding or estimate of the half-life of a chemical or its metabolite (the toxi-cokinetics) is essential to the design of the study protocol. In a controlled occupational setting where exposures occur over a set working shift it is possible to take biological specimens with the maximum circulating levels in blood or excreted in urine. However, as environmental exposures are not as well defined temporally, it is not usually possible to take samples at an optimum time.

Metabolites with short half-lives reflect exposure over a short period of time often only the previous day (e.g. phthalates and organophosphorus pesticides) whereas for persistent compounds (i.e. dioxins, organochlorine pesticides) levels detected in blood, fat, or milk are a reflection of a longer-term exposure.

The UK Health and Safety Laboratory and the German Research Foundation (DFG, Deutsche Forschungsgemeinschaft) produce detailed protocols for the determination of human exposure and uptake markers of occupational exposures. These are a valuable template to consider when developing a study design for environmental exposures. A detailed discussion of the study design is beyond the scope of this chapter.

The specificity of the biomarker also has to be considered, i.e. if the biomarker reflects exposure to one compound only or is a more general marker.

4.4.3 Sample collection storage and analysis

The choice of sample is dependent on the toxicodynamics, i.e. in which part of the body you would expect to detect the compound or its metabolites. The optimal time to take the sample has been discussed above. The appropriate sample collection protocol will include the type of container, the optimum storage, and sample processing requirements to meet all quality criteria.

The most frequently used tissues in population-based studies are blood and urine (Table 4.1, referenced with examples of population-based studies). However, other tissues such as fat, milk etc., have their own advantages and disadvantages. There are many studies that investigate tissues such as brain, liver, and kidney (post-mortem). Such studies are useful to develop the evidence base but of little obvious value to population studies (Chu et al. 2003).

4.4.4 Confounding factors

There are many confounding factors that may affect the level of biomarker detected or the interpretation of the data. These confounding factors include age, gender, metabolic capacity, ethnic origin, socio-economic status, and life-style. This is a non-exhaustive list.

4.4.5 Communication

Communication is a dynamic task and requires the development of tailored material for different groups of stakeholders (Sepai et al. 2008). These include the volunteers, the public in general, and health professionals. The key aspect to communication is the understanding of our ability to interpret human biomonitoring data and to be able to place the biomarker

Table 4.1 Common biomonitoring matrices used in population-based studies

Sample	Sample type	Exposure timeframe	Biomarker category	Example
Blood	Invasive	Medium to long term	Exposure, effect	Heavy metals,[1] organic compounds
Blood fat	Invasive	Longer term: months to years	Exposure uptake	Dioxins, PCBs[2]
Urine	Non-invasive	24–48 hours	Exposure, effect	Phthalates[3]
Milk	Non-invasive	Reflection of longer term exposure	Exposure	Dioxins, PCBs[4]
Exhaled air	Non-invasive	Short-term: hours	Exposure	Organic solvents (styrene[5])
Hair	Non-invasive	Exposure at a given time, but reflected in the growth of hair	Exposure	Heavy metals (arsenic[6]) organics[7]
Nails	Non-invasive	Exposure at a given time, but reflected in the growth of nail	Exposure	Heavy metals (arsenic[8])
Saliva	Non-invasive	Short to medium term	Exposure and effect	Mercury,[9] atrozine[10]
Post-partum umbilical (cord) blood	Non-invasive	Same as blood	Exposure and effect	Same as blood[11]

1. Wilhelm et al. 2004; 2. Schwenk et al. 2002; 3. Koch and Angerer 2007; 4. Bordajandi et al. 2008; 5. Somorovská et al. 1999; 6. Gebel et al. 1998; 7. Schramm 1997; 8. Wilhelm et al. 2005; 9. Zimmer et al. 2002; 10. Denovan et al. 2000; 11. Elwood et al. 2005).

into one of the categories described in section 4.3 on biomarker utility. Whether individual results or population averages are reported will of course depend on the study. However, these decisions need to be taken at the design stage of a study and it may be necessary to seek ethical approval.

4.5 Ethical issues

The collection and analysis of human samples for the evaluation of environmental pollutants requires careful consideration of the ethical issues. These issues include the rights of volunteers and data protection issues as well as the need for follow-up and communication of results. The NHS Research Ethics Committees (REC) is generally thought to focus on clinical trials and patient-based studies. However, it is unethical to carry out human exposure studies without due consideration of the ethical aspects of the study and, where appropriate, securing REC approval.

4.6 Summary

The use of human biomonitoring in the assessment of environmental exposure is not just an analytical exercise. The continuum from exposure to disease potentially includes biomarkers of exposure and uptake, of effect and of susceptibility. The study design must include consideration of the study population, the sampling regime, and the current knowledge base with regard to chemical toxicity, toxicokinetics, and the analytical sensitivity and specificity. Finally, every population-based human biomonitoring study will have to seek REC approval where appropriate; this approval includes a description of the communication strategy.

4.7 References

Becker K, Seiwert M, Angerer J, Kolossa-Gehring M, Hoppe H-W, Ball M, Schulz C, Thumulla J, Seifert B. (2006) GerES IV Pilot Study: assessment of the exposure of German children to organophosphorus and pyrethroid pesticides. *Int J Hyg Environ Health* **209**:221–233.

Boogart, P. (2007) Human biomonitoring activities–Programmes by industry. *Int J Hyg Environ Health* **210**:259–261.

Bordajandi L, Abad E, González M. (2008) Occurrence of PCBs, PCDD/Fs, PBDEs and DDTs in Spanish breast milk: Enantiomeric fraction of chiral PCBs. *Chemosphere* **70**:567–575.

Burke T, Anderson H, Beach N, Colome S, Drew RT. (1992) Role of exposure databases in risk management. *Arch Environ Health* **47**(6):421–429.

CDC. (2005) *Third National Report on Human Exposure to Environmental Chemicals*. Centers for Disease Control and Prevention, Atlanta, GA.

Chu S, Covaci A, Schepens P. (2003) Levels and chiral signatures of persistent organochlorine pollutants in human tissues from Belgium *Environ Res* **93**(2):167–176.

Denovan L, Lu C, Hines C, Fenske R. (2000) Saliva biomonitoring of atrazine exposure among herbicide applicators. *Int Arch Occup Environ Health* **73**(7):457–462.

Elwood P, Jones M, James K, Toothill C. (2005) Evidence of a fall in cord blood lead levels in South Wales 1984–85. *Environ Geochem Health* **12**:235–257.

Gebel T, Suchenwirth R, Bolten C, Dunkelberg H. (1998) Human biomonitoring of arsenic and antimony in case of an elevated geogenic exposure. *Environ Health Perspect* **106**:33–39.

Koch H, Angerer J. (2007) Di-iso-nonylphthalate (DINP) metabolites in human urine after a single oral dose of deuterium-labelled DINP. *Int J Hyg Environ Health* **210**:9–19.

NRC. (1987) Biologic markers in environmental health research. *Environ Health Perspect* **74**:3–9.

Schramm K. (1997) Hair: a matrix for non-invasive biomonitoring of organic chemicals in mammals. *Bull Environ Contam Toxicol* **59**(3):396–402.

Schwenk M, Gabrio T, Päpke O, Wallenhorst T. (2002) Human biomonitoring of polychlorinated biphenyls and polychlorinated dibenzodioxins and dibenzofuranes in teachers working in a PCB-contaminated school. *Chemosphere* **47**:229–233.

Sepai O, Collier C, Van Tongelen B, Casteleyn L. (2008) Human biomonitoring data interpretation and ethics, obstacles or surmountable challenges? *Environ Health* **13**.

Somorovská M, Jahnová E, Tulinská J, Zámecníková M, Sarmanová J, Terenová A, Vodicková L, Lísková A, Vallová B, Soucek P, Hemminki K, Norppa H, Hirvonen A, Tates AD, Fuortes L, Dusinská M, Vodicka P. (1999) Biomonitoring of occupational exposure to styrene in a plastics lamination plant. *Mutat Res Fund Mol M* **428**(1–2):255–269.

WHO. (2001) Biomarkers in Risk Assessment: Validity and Validation. *Environmental Health Criteria*. World Health Organization, Geneva.

Wilhelm M, Ewers U, Schulz C. (2004) Revised and new reference values for some trace elements in blood and urine for human biomonitoring in environmental medicine. *Int J Hyg Environ Health* **207**:69–73.

Wilhelm M, Pesch B, Wittsiepe J, Jakubis P, Miskovic P, Keegan T, Nieuwenhuijsen M, Ranft U. (2005) Comparison of arsenic levels in fingernails with urinary As species as biomarkers of arsenic exposure in residents living close to a coal-burning power plant in Prievidza District, Slovakia. *J Expo Anal Environ Epidemiol* **15**(1):89–98.

Zimmer H, Ludwig H, Bader M, Bailer J, Eickholz P, Staehle H, Triebig G. (2002) Determination of mercury in blood, urine and saliva for the biological monitoring of an exposure from amalgam fillings in a group with self-reported adverse health effects. *Int J Hyg Environ Health* **205**:205–211.

Section 2

Applications of Toxicology

Chapter 5

Sources of toxicological information

Robie Kamanyire and Nicholas Brooke

Learning outcomes

At the end of this chapter and any recommended reading the student should be able to:

1. explain the importance of the accurate identification of potentially toxic agents and the use of chemical identification numbers;

2. navigate their way though the wide array of available toxicological information sources;

3. take a critical approach to information resources, and

4. apply acquired knowledge in the analysis and management of hazardous situations.

5.1 Introduction

The environment is increasingly recognized as having an impact on human and ecological health, as well as on specific types of human morbidity, mortality, and disability.

As environmental health concerns continue to increase, it is important for health professionals and other communities to have ready access to information resources. There is a large and diverse potential audience for toxicology and environmental health information, ranging from emergency department physicians to local community advocates attempting to determine the environmental health hazards faced by their communities. Although the user communities in this broad spectrum have diverse information needs, it should not be impossible to provide relevant information resources effectively and efficiently.

This chapter aims to provide the tools to direct health professionals through the wide array of information resources that are available for toxicology. Access to the right information at the right time is a crucial ingredient of modern health care. The rapid growth of biomedical knowledge and the resulting increase in the number of scientific journals that have inundated health professionals have made it important to define key sources of such information from the available mass. Improving access to information is an important goal for all health professionals as well as the public.

Toxicology, at its simplest, is the study of the nature and mechanism of the potential effects of substances on living organisms and other biological systems. The assessment of the health hazards of industrial chemicals, environmental pollutants, and other substances represents an important element in the protection of the health of workers and members of communities.

5.2 Chemical identification

One of the key factors for obtaining good quality toxicology information is to ensure an accurate identification of the chemical or compound of interest. There has been a phenomenal growth in the number of chemical compounds being synthesized (or isolated) and then reported in the scientific literature. By June 2011, CAS had formally identified over 62 million chemical compounds. The names of many of these compounds are often complex and hence not very easy to remember or cite accurately. Also it is difficult to keep track of them in the literature. Several international organizations like the International Union of Pure and Applied Chemistry (IUPAC) and CAS have initiated steps to make such tasks easier. CAS provides an abstracting service of the chemical literature, consisting of a numerical identifier, known as the CAS registry number, for each chemical substance that has been reported in the chemical literature. Establishing accurate identification of a compound of concern allows accurate access to sources of toxicology information.

Other systems of chemical identification numbers exist such as the EC number, a seven-digit code allocated by the Commission of the European Communities for commercially available chemical substances within the European Union. The EC number designation supersedes the older European Inventory of Existing Commercial Chemical Substances Information System (EINECS) and European List of Notified Chemical Substances (ELINCS) designations which were required on the label and the packaging of dangerous substances.

The United Nations (UN) Committee of Experts on the Transport of Dangerous Goods assigns four-digit UN numbers that identify hazardous substances and articles (such as explosives, flammable liquids, toxic substances, etc.) in the framework of international transport. Some hazardous substances have their own UN numbers, while sometimes groups of chemicals or products with similar properties receive a common UN number (e.g. flammable liquids, not otherwise specified, are UN1993). A chemical in its solid state may receive a different UN number than its liquid phase if the hazardous properties differ significantly; substances with different levels of purity (or concentration in solution) may also receive different UN numbers.

5.3 Sources of information

Once a chemical has been correctly identified it is then necessary to obtain suitable information on its toxicity. Sources of information can be broadly classified into primary, i.e. toxicology journals, or secondary, i.e. searchable databases or books. It is usually not necessary for the vast majority of queries to use a primary source to obtain toxicology information. Secondary sources have a longstanding tradition of use in toxicology, originally handbooks or textbooks and more recently databases delivered via the internet. This chapter will concentrate on a few key textbooks and databases which should be easily accessible from most libraries or via the internet. This summary is not intended to be an exhaustive list but should provide a basis for initiating a search for information, which often leads to further resources.

5.3.1 Textbooks

Sax's Dangerous Properties of Industrial Materials (3 vols, 11th edn, 2004) covers over 26,000 toxic, carcinogenic, mutagenic, highly flammable, or potentially explosive substances. Included are health-related and physical property data. There are many pages of synonyms in several languages to assist users and it also includes a CAS Registry Number index. A CD-ROM version is also available.

Patty's Industrial Hygiene and *Patty's Toxicology*, now in its 6th edition, collectively cover general principles, toxicology, and theory and rationale. The focus of these texts in recent editions has been extended beyond the industrial workplace to environmental safety and hazard control. Both books contain comprehensive toxicological data for industrial compounds from metals to synthetic polymers. Information for each compound includes CAS numbers, Registry of Toxic Effects of Chemicals (RTECS) numbers, physical and chemical properties, threshold limit values (TLVs), permissible exposure limits (PELs), maximum workplace concentrations (MAK), and biological tolerance values for occupational exposures.

Ellenhorn's Medical Toxicology: Diagnosis and Treatment of Human Poisoning, (3rd edn, 2003) by Williams and Wilkins, published posthumously, has over 300 chapters with more than 13,000 references. The text, organized into six sections, gives a national and international approach to principles of poison management, individual drugs, intoxicants in the home, chemical poisons, natural toxins, and mass incidents.

Goldfrank's Toxicologic Emergencies (8th edn, 2006) uses a case-study approach to medical toxicology. This comprehensive reference has 135 chapters covering toxicological emergencies, related environmental problems, and issues affecting emergency departments, the poison centres and the poisoned patient. In addition, an accompanying study guide provides several case studies as well as a questions and answer section.

Textbooks have evolved from print-based materials to electronic internet-based resources, including some of the texts listed above.

5.3.2 Internet resources

When accessing toxicology resources on the internet care must be taken as there are numerous sites and it is important to access reputable or 'accredited' sources.

Individuals vary in their ability to conduct internet searches for reliable information. When using internet resources it is important to ensure that the material found has been critically appraised and validated, from an authoritative source or subject to independent peer review. A small selection of authoritative sites is presented below.

5.3.2.1 Compendium of Chemical Hazards, Health Protection Agency

The Health Protection Agency's (HPA) Chemical Hazards and Poisons Division produces as part of its information resource a series entitled a ***Compendium of Chemical Hazards***. The aim is to produce an online information resource for the public and professionals who may be involved in advising and responding to chemical incidents, especially public health professionals and emergency services. The *Compendium of Chemical Hazards* is split into three sections:

- *general information*, which provides background information on the compound, including its uses and frequently asked questions, and aims to be accessible for those from a non-toxicological background;

- *incident management* focuses on information that may be needed during chemical incidents, such as physicochemical properties, health effects and decontamination;

- *toxicological overview* provides more in-depth toxicology of the compound, summarizing the most relevant human and animal studies from the literature;

5.3.2.2 INCHEM, International Program on Chemical Safety

The International Program on Chemical Safety (IPCS) produces **INCHEM** as a co-operative program, which is an invaluable tool for those concerned with chemical safety and the proper management of chemicals. IPCS INCHEM directly responds to one of the Intergovernmental Forum on Chemical Safety (IFCS) priority actions to consolidate current, internationally peer-reviewed chemical safety-related publications and database records from international bodies for public access. IPCS INCHEM offers rapid access to internationally peer-reviewed information on chemicals commonly used throughout the world, which may also occur as contaminants in the environment and food. The site provides quick and easy electronic access to thousands of searchable full-text documents on chemical risks and the sound management of chemicals:

- Concise International Chemical Assessment Documents (CICADS);
- Environmental Health Criteria (EHC) Monographs;
- Joint Expert Committee on Food Additives (JECFA)—Monographs and Evaluations;
- Health and Safety Guides (HSGs);
- International Agency for Research on Cancer (IARC)—Summaries and Evaluations;
- International Chemical Safety Cards (ICSC);
- Joint Meeting on Pesticide Residues (JMPR);
- Pesticide Data Sheets and Documents (PDSs);
- Screening Information Data Set (SIDS) for High Production Volume Chemicals.

5.3.2.3 TOXNET, National Library of Medicine

The US National Library of Medicine (NLM) toxicology data service **TOXNET** is a free service with access to a range of free toxicology databases. Included are:

- Toxicology Data Search for factual information in the databases HSDB (see below), Gene-Tox, CCRIS (carcinogenesis), IRIS (the US Environmental Protection Agency's (EPA) risk assessment database) and the Registry of Toxic Effects of Chemical Substances (RTECS);

- Toxicology Literature Search for bibliographic records from TOXLINE and the genotoxic/reproductive database DART/ETIC;

◆ Toxic Release Inventory (TRI) Search, reporting EPA's annual estimate of releases of toxic substances into the environment;

◆ Chemical Information Search for identification of substances by name, structure, etc. (ChemIDplus contains >367,000 records and >182,000 structures; HSDB: >4500 records; and NCI-3D: >213,000 substances).

5.3.2.4 Hazardous Substances Data Bank

The **Hazardous Substances Data Bank** (HSDB, available through TOXNET) contains over 6000 chemical records, each of which can have as many as 150 data fields covering human health effects, emergency medical treatment, animal toxicity studies, metabolism/pharmacokinetics, pharmacology, environmental fate and exposure, environmental standards and regulations, chemical/physical properties, chemical safety and handling, occupational exposure standards and more. HSDB is peer-reviewed by a committee of experts, the Scientific Review Panel (SRP).

5.3.2.5 Integrated Risk Information System, US Environmental Protection Agency

The **Integrated Risk Information System** (IRIS) is prepared and maintained by the US Environmental Protection Agency (US EPA), and is an electronic database containing information on human health effects that may result from exposure to various chemicals in the environment. The information in IRIS is intended for those without extensive training in toxicology, but with some knowledge of health sciences. The dataset contains descriptive and quantitative information in the following categories:

◆ oral reference doses and inhalation reference concentrations (RfDs and RfCs, respectively) for chronic non-carcinogenic health effects;

◆ hazard identification, and oral and inhalation unit risks for carcinogenic effects.

5.3.2.6 Pocket Guide to Chemical Hazards, National Institute for Occupational Safety and Health

The *NIOSH Pocket Guide to Chemical Hazards* is intended as a source of general industrial hygiene information for workers, employers, and occupational health professionals. The *Pocket Guide* presents key information and data in abbreviated tabular form for 677 chemicals or substance groupings (e.g. manganese compounds, tellurium compounds, inorganic tin compounds, etc.) that are commonly found in the work environment. The industrial hygiene information found in the *Pocket Guide* should help users recognize and control occupational chemical hazards. The chemicals or substances contained in this revision include all substances for which the National Institute for Occupational Safety and Health (NIOSH) has recommended exposure limits (RELs).

5.3.2.7 Agency for Toxic Substances and Disease Registry

The **Agency for Toxic Substances and Disease Registry** (ATSDR) is the principal federal public health agency charged with responsibility for evaluating the human health effects of exposure to hazardous substances. The United States Congress requires ATSDR to provide toxicological profiles to state health and environmental agencies and to make them available to other interested parties. The toxicological profiles are summaries of ATSDR's evaluations concerning whether and at what levels of exposure adverse health effects occur and levels at which no adverse effects occur. The profiles include information about exposure and environmental fate that may help readers determine the significance of levels found in the environment. Toxicological profiles also provide interpretations of data, which distinguishes them from ordinary reviews. Interpretations are useful for those health professionals who may not have the resources to gather and consider all the toxicological data themselves.

5.3.2.8 European Centre for Ecotoxicology and Toxicology of Chemicals

European Centre for Ecotoxicology and Toxicology of Chemicals (ECETOC) was established in 1978 as a scientific, non-profit, non-commercial association. It is financed by leading companies with interests in the manufacture and use of chemicals. A stand-alone organization, it was established to provide a scientific forum through which the extensive specialist expertise in the European chemical industry could be harnessed to research, review, assess, and publish studies on the ecotoxicology and toxicology of chemicals. ECETOC produces a range of peer-reviewed technical reports and monographs reviewing generic topics or issues fundamental to the application of sound science in evaluating the hazards and risks of chemicals to human health and the environment.

5.3.3 UK independent advisory committees

5.3.3.1 Committee of Carcinogenicity and Committee on Mutagenicity

The Committee of Carcinogenicity (CoC) and the Committee on Mutagenicity (CoM) are independent advisory committees that provide advice to UK government departments and agencies on matters concerning the potential carcinogenicity or mutagenicity of chemicals ranging from natural products to new synthetic chemicals used in pesticides or pharmaceuticals. The committees consist of a panel of independent doctors and scientists recruited for their individual expertise from universities and research institutes and, in some cases, industry. The committees are tasked with providing advice on a range of issues related to the carcinogenicity or mutagenicity of chemicals.

5.3.3.2 Committee on Medical Effects of Air Pollution

The Committee on Medical Effects of Air Pollution (COMEAP) is an advisory committee of independent experts that provides advice to UK government departments and agencies on all matters concerning the potential toxicity and effects on health of air pollutants.

5.3.4 UK agency guidance

5.3.4.1 Environment Agency: Contaminated Land Exposure Assessment

The Department for Environment, Food and Rural Affairs (Defra) and the Environment Agency has published a series of reports that provide a scientifically based framework for the assessment of risks to human health from land contamination. The health criteria values and the soil guideline values (SGVs) published through the Contaminated Land Exposure Assessment (CLEA) programme are developed through an extensive process of consultation between independent experts, peer reviewers, and regulatory authorities. Authoritative health criteria values for each contaminant are established through a review of scientific literature; the health criteria values are protective of human health and are used in the derivation of SGVs and can be used for site-specific risk assessment.

5.3.4.2 Health and Safety Executive

The UK's Health and Safety Commission's Advisory Committee on Toxic Substances (ACTS) advises the Health and Safety Executive on matters relating to the prevention, control, and management of hazards and risks to the health and safety of persons arising from the supply or use of toxic substances at work, with due regard to any related risks to consumers, the public, and the environment. The ACTS is sub-divided into a number of sub-committees to cover issues such as workplace exposure limits and packaging hazards.

5.3.5 World Health Organization

5.3.5.1 Air quality

The WHO Air Quality Guidelines for Europe aim to provide a basis to protect public health from the adverse effects of air pollutants, and to eliminate, or reduce to a minimum, pollutants that are known or are likely to be hazardous to human health and well-being. In providing pollutant levels below which lifetime exposure or exposure for a given averaging time does not constitute a health risk, they form a basis for setting national standards for air pollution.

5.3.5.2 Water quality

The WHO Guidelines for Drinking-water Quality include facts sheets and comprehensive review documents for many individual chemicals. The guidelines are addressed primarily to water and health regulators, policymakers, and their advisors to assist in the development of national standards. The guidelines and associated documents are also used by many others as a source of information on water quality and health, and on effective management approaches.

5.4 Summary

This chapter summarizes a few key resources in the field of toxicology which should enable anyone involved in health protection to access the information they require to answer questions relating to the exposure of a population to noxious chemicals using authoritative secondary sources.

5.5 Further reading

Advisory Committee on Toxic Substances (ACTS). UK Health and Safety Commission. http://www. hse.gov.uk/aboutus/meetings/iacs/acts/.

Agency for Toxic Substances and Disease Registry (ATSDR). US Centres for Disease Control and Prevention http://www.atsdr.cdc.gov/.

Centre for Radiation, Chemicals and Environmental Hazards (CRCE). *Chemical Compendium*, UK Health Protection Agency. http://www.hpa.org.uk/chemicals/compendium/default.htm.

Chemical Abstract Service (CAS). American Chemical Society. http://www.cas.org/.

Committee on Carcinogenicity of Chemicals in Food, Consumer Products and the Environment (COC). UK Department of Health. http://www.iacoc.org.uk/.

Committee on Mutagenicity of Chemicals in Food, Consumer Products and the Environment (COC). UK Department of Health. http://www.iacom.org.uk/.

Committee on the Medical Effects of Air Pollutants (COMEAP). UK Department of Health. http://comeap.org.uk/.

Contaminated Land Exposure Assessment (CLEA). UK Environment Agency. http://www.environment-agency.gov.uk/research/planning/33714.aspx.

European Centre for Ecotoxicology and Toxicology of Chemicals (ECETOC). http://www.ecetoc.org/.

Hazardous Substances Database Network (HSDN), Toxicology Data Network (TOXNET). http://toxnet.nlm.nih.gov/cgi-bin/sis/htmlgen?HSDB.

INCHEM, International Programme on Chemical Safety. http://www.inchem.org/.

Integrated Risk Information System (IRIS). US Environmental Protection Agency. http://www.epa.gov/IRIS/.

National Institute for Occupational Safety and Health (NIOSH). *Pocket Guide to Chemical Hazards*, US Centres for Disease Control and Prevention. http://www.cdc.gov/niosh/npg/pgintrod.html.

Toxicology Data Network (TOXNET). http://sis.nlm.nih.gov/enviro.html.

United Nations Committee of Experts on the Transport of Dangerous Goods, UN Economic Commission for Europe (UNECE). http://www.unece.org/trans/welcome.html.

World Health Organization (2002) WHO Air Quality Guidelines for Europe, 2nd edition, World Health Organization http://www.who.int/phe/air/pheair/en/.

World Health Organization. WHO Guidelines for Drinking-water Quality, World Health Organization http://www.who.int/water_sanitation_health/dwq/en/.

Chapter 6

Medical management of chemical incidents

Simon F.J. Clarke and Nicholas Castle

Learning outcomes

At the end of this chapter and any recommended reading the student should be able to:

1. explain how the state of the patient is assessed following toxic exposure;
2. describe and discuss the supportive and symptomatic management of poisoned patients;
3. describe and discuss decontamination techniques, methods used to reduce absorption of toxic substances, antidotes, and the enhancement of the elimination of toxic substances;
4. explain the roles of the various agencies involved, including the prehospital emergency services and hospital emergency departments;
5. critically discuss the protocols used in the management of the poisoned patient, e.g. in the prevention of secondary contamination, and
6. apply acquired knowledge in the analysis and management of acute chemical incidents.

6.1 Introduction

Toxicology has been defined as the study of the adverse effects of xenobiotics (extraneous chemicals) on biological systems. If this definition is applied to human medicine, it can be seen that it incorporates a number of scenarios involving pharmaceuticals (adverse drug reactions, interactions, and overdose) and exposure to non-pharmaceuticals (domestic and industrial chemicals, and chemical warfare agents). Although poisoning by pharmaceuticals is more commonly encountered in clinical medicine, exposure to non-pharmaceutical chemicals during chemical incidents is more important from the health protection perspective. This is due to the potential for spread of contamination to other individuals (both members of the public and healthcare staff) and the environment, as well as disruption to infrastructure.

Toxins can be absorbed via the gastrointestinal tract (ingested), absorbed across the lungs (inhaled), or absorbed across the skin or eyes.

This chapter will focus on the medical management of chemical incidents. The issues that will be discussed include:

- the risk of *secondary contamination* of healthcare staff and facilities, and systems used to reduce that risk (*containment*);
- the diagnostic challenges presented by exposure to chemicals;
- the treatment strategies available, such as:
  - reducing absorption of chemical (decontamination),
  - *promoting elimination* of any toxin that has been absorbed,
  - specific therapies for individual chemicals (*antidotes*), and
  - the *symptomatic and supportive* approach, which is the mainstay of clinical toxicology;
- sources of expert help for both clinicians and public health practitioners.

6.2 Secondary contamination

The main feature that sets chemical incidents apart from other causes of presentation to emergency departments (EDs) is the fact that there is a risk that healthcare staff and facilities may themselves become affected by the chemicals. There are many reported cases where casualties have caused significant disruption to EDs, operating theatres and intensive care units (Burgess 1999; Geller et al. 2001; Harrison et al. 2002; Stewart et al. 2003; Davey and Moppet 2004; Stacey et al. 2004). Even single patients have caused significant disruption; however, the most widely reported incident was the sarin attack on the Tokyo subway in 1996 where 10–20% of emergency responders and healthcare staff developed clinical features of sarin poisoning (Okumura et al. 1996; Nozaki et al. 1997; Ohbu et al. 1997), many of whom required medical treatment, and some of whom suffered from persistent symptoms for at least 7 years after the incident (Miyaki et al. 2005).

Secondary contamination can occur from a number of sources:

- Residues can be brought in on the patients' clothes and skin. This can be transferred to other individuals either by direct splashing onto their skin or in their eyes or by inhalation in the case of volatile chemicals and particulates.
- Volatile agents may be found in significant concentrations in the casualty's expired air (*respiratory off-gassing*). These can be inhaled by other individuals nearby, particularly those who are managing the patient's breathing.
- Chemicals may be present in body fluids; in particular, ingested toxins can be present in high concentrations in vomitus. Again, these pose a risk of skin or eye contamination for members of staff treating the patient, or an inhalational risk if the body fluids contain volatile agents.

The risk of secondary contamination depends upon a number of chemical properties (Cox 1994; Horton et al. 2003; Brennan et al. 1999; Moles and Baker 1999; Baker 1999):

- *Volatility*: this indicates how rapidly an agent evaporates. Such agents may present an immediate risk of inhalation injury but they disperse rapidly; external decontamination does not eliminate the risk of secondary contamination because the patients may continue to 'off-gas' (continuing evaporation of chemical after external decontamination) from their expired breath, but the risk is relatively short-lived in a well-ventilated environment.

◆ *Persistence*: this is the inverse of volatility. These agents pose more of a risk from direct contact, although the risk can be eliminated by efficient external decontamination.

◆ *Toxicity*: this is the potential for a chemical to cause harm to biological systems. Chemical warfare agents have been specifically designed to have a particularly high degree of toxicity, which means that small doses can cause harm.

◆ *Latency*: this is the period of time between exposure and the onset of symptoms; it is of particular concern if there is a delay in symptoms becoming apparent as the casualties may not realize that they are being exposed and therefore do not seek to escape from the area and minimize contamination.

◆ *Corrosiveness*: strong acids and alkalis produce tissue damage by a variety of mechanisms; in addition, some chemicals, such as certain elemental metals, react violently with moisture on the skin and can produce thermal burns. Agents such as phosgene react with metals in a moist environment, which can damage equipment such as metal valves in breathing systems: strong acids can degrade plastic material.

The risk of secondary contamination can be minimized by early recognition that a chemical incident has occurred, appropriate use of personal protective equipment (PPE), and adequate decontamination of the patient. It is important for each healthcare facility to have a single, generic, well-rehearsed protocol for dealing with such incidents (Burgess et al. 1999; Tan et al. 2002; Timm and Reeves 2007) using the following principles:

◆ recognition

◆ containment

◆ decontamination with life support measures

◆ definitive care.

These will be discussed in the following section.

6.3 Management of a chemical incident

6.3.1 Recognition

Chemical substances can be released overtly or covertly. In many cases it is obvious that a chemical incident has occurred. Ideally the ED will receive a formal warning from the emergency services or directly from an industrial site. Patients may allege that they have been involved in a chemical incident, arrive obviously contaminated, or attend complaining of feeling ill after smelling a 'funny' or 'chemical' odour. It should be noted that the ability to smell certain chemicals is genetically determined and not everyone has the ability to detect them; in addition, odour may only be detected at a level that exceeds the toxic threshold, which is important when staff members notice the smell.

Unfortunately, recognition that a chemical incident has occurred may not be so obvious and a degree of vigilance is necessary by emergency services or healthcare staff.

Box 6.1 Step 1-2-3 system

Step 1. One casualty: approach using normal procedures.
Step 2. Two casualties: approach with caution, consider all options. Report on arrival and update Control.
Step 3. Three or more casualties:
Do NOT approach
Withdraw
Contain
Report
Isolate yourself and SEND for SPECIALIST HELP

Multiple patients may arrive unannounced with similar symptoms (e.g. respiratory or neurological symptoms) from the same geographical location. This is the basis of the Step 1-2-3 protocol used by the emergency services (see Box 6.1).

Patients may present with certain toxidromes, which are clusters of symptoms and signs suggestive of exposure to chemicals (see Table 6.1). A good example of the value of toxidromes as an indicator of toxic exposure comes from Japan, where clinicians who had treated patients from the Matsumoto sarin release were amongst the first to recognize the features of sarin poisoning whilst watching news footage of the later Tokyo attack (Murakami 2003).

6.3.2 Containment

A number of protocols have been devised to reduce the risk of secondary contamination.

- The hospital needs to be *'locked down'*, which means that all of the entrances are secured except the one where patients enter the ED and a separate access point for staff.

- The air conditioning must be isolated to prevent the spread of volatile agent to other parts of the hospital.

- Patients who present to an ED following a chemical incident should be asked to go outside, where they should be assessed by a senior clinician. A rapid risk assessment will need to be undertaken as to whether the waiting room should be evacuated and ventilated. In most instances the risk of secondary contamination from a single, ambulant casualty is minimal.

Not every chemical presents a risk of secondary contamination, for example patients exposed to gases may be free of residual contamination. Although both fire and ambulance services have the capability to detect and identify the chemicals at the scene of release, precise information about the nature of the chemical is unlikely to be rapidly available. Also the current generation of detection and identification monitors available to EDs are based on military models that were designed for battlefield identification of chemical warfare agents (CWAs). Unfortunately, they do not identify most toxic industrial chemicals (TICs) and provide false positive readings in the presence of ethanol, alcohol hand gel and some perfumes. Therefore, the safest default option is to assume that all patients presenting from the scene of an incident pose a risk until definite information is available.

6.3.3 Decontamination

6.3.3.1 External decontamination

The process Decontamination is the process of removing a chemical from the patient before it is absorbed. External decontamination describes the method of removing a chemical from the patient's skin, hair, eyes, and any wounds.

Table 6.1 Toxidromes of chemical warfare agents (see also Chapter 17)

Agents	Odour	Onset	Symptoms	Signs	Differential diagnosis
Nerve agents	Fruity	Rapid	Weakness, dyspnoea, runny nose, blurred vision, painful eyes	Muscle fasciculations, miosis, wheeze, copious secretions, altered mental state, collapse	Organo-phosphate/ carbamate pesticides cyanide, myasthenia gravis
Blister agents	Mustard/garlic/ horseradish	Mustard: hours Lewisite: minutes	Burning/itchy skin, sore throat/painful eyes	Erythema/blisters, haemoptysis/ pulmonary oedema	Contact with caustics, sodium hydroxide, and ammonia
Choking agents	Chlorine: characteristic smell Phosgene: hay/mown grass	Chlorine: rapid onset mild ➜ more severe over hours Phosgene: 1–24 hours	Sore throat/ painful eyes, throat/chest tightness, dyspnoea, wheeze	Laryngeal oedema/ inflamed throat, pulmonary oedema	Upper airway sepsis
Cyanide	Bitter almonds	Rapid	Painful eyes, dizziness/ headache, dyspnoea, collapse	Convulsions, hypotension, rapid, deep respirations, metabolic acidosis, and high venous oxygen content	Nerve agents, carbon monoxide, hydrogen sulphide
Ricin	None	18–24 hours (ingestion) 8–36 hours (inhalation)	Ingestion: diarrhoea/ vomiting/ abdominal pain Inhalation: cough/tight chest, fever, nausea, weakness	Combined acute pulmonary and gastrointestinal signs	Atypical infections/ biological weapons (tularaemia, plague, Q-fever) Phosgene

The aims of decontamination are:

- to stop ongoing exposure for the patient and reduce their absorbed toxic dose; and
- to reduce the risk of secondary contamination of healthcare facilities and staff.

There are a number of different possible methods of undertaking decontamination: firstly, physically removing the chemical by washing with soap and water (or brushing for dry powders); secondly, inactivating the chemical, such as using hypochlorite solution to inactivate organophosphorous compounds (Duirk and Colette 2006); thirdly, using adsorbents such as Fuller's earth (Taysse et al. 2007); lastly, chelating agents such as diphoterine (Nehles et al. 2006) have been recently advocated to bind chemicals. Wet decontamination using soap and water is currently recommended in the UK (Heptonstall and Gent 2007; Morgan et al. 2007) primarily for logistical reasons, since water is universally available. It should be remembered that external decontamination does not reduce the damage that is caused by chemicals that have already been absorbed (Hall and Maibach 2006), therefore it is imperative that it must be undertaken as soon as possible after exposure has occurred. Resources have recently been allocated to the blue light services to allow rapid deployment of decontamination equipment to the scene of the incident (Communities and Local Government 2008).

The patients disrobe and are then decontaminated following the 'rinse-wipe-rinse' system:

- *Rinse 1*. The patient is drenched under the shower. This removes particulate matter and water-soluble substances.
- *Wipe*. Detergent solution (10 ml in a bucket of water) is applied with a soft brush/sponge. This removes organic chemicals.
- *Rinse 2*. The patient is drenched again under the shower. This removes the detergent and chemicals.

Particular attention should be paid to the patient's face and the process should be repeated if there is any visible residual contamination. In addition, wounds should be thoroughly irrigated. Water should be lukewarm; there is a known risk of inducing hypothermia in the patients (Black 2003) if it is too cold, while there is a theoretical risk that water that is too warm may promote transcutaneous absorption of chemical (Moody and Maibach 2006; Renshaw 1947). Eyes should be thoroughly irrigated with 1–2 litres of normal saline or Hartmann's solution (two common forms of intravenous rehydration therapy). Contact lenses should be removed. In the case of mustard gas, irrigation should continue for at least 30 minutes (Department of Health 2003). If an acid or alkali has contaminated the patient's eyes, irrigation should continue until a neutral pH has been achieved.

Limitations of decontamination

1. *Difficulties in achieving adequate decontamination*. The process of external decontamination is not as simple as it seems. Exercises have indicated that removal of contamination may not always be complete (Al-Damouk and Bleetman 2005). However, decontamination procedures are currently the subject of a series of studies (Chilcott 2009) and

the first published report has indicated that use of a washcloth during the standard protocol described above may result in a 20% increase in removal of contaminant (Amlôt 2010).

2. *Respiratory off-gassing.* It must be remembered that the process described above only removes chemical from the patient's exterior (Lavoie et al. 1992; Schultz et al. 1995; Al-Damouk and Bleetman 2005). Some chemicals may be present in significant concentrations in the patient's expired air; this is called *'respiratory off-gassing'*. There are a number of case reports where staff have become clinically affected by breathing in these contaminated gases. Most of these cases involved anaesthetists who intubated the patients and were therefore close to the patient's breathing zone (Harrison et al. 2002; Davey and Moppet 2004). However, one case (incident 3 in Harrison et al. 2002) involved the secondary contamination of an intensive care unit nurse who was looking after a patient who had been exposed to trichlorethylene, a volatile chemical that is excreted via the lungs. The patient's expired breath was heavily contaminated with the chemical and this was vented out of the back of the ventilator into the area where the nurse was working. The problem was solved by moving the patient to an operating theatre where the ventilators were attached to a *scavenging system*, where the expired gases were removed to a safe area outside the building by low-pressure suction.

The risk of secondary contamination by respiratory off-gassing can be reduced by simple measures such as regularly rotating staff out of the area and keeping the resuscitation room well ventilated i.e. keep the external doors open (Okumura et al. 1996).

3. *Contaminated body secretions.* Vomitus may contain ingested chemical (Stacey et al. 2004) and should be cleared up quickly into sealed bags. In the case of vesicant agents, blisters should be kept intact until the responsible agent is formally identified because blisters caused by Lewisite will contain active chemical (Chilcott 2007), unlike those due to mustard gas or TICs with a blistering action.

4. *Gaps in capacity.* Ambulance services and fire brigades both have equipment that can cope with decontaminating large numbers of casualties. However, there are concerns about the capacity of the current decontamination equipment supplied to hospitals (Malpass and Blunden 2003); although plans are in place to upgrade hospital facilities, there is currently a possible gap in resilience that needs to be addressed locally at the planning stage (e.g. developing agreements with the local fire service to provide tenders to the hospital to rapidly wash large numbers of self-presenting casualties) (Clarke et al. 2008).

Treatment prior to decontamination PPE limits dexterity and restricts patient assessment of visual clues before decontamination is undertaken. Until recently, it was accepted practice for medical care to be started only once the casualties had been removed from the contaminated area (the 'hot zone'); this has recently been questioned (primarily due to length of time required to decontaminate an individual patient) and it is becoming recognized that earlier medical intervention in the hot zone may be life saving (DJ Baker, personal communication; Byers et al. 2008). A series of studies looking at resuscitation skills that can be performed whilst wearing PPE has been undertaken (Castle et al. 2009, 2010a–c) and is described in the PPE and definitive treatment sections below.

6.3.3.2 Gastrointestinal decontamination

There are a number of techniques available to try to prevent absorption of ingested drug. However, these techniques are limited because to be effective they need to be administered before a significant amount of drug has been absorbed. Although the evidence base for these techniques is limited, expert consensus has agreed that they must be performed within 1 hour of ingestion in most situations.

Activated charcoal (AC) (American Academy of Clinical Toxicology 2005): AC binds drug in the bowel lumen, which prevents it from being absorbed. Unfortunately, AC is not palatable and it is often difficult to persuade the patient to take it. It may be given via a wide-bore nasogastric tube but this can precipitate vomiting in the conscious patient and the airway must be secured in those with reduced conscious levels to prevent aspiration. Certain agents are not adsorbed onto AC:

- metals (e.g. iron, lithium, mercury)
- acids and alkalis
- hydrocarbons.

Whole bowel irrigation (WBI) (American Academy of Clinical Toxicology 2004a): The aim of this treatment is to flush the bowel lumen so that the drug passes through without being absorbed. The patient is required to drink 1.5–2 litres of polyethylene glycol per hour, or it can be administered via a nasogastric tube. This is continued until the rectal effluent is clear. It is particularly useful for substances not adsorbed onto AC, for slow-release formulations of medicines, or for well-wrapped packets of illicit drugs swallowed for the purposes of smuggling.

Induced emesis and gastric lavage (American Academy of Clinical Toxicology 2004b,c): Neither of these techniques is recommended because of the lack of evidence of efficacy and the unacceptable risk of serious complications, such as injury to the patient's oesophagus or aspiration of stomach contents.

6.3.4 Personal protective equipment

6.3.4.1 Levels of PPE

There are four levels of PPE (see Table 6.2) and currently all UK EDs and ambulance services have been issued with standardized level C PPE. The UK standardized level C suit provides the highest level of protection achievable at level C as it is a fully encased suit that provides filtered air via an electric motor, which reduces the work of breathing and cools the suit. However, a level C suit can only be utilized where the atmospheric oxygen content is not depleted. Currently only the fire service and specialist ambulance teams (hazardous area response teams) are trained to work in areas with low levels of oxygen using higher levels of PPE with self-contained breathing systems.

Table 6.2 Levels of PPE

Level	Description	Advantages	Disadvantages
A	Completely encapsulated suit with self-contained breathing apparatus	Highest level of protection possible	Expensive and requires significant training to use safely and typically limited to specialist teams
			Air supply limited and heavy, affecting mobility
B	Encapsulating suit, air supplied via a hose or breathing apparatus	A high level of protection, air supplied via hose reduces weight and increases availability of air supply	Dependence on external air supply
C	Splash suit and filtered air UK NHS suit is fully encapsulated (maximizing protection) and provides air via a motor, minimizing work of breathing	More light weight, less training required UK version does not need 'fit testing of the respirator' and easier to put on Less expensive than level A and B equipment	Not suitable for use in low oxygen environments

Levels A–C are all hot and cumbersome, with levels A and B being more cumbersome and hotter than level C.

Level	Description	Advantages	Disadvantages
D	Normal clothing with splash protection (plastic apron), gloves and face masks (not theatre masks but FFP3 mask that filters 99% of atmospheric particles)	Cheap, easy to wear, limited impact on mobility	Not suitable for chemical protection, but useful for some degree of biological, e.g. pandemic flu FFP3 masks do require a degree of training for effective use

Adapted from Hick et al., Protective equipment for health care facility decontamination personnel: Regulations, risks, and recommendations, *Annals of Emergency Medicine*, **42**(3) 370–80, 2003, with permission from Elsevier.

6.3.4.2 Performing skills whilst wearing PPE

All PPE adversely affects skill performance as it is designed to ensure wearer protection and not optimal skill performance. Level A–C suits affect vision and motor dexterity, and reduce (or eliminate totally) tactile sensation. Krueger (2001) noted that hand steadiness reduced by 30%, two-handed fine dexterity by 55% and single-handed dexterity by 30%. This loss of dexterity was primarily due to the butyl gloves worn as part of the PPE. Therefore only life-saving skills should be performed prior to decontamination, with those patients with less time-critical injuries/symptoms waiting until after decontamination. **It is important to remember that decontamination is a form of treatment.**

This loss of dexterity and tactile sensation will affect the performance of resuscitation skills. Castle et al. (2009) noted that the more dextrous a skill the longer it took to perform whilst wearing level C PPE; this will be discussed in more detail in the definitive care section below.

6.3.4.3 Training in PPE

PPE training should consist of individual familiarization, team working in putting on/removing the chemical suits, and specialist skills performance. Northington et al. (2007) noted poor skill retention with regards donning/removing PPE when paramedics were retested at 6 months with less than 15% of paramedics able to complete donning/removing PPE without performing a critical error. An important part of training is suit familiarization. PPE is generally well tolerated, with Castle and colleagues (Castle 2010b,c) recruiting 156 participants with only one episode of claustrophobia, although Carter and Cammermeyer (1985) reported seven episodes of failure to wear PPE out of 105 participants utilizing military PPE. However participants in the Carter and Cammermeyer (1985) study wore PPE for at least 1 hour and it must be remembered that PPE can be hot and uncomfortable to wear.

A learning curve exists with regard to the performance of clinical skills whilst wearing PPE (Castle 2009, 2010b) even if the clinician is used to performing those skills in normal practice. In addition, new practical procedures may have to be learnt or practised, such as new techniques for securing endotracheal tubes, because traditional methods may not be practicable while wearing PPE (Castle 2010c). Training needs to concentrate on emergency drills, allowing clinicians to practise established and new emergency skills whilst being as realistic as possible. This will allow clinicians to become accustomed to the difficulties of skill completion whilst wearing PPE (Carter and Cammermeyer 1985; Krueger 2001).

6.3.5 Definitive care

6.3.5.1 Symptomatic and supportive therapy

There are more than 56 million organic and inorganic substances registered with the Chemical Abstract Service (CAS 2010); clearly it is not possible to have individual treatments for each chemical.

Patients should be managed using a standard ('A-B-C-D-E') approach, which ensures that the most rapidly dangerous clinical problems are identified first. As a physiological abnormality is identified, appropriate treatment measures are implemented to try to reverse the problem before moving on with the assessment. In reality, these patients are likely to be looked after by a clinical team, individual members of which will be responsible for each of the areas outlined below, so a number of assessments will continue concurrently.

Airway Ensure that the airway is clear and that a gag reflex is present (taking care not to stimulate vomiting). There are a number of techniques that can be used to open a patient's airway, but the definitive method is to insert a tube into the patient's trachea (endotracheal intubation), usually assisted by the administration of anaesthetic drugs. However, intubation is a highly specialized skill and it is becoming accepted practice to use supra-glottic airway devices such as the laryngeal mask airway (LMA) to establish an open airway rapidly. These are easier to use and their use is supported by the international resuscitation communities (Nolan 2010). Castle et al. (2009) noted that LMA insertion requires less dexterity than formal endotracheal intubation so recommend that it is the technique of choice for managing the airway when the clinician is wearing PPE. They also noted that skills performance varied by speciality with anaesthetists being the fastest and the most successful at both intubation and LMA insertion.

In normal clinical practice when a patient requires intubation (e.g. while having an anaesthetic before an operation or even as an emergency procedure in the resuscitation room) the ideal position for ease of intubation is to have the patient lying on a trolley at waist height. An additional advantage of LMA was reported by a further study by Castle et al. (2010a) which showed that LMA use while wearing PPE was not affected by patient position to the same degree as intubation. Therefore it should be the procedure of choice at the scene of an incident where patients are likely to be on the floor rather than on a trolley in a resuscitation room.

Once the patient has been externally decontaminated and moved into a safer area, then they can be intubated by a suitably skilled clinician with the patient in the optimal position on a trolley.

Breathing Look for central cyanosis (blue discolouration of the lips, tongue, and fingernails due to lack of oxygen), count the respiratory rate, look at the pattern of respiration, and attempt to assess depth of breathing. Monitor the patient's oxygen saturations using a pulse oximeter. The simplest treatment of inadequate respiration is the administration of supplemental oxygen. More profound ventilatory failure may require the patient to be intubated and artificial ventilation to be instituted.

Circulation Measure pulse rate and blood pressure. Intravenous access should be established. Cannulation of a vein has been the standard means of administering fluids and drugs in the emergency situation. However, it is a skill that requires fine motor skills and can be difficult to achieve rapidly in very sick patients. Recently, an alternative technique has gained favour for rapid vascular access in unconscious patients, particularly those who are in cardiac arrest: intraosseous (IO) access involves drilling a needle into a superficial bone such as the shin. It requires a lower degree of dexterity than cannulation of a vein and Castle et al. (2009) showed that it is relatively easy to perform while wearing PPE.

Hypotension often responds to intravenous administration of fluids. Rarely, drug therapy to support the circulation may be necessary, but this should be undertaken with advice from the National Poisons Information Service (NPIS) and once invasive monitoring (arterial and central venous pressures) has been set up. Slow heart rates are often well tolerated by patients but some casualties may need atropine or even application of temporary pacemakers to maintain a satisfactory heart rate. Fast heart rates (tachyarrhythmia) may need drug therapy but again this should only be started after advice from the NPIS because in some cases of poisoning these drugs may exacerbate the arrhythmia. Administration of antidotes/drugs is also adversely affected by PPE, mainly due to the loss of dexterity. The use of pre-filled emergency syringes and/or pre-drawn up drugs will increase the speed of drug administration and accuracy, and minimize the risk of needle stick injury to the rescuer (Castle 2010b). Wherever possible glass ampoules should be avoided as they are difficult to break and may damage PPE (Castle 2010b).

Disability Assess the conscious level of the patient; there are two standard methods:

AVPU (**A**lert; responds to **V**oice, responds to **P**ainful stimulus, **U**nresponsive)

Glasgow Coma Scale (GCS—see Box 6.2) (Teasdale and Jennett 1974).

Although neither of these assessment tools has been formally validated for toxicological causes of impaired consciousness, there are currently no other systems available and it seems reasonable to continue to use them. In addition to meticulous attention to the airway, breathing, and circulation, the patient's blood glucose level should be monitored closely.

Exposure This involves removing the patient's clothes and undertaking a 'top-to-toe' examination. Again, problems that are identified should be treated as necessary.

The importance of this approach cannot be overemphasized; during the Moscow theatre siege in 2002 (BBC 2002) patients died as a result of inadequate basic airway management, not due to delays in identifying the chemical agents involved or administering specialized treatments.

Agent-specific therapies (antidotes) are available for only a small number of toxins. They should be given if there is strong clinical suspicion (from the presence of toxidromes—see Table 6.1) as to the identity of the causative agent or after chemical analysis from the scene.

Box 6.2 Glasgow Coma Scale

Eye opening

Spontaneously	4
To verbal command	3
To painful stimulus	2
Not opening	1

Verbal response

Orientated	5
Disorientated but converses	4
Inappropriate words	3
Incomprehensible words	2
No response	1

Motor response

Obeys commands	6
Localizes pain	5
Flexion (withdraws from pain)	4
Abnormal flexion	3
Abnormal extension	2
No response	1

Reproduced from Teasdale and Jennett, Assessment of coma and impaired consciousness, *The Lancet*, Vol. 304, Issue 7872, pp. 81–4, 1974, with permission from Elsevier.

6.3.5.2 Enhanced elimination techniques

In some circumstances, the elimination of absorbed toxins can be encouraged. The simplest method is to ensure that the patient is well hydrated, which increases the glomerular filtration rate (the volume of blood that is filtered by the kidneys per unit time). This promotes elimination of renally excreted drugs or metabolites of drugs. In a limited number of cases, more specialized techniques are available to increase the rate of elimination of certain drugs. To be successfully eliminated, substances must have a low volume of distribution (they are located primarily in the bloodstream) and be poorly bound to plasma proteins.

Urinary alkalinization (Morgan and Polak 1971; Prescott et al. 1982): Administration of bicarbonate promotes excretion of weakly acidic drugs; they form the ionized form in the kidney, which prevents reabsorption back into the bloodstream and hence promotes excretion in the urine. This technique may be useful for poisoning by the herbicide 2,4-dichlorophenoxyacetic acid.

Extracorporeal techniques: Haemoperfusion, haemofiltration, and haemodialysis may be useful for eliminating a small number of substances. These techniques require specialized equipment and are usually only available on critical care units (haemofiltration) or renal units (haemoperfusion and dialysis). Filtration and dialysis may also be used to support failing kidneys.

Artificial ventilation: Some volatile chemicals are excreted via the lungs. In theory, by intubating and artificially ventilating the patient, the depth and rate of respiration can be intentionally increased to speed up the elimination of the chemical.

6.3.5.3 Antidotes

Antidotes are treatments that are specific to individual toxins. There are relatively few, some of which are held in regional centres so are not readily available to EDs Therefore, the emphasis on acute treatment is based on the symptomatic, supportive approach described above.

The non-pharmaceutical chemicals which have known antidotes include the following:

- *Cyanide*: There are a number of antidotes which bind cyanide and form non-toxic compounds. These include dicobalt edetate, sodium nitrite, sodium thiosulphate, and hydroxocobalamin. All of these have significant side-effects if given in the absence of cyanide exposure, with the possible exception of hydroxocobalamin. However, there is little information about the use of hydroxocobalamin with hydrogen cyanide and large volumes have to be given, so currently dicobalt edetate is recommended as the first-line treatment and has been stockpiled by the Department of Health (Department of Health 2003).

- *Organophosphate compounds (including nerve agents)*: Atropine is used to counteract the cholinergic effects of these compounds. Pralidoxime is used to reactivate the inhibited enzyme, cholinesterase. Both of these agents have been stockpiled by the Department of Health.

- *Heavy metals*: There are a number of antidotes, including sodium calcium edetate and succimer (DMSA), both particularly useful for lead poisoning, Unithiol (DMPS) and dimercaprol are used for mercury poisoning. Heavy metal poisonings are relatively rare conditions and use of the antidotes should be supervised by a clinical toxicologist and advice sought from the NPIS.

◆ *Thallium*: The antidote is Prussian Blue, and again this should be used under the supervision of a clinical toxicologist and advice sought from the NPIS.

A full list of all antidotes available in the UK can be found on the website of the College of Emergency Medicine (College of Emergency Medicine 2008).

6.4 Sources of information: role of the NPIS and the Centre for Radiation, Chemical and Environmental Hazards of the Health Protection Agency

There are a number of sources of information for clinicians when faced with poisoned patients. Toxbase is an online information resource developed by the NPIS and widely used as the first source of information for acute clinicians. It is found at www.spib.axl. co.uk and an institutional password is needed to access this site.

The NPIS, a service commissioned by the Health Protection Agency (HPA), runs a telephone advice service and is able to give advice about the clinical treatment of individual patients and other aspects of management when the chemical has been identified. Some of the individual poisons units that comprise the NPIS hold regional stocks of some antidotes and also have laboratories that can undertake certain toxicological analyses. Lists of accredited toxicological laboratories can also be found on the website www.assayfinder.com.

During an acute chemical incident, the Centre for Radiation, Chemical and Environmental Hazards (CRCE) of the HPA can provide information about the toxic effects of chemicals, but will also liaise with the local Health Protection Unit (HPU), assist the emergency services in identifying the chemical(s), and advise other agencies, such as the utilities and local authority. CRCE undertakes surveillance of acute chemical incidents and therefore should be informed of all such events. Both CRCE and the NPIS provide a 24-hour service.

6.5 Planning and preparation

All EDs should have developed a Chemical Incident Plan, which should be separate from, but dovetails into, the Major Incident Plan. This should use the above system but be adapted to the specific facilities and geography. An assessment of the risks in the catchment area of the hospital should be made, including local industry, including Control of Major Accident Hazards (COMAH) sites (Control of Major Accident Hazards Regulations 2005), transport systems (motorways, railways, and airports), and possible terrorist targets.

The plan should include contact details of sources of information, which should include:

◆ NPIS

◆ CRCE

◆ local HPUs

◆ institutional password for Toxbase.

It is helpful if an individual or group of members of staff have responsibility for updating the plan and organizing appropriate training. It is useful if that group establishes links with those responsible for chemical response in the blue light services and with the local health emergency planning advisors. The plan should be tested and specific aspects, such as setting up the decontamination equipment and donning PPE, should be practised regularly. In particular, each hospital should determine in advance who will be undertaking decontamination; there are pros and cons to using clinical and non-clinical staff.

6.6 Summary

Treatment of all types of poisoning is primarily symptomatic and supportive, with gut decontamination, enhanced elimination techniques, and antidotes only being suitable for relatively few cases.

In chemical incidents, risk of secondary contamination can be reduced by external decontamination of casualties and appropriate use of PPE by staff who come into contact with patients before and during decontamination.

Advice should be sought from the NPIS and CRCE should be informed.

Chemical incident plans should be developed by all EDs and these should be thoroughly tested and practised.

6.7 References

Al-Damouk M and Bleetman A. (2005) Impact of the Department of Health initiative to equip and train acute trusts to manage chemically contaminated casualties. *Emerg Med J* 22:347–350.

American Academy of Clinical Toxicology. (2004a) European Association of Poisons Centres and Clinical Toxicologists. Position paper: whole-bowel irrigation. *J Toxicol Clin Toxicol* 42:843–854.

American Academy of Clinical Toxicology. (2004b) European Association of Poisons Centres and Clinical Toxicologists. Position paper: ipecac syrup. *J Toxicol Clin Toxicol* 42:133–143.

American Academy of Clinical Toxicology. (2004c) European Association of Poisons Centres and Clinical Toxicologists. Position paper: gastric lavage. *J Toxicol Clin Toxicol* 42:933–943.

American Academy of Clinical Toxicology. (2005) European Association of Poisons Centres and Clinical Toxicologists. Position paper: single-dose activated charcoal. *J Toxicol Clin Toxicol* 43:61–87.

Amlôt R, Larner J, Matar H, Jones DR, Carter H, Turner EA, Price SC, Chilcott RP. (2010) Comparative analysis of showering protocols for mass-casualty decontamination. 25:435–439.

Baker D. (1999) Management of respiratory failure in toxic disasters. *Resuscitation* 42:125–131.

BBC. (2002) *Moscow theatre siege*. British Broadcasting Association. http://news.bbc.co.uk/2/hi/europe/2362609.stm.

Black J. (2003) Exercise Alex. *Chemical Incident Response* 28:16–19.

Brennan R, Waerckerle J, Sharp T, Lillibridge S. (1999) Chemical warfare agents: emergency medical and emergency public health issues. *Ann Emerg Med* 34:191–204.

Burgess J. (1999) Hospital evacuations due to hazardous materials incidents. *Am J Emerg Med* 17:50–52.

Burgess J, Kirk M, Borron S, Cisek J. (1999) Emergency department hazardous materials protocol for contaminated patients. *Ann Emerg Med* 34:205–212.

Byers M, Russell M, Lockey D. (2008) Clinical care in the 'Hot Zone'. *Emerg Med J* 25:108–112.

Carter BJ, Cammermeyer M. (1985) Biopsychological responses of medical unit personnel wearing checial defense ensemble in a simulated chemical environment. *Mil Med* 150(5):239–249.

CAS (Chemical Abstract Service Registry). www.cas.org/expertise/cascontent/registry/index.html Accessed December 2010.

Castle N, Owen R, Clarke S, Hann M, Reeves D, Gurney I (2009) Impact of Chemical, Biological, Radiation and Nuclear Personnel Protective Equipment on the performance of low- and high-dexterity airway and vascular skills. *Resuscitation* **80**:1290–1295.

Castle N, Owen R, Clarke S, Hann M, Reeves D, Gurney I (2010a) Does position of the patient adversely affect successful intubation whilst wearing CBRN-PPE? *Resuscitation* **81**:1165–1171.

Castle N, Bowen J, Spencer N (2010b) Does wearing CBRN-PPE adversely affect the ability for clinicians to accurately, safely, and speedily draw up drugs? *Clin Toxicol* **48**:522–527.

Castle N, Owen R, Clark S, Hann M, Reeces D, Gurney I (2010c) Improving the technique of securing an endotracheal tube while wearing chemical, biological, radiological, or nuclear protection: a manikin study. *Prehosp Disaster Med* **25**:589–594.

Chilcott R. (2007) Dermal effects of chemical warfare agents. In: Marrs TC, Maynard RL, and Sidell FR. Chemical warfare agents: toxicology and treatment, 2nd edn. John Wiley & Sons, New York.

Chilcott RP (2009) An overview of the Health Protection Agency's Research and Development Programme on Decontamination. *Chemical Hazards and Poisons Report* **15**:26–28.

Clarke SFJ, Chilcott RP, Wilson JC, Kamanyire R, Baker DJ, Hallett A. (2008) Decontamination of multiple casualties who are chemically contaminated: a challenge for acute hospitals. *Prehospital Disast Med* **23**:175–181.

College of Emergency Medicine. (2008) Clinical Guidelines, CEC Best Practice Guidelines, CEM Antidotes Guidelines. Available at: www.collemergencymed.ac.uk/Shop%2DFloor/Clinical%20Guidelines/Clinical%20Guidelines. Accessed December 2010.

Communities and Local Government. (2008) *New Dimensions mass decontamination programme.* Available at: http://www.communities.gov.uk/fire/resilienceresponse/newdimensionequipping/. Accessed February 2008.

Control of Major Accident Hazards (Amendment) Regulations. (2005) Statutory Instrument No. 1088. HMSO, London.

Cox R. (1994) Decontamination and management of hazardous materials exposure victims in the Emergency Department. *Ann Emerg Med* **23**:761–770.

Davey A, Moppett I. (2004) Postoperative complications after CS spray exposure. *Anaesthesia* **59**:1219–1220.

Department of Health (2003) Expert Group on the Management of Chemical Casualties Caused by Terrorist Activity. First report. Treatment of poisoning by selected chemical compounds. Department of Health, London.

Duirk S, Collette T. (2006) Degradation of chlorpyrifos in aqueous chlorine solutions: pathways, kinetics, and modeling. *Environ Sci Tech* **40**:546–551.

Geller R, Singleton K, Tarantino M, Drenzel C, Toomey K. (2001) Nosocomial poisoning associated with Emergency Department treatment of organophosphate toxicity—Georgia, 2000. *J Toxicol Clin Toxicol* **39**:109–111.

Hall A, Maibach H. (2006) Water decontamination of chemical skin/eye splashes: a critical review. *Cutaneous Ocular Toxicol* **25**:67–83.

Harrison H, Clarke S, Wilson A, Murray V. (2002) Chemical contamination of healthcare facilities and staff. *Chemical Incident Report* **25**:2–5. Available at: www.hpa.org.uk/web/HPAwebFile/HPAweb_C/1194947350265.

Heptonstall J, Gent N. (2007) Generic Incident Management. CBRN incidents: clinical management and health protection. Version 2. Health Protection Agency. Available at: www.hpa.org.uk/emergency/pdfs/generic.pdf.

Hick JL, Hanfling D, Burstein J, Markham J, Macintyre AG, Barbera JA. (2003). Protective equipment for health care facility decontamination personnel: Regulations, risks and recommendations. *Ann Emerg Med* **42**:370–380.

Horton D, Berkowitz Z, Kaye W. (2003) Secondary contamination of ED personnel from hazardous materials events, 1995–2001. *Am J Emerg Med* **21**:199–204.

Krueger G. (2001) Psychological and performance effects of chemical Biological Protective clothing and equipment. *Mil Med* **166** (suppl 2):41–43.

Lavoie F, Coomes T, Cisek, J, Fulkerson L. (1992) Emergency Department external decontamination for hazardous chemical exposures. *Vet Hum Toxicol* **34**:61–64.

Malpass T, Blunden M. (2003) Deployment of PPE in the event of a chemical incident. The importance of pre-planning and estimating capacity. *Chemical Hazards and Poisons Report* **1**:23–24.

Miyaki K, Nishiwaki Y, Maekawa K, Ogawa Y, Asukai N, Yoshimura K, Etoh N, Matsumoto Y, Kikuchi Y, Kumagai N, Omae K. (2005) Effects of sarin on the nervous system of subway workers seven years after the Tokyo subway sarin attack. *J Occup Health* **47**:299–304.

Moles T, Baker D. (1999) Clinical analogies for the management of toxic trauma. *Resuscitation* **42**:117–124.

Moody R, Maibach H. (2006) Skin decontamination: Importance of the wash-in effect. *Food Chem Toxicol* **44**:1783–1788.

Morgan A, Polak A. (1971) The excretion of salicylate in salicylate poisoning *Clin Sci* **41**:475–484.

Morgan D, Said B, Walsh A, Murray V, Clarke S, Lloyd D, Gent N. (2007) Initial investigation and management of outbreaks and incidents of unusual illnesses: A guide for health professionals. Health Protection Agency. Available at: www.hpa.org.uk/infections/topics_az/deliberate_release/unknown/Unusual_Illness.pdf.

Murakami H. (2003) Underground. The Tokyo gas attack and the Japanese psyche. Vintage Books, New York.

Nehles J, Hall A, Blomet J, Mathieu L. (2006) Diphoterine for emergent decontamination of skin/eye chemical splashes: 24 cases. *Cutaneous Ocular Toxicol* **25**:249–258.

Northington WE, Mahoney M, Hahn ME, Suyama J, Hostler D (2007) Training retention of level C personnel protective equipment used by emergency medical services personnel. *Acad Emerg Med* **14**(10):846–849.

Nozaki H, Hori S, Shinozawa Y, Fujishima S, Takuma K, Sagoh M, Kimura H, Ohki T, Suzuki M, Aikawa N. (1997) Secondary exposure of medical staff to sarin vapor in the emergency room. *Intes Care Med* **21**:1032–1035.

Ohbu S, Yamashina A, Takasu N, Yamaguchi T, Murai T, Nakano K, Matsui Y, Mikami R, Sakurai K, Hinohara S. (1997) Sarin poisoning on Tokyo subway. *South Med J* **90**:587–593.

Okumura T, Takasu N, Ishimatsu S, Miyanoki S, Mitsuhashi A, Kumada K, Tanaka K, Hinohara S. (1996) Report on 640 victims of the Tokyo subway sarin attack. *Ann Emerg Med* **28**:129–135.

Prescott L, Balali-Mood M, Critchley J, Johnstone A. (1982) Diuresis or urinary alkalinisation for salicylate poisoning? *Brit Med J* **285**:1383–1386.

Renshaw B. (1947) Observations on the role of water in the susceptibility of human skin to injury by vesicants. *J Invest Dermatol* **9**:75–85.

Schultz M, Cisek J, Wabeke R. (1995) Simulated exposure of hospital emergency personnel to solvent vapors and respirable dust during decontamination of chemically exposed patients. *Ann Emerg Med* **26**:324–329.

Stacey R, Morfey D, Payne S. (2004) Secondary contamination in organophosphate poisoning: analysis of an incident. *Q J Med* **97**:75–80.

Stewart A, Whiteside C, Tyler-Jones V, Ghebrehewet S, Reid J, McDonald P, Kennedy C, Pennycock A, Gent N, Seddon D. (2003) Phosphine suicide. *Chemical Incident Report* **27**:23–25.

Tan G et al. (2002) Chemical-Biological-Radiological (CBR) response: a template for hospital Emergency Departments. *Med J Australia* **177**:196–199.

Taysse L, Daulon S, Delamanche S, Bellier B, Breton P. (2007) Skin decontamination of mustards and organophosphates: comparative efficiency of RSDL and Fuller's earth in domestic swine. *Hum Exp Toxicol* **26**:135–141.

Teasdale G, Jennett B. (1974) Assessment of coma and impaired consciousness. A practical scale. *Lancet* **2**:81–84.

Timm N, Reeves S. (2007) A mass casualty incident involving children and chemical decontamination. *Disaster Management & Response* **5**:49–55.

Chapter 7

Susceptibility to environmental hazards

David Baker and Ishani Kar-Purkayastha

Learning outcomes

At the end of this chapter and any recommended reading the student should be able to:

1. discuss how risks to human health from chemicals are assessed;

2. identify susceptible or vulnerable population groups, and explain why they are more susceptible;

3. explain how a hazardous chemical affects human health using a source-pathway-receptor model;

4. discuss aspects of susceptibility/vulnerability using examples, and

5. apply acquired knowledge in the analysis and management of hazardous situations.

7.1 Introduction

Risk to human health from exposure to potentially hazardous environmental chemicals is assessed on the basis of the best available data. Only rarely are there adequate toxicology data for exposure to environmental chemicals available from human populations. Therefore, many toxicological risk assessments will largely use experimental animal data with added uncertainty factors to allow inter-species variability (between animals and humans) and for intra-species variability (between different groups within the same species). (See Chapter 3: Experimental methods for investigating the toxicity of chemicals).

Better understanding of the factors resulting in human disease and of the variation in human susceptibility to disease induced by chemicals has lead to the approach of risk assessments being directed towards specific groups, such as children and the elderly. An example of this is in the USA, where the 1996 Food Quality Protection Act mandated the use of an additional safety (or uncertainty) factor to account for differences between adults and children when risk assessing pesticides. This was undertaken to account for developmental risks and incomplete data when considering a pesticide's effect on infants and children and any special sensitivity and exposure to pesticide chemicals that infants and children may have. More recently, the UK Committee on the Toxicity of Chemicals in Food, Consumer

Products and the Environment (COT) published a report on variability and uncertainty in the toxicology of chemicals, which gives detailed consideration of vulnerable subgroups, including children (COT 2007). The working group was specifically asked to consider the appropriateness of the uncertainty factors usually used to extrapolate toxicological data from animals to humans and for variability in the human population, including children. They found that the current approaches and uncertainty factors are adequate in the case of interspecies extrapolation and generally appropriate in the case of variability in the human population, but recommended that the area be kept under review.

7.2 Understanding susceptibility

Specific subgroups within a general population, who might be particularly vulnerable to exposure to chemicals due to some deviation from the 'normal' exposed person, can be considered in the following three ways:

- **A subgroup of a population is considered to be more susceptible than the population as a whole to a chemical hazard assuming that there are no other confounders or biasing factors,** i.e. exposure to a chemical at a particular dose will elucidate a harmful effect in the susceptible person, where no effect would be noticed in a 'normal' person.

- **The level of exposure to a hazard (or dose) that is needed to elucidate an adverse response in the susceptible group compared to the population as a whole,** i.e. the susceptible person will require a smaller exposure compared to a 'normal' person for an adverse response to occur.

- **The time period before the adverse effect manifests in different equally exposed groups,** i.e. the adverse effect will occur much earlier in time in the susceptible person, compared to the 'normal' person.

Some population subgroups may be innately more susceptible to the effects of exposure to pollutants than others due to genetic predisposition or to incomplete development of normal (adult) physiological functions. Individuals who have specific genetic or immunological variations from the 'normal' are likely to be vulnerable throughout their lives. On the other hand, some population groups may be particularly vulnerable at specific times during their lives, such as during pregnancy, childhood, or old age (Risk Assessment and Toxicology Steering Committee 1999). Also important are those who become more susceptible as a result of environmental or social factors, or personal behaviour (acquired susceptibility) and those who are simply exposed to unusually large amounts of pollutants. Members of the last group may well be more vulnerable by virtue of the magnitude of exposure rather than as a result of individual susceptibility, for example by living near a busy road or through occupational exposure.

Susceptible subgroups of the population can be split into three main groups based on biological, socio-cultural, or ethnic characteristics that may affect their vulnerability to adverse effects resulting from environmental exposure to a particular hazardous chemical, shown in Table 7.1. However, it is important to remember that susceptibility will vary with different chemicals.

Table 7.1 Factors affecting vulnerability to an environmental hazard

Biological	Sociocultural	Ethnic
Age group (e.g. infant, elderly)	Diet	Genetic
Gender	Smoking status	Social (e.g. diet)
Disease state/medication	Alcohol, drugs	
Genetic susceptibility	Socioeconomic deprivation	
Pregnancy (e.g. foetal development)	Religion	
Physiological variation (e.g. height, weight)	Housing quality	
	Housing location	
	Occupation	

Data from Risk assessment strategies in relation to population subgroups, Institute for Environment and Health, 1999 available from http://ieh.cranfield.ac.uk/ighrc/cr3.pdf (accessed 17.08.11)

The following groups are considered in more detail later in the chapter:

- developing foetuses, infants, and very young children;
- the elderly;
- groups of people with genetic polymorphisms;
- those who are socially and economically deprived.

7.3 Source-pathway-receptor model

Three essential factors determine the risk from a hazardous chemical present in the environment to human health. These are (i) the **source** of the chemical of concern, (ii) the **pathway** by which it can come into contact with the public, including air, water, land, and food, and (ii) the **receptor**—in this case the person or group of people.

Other factors which must be taken into account are:

- age at time of exposure, e.g. infancy, childhood;
- duration of exposure: brief, intermittent, or over a long period of time;
- level of exposure: a high or low dose;

This is simplified into the source-pathway-receptor model (Figure 7.1).

7.4 Increased susceptibility of developing foetuses, infants, and very young children

In 2009, the HPA published *A Children's Environment and Health Strategy for the UK* at the request of the Department of Health, which clearly set out the unique aspects of environmental and other influences on health faced by children (Health Protection Agency 2009). Children are considered to be particularly susceptible to environmental chemicals compared to the general population of adults because of their fundamental differences from adults, which may lead to an unusual pattern of exposure (see Table 7.2). Young children also spend the majority of their time within the home, with one estimate of an average of 19.3 hours per day in the UK (Farrow and Golding 1997). The home environment

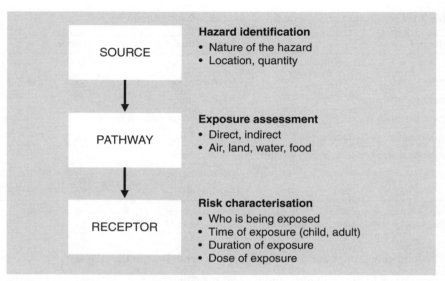

Fig. 7.1 Illustrating the source-pathway-receptor model.

is a unique environment known to accumulate air pollutants at a higher concentration than outdoors (Whitmore et al. 1994). Children also have a longer expected length of life left which all lead to a potentially greater exposure to toxic chemicals.

7.4.1 Physical differences

Children are much smaller than adults, which means that they tend to be in much closer contact with the ground. Proportionally they have a larger surface area of skin compared to their body size, which increases the potential for exposure and the absorption of chemicals through their skin. Proportional to body weight, children breathe more air, drink more water and eat more food than adults do. The amount of air breathed in by a child while resting, per unit time on a weight-by-weight basis, may be nearly three times that of an adult.

7.4.2 Time windows

Children are both growing and developing rapidly, with their internal structures constantly developing and maturing. This is vital for the correct functioning of their bodies, for example their ability to produce specific hormones. Exposure during critical 'time windows' in development may cause irreparable damage and render the body unable to function properly. The organs that are particularly sensitive to chemical damage during development include the brain and central nervous system, the immune system, and the reproductive system.

7.4.3 Metabolic pathways

Some internal functions of infants and young children differ from adults, making children more vulnerable to exposure. Their mechanisms for detoxifying and excreting environmental chemicals are immature and less efficient. Metabolic pathways may not yet include the same enzymes, or the same amount of a particular enzyme, which an adult would use to metabolize and detoxify the chemicals that enter their bodies (Eskenazi et al. 1999). This means that a dose of a specific chemical, which an adult body could quickly eliminate before damage is caused, has the potential to cause harm to a child.

7.4.4 Behavioural patterns

Younger children have age-specific behaviours that may increase their exposure to hazardous chemicals. For example, playing close to the ground and crawling can increase potential exposure through the skin. Children also have a higher ratio of skin surface area to body weight compared to adults. Younger children routinely explore their environment by putting fingers, toys, and other objects into their mouths, and contact with floors, carpets, lawns, and other surfaces during crawling may lead to enhanced exposure via hand-to-mouth and object-to-mouth transfer. Some children exhibit pica behaviour, which is the deliberate ingestion of non-food items.

Table 7.2 Differences between children and adults

Factor	How children differ from adults
Exposure to hazard	Sources of exposure (e.g. industry, use in gardens)
	Pathways of exposure (e.g. dust, water, soil)
	Routes of exposure (e.g. dermal, inhalation, ingestion)
	Greater intake of air/food/water per unit body
	Increased surface area to weight ratio
Physiological factors	Greater rate of circulation
	Higher cell growth in many organs
	Shorter height
	Lighter weight
	Faster rate of respiration
Pharmacokinetics	Greater intake through the gut in the very young
	Higher rate of intake through the lungs
	Reduced ability to break down harmful chemicals in the very young
	Higher membrane permeability affecting oral absorption of chemicals in the very young
	Undeveloped ability to bind and store chemicals
	Increased bioavailability in body
	Decreased excretion from the body in the very young
Pharmacodynamics	Immature immune system
	Different extent of effect and response to toxic substances in the very young (may be increased or decreased sensitivity depending on substance)
	Increased sensitivity of particular organs

7.5 Increased susceptibility in the elderly

This susceptibility is most often the result of disease states that are more common in older people compromising their physiological reserves and the ability to withstand stress. Diseases such as heart disease or high blood pressure reduce the ability to compensate for the changes in blood volume or falls in blood pressure or the risk of disturbances of heart rhythm that may follow toxic exposures.

The alteration in the structure of blood vessels, such as thickening of the walls of the arteries with age-related arteriosclerosis, will prevent compensatory increases in blood flow that may be necessary (due to loss of elasticity) to prevent ill-health following toxic exposures. Similarly, chest or respiratory diseases such as emphysema or chronic bronchial asthma may prevent compensatory respiratory mechanisms coming into effect if respiration is compromised by toxic exposures.

The elderly and those who have been exposed previously or concurrently to relatively high levels of other xenobiotics, such as therapeutic drugs, may have altered functions of vital organs which would prevent the normal body compensatory mechanisms coming in to effect following toxic exposures. An example is an individual who is treated with a drug to slow the heart rate. The presence of such a drug will diminish the ability of the heart to increase the rate as a compensatory response.

7.6 Increased susceptibility due to genetic polymorphisms

Genetic polymorphisms often affect the qualitative and quantitative functions of enzymes needed for the inactivation or detoxification of toxic chemicals. One of the better known examples is the absence of the enzyme to metabolize alcohol in some population groups. This enzyme—alcohol dehydrogenase—is absent in nearly 20% of the Japanese population and such individuals develop adverse effects after even minimal doses of alcohol. Similarly the genetic polymorphisms associated with metabolizing enzymes (e.g. acetyltransferase and cholinesterase) produce variations in the ability to inactivate many xenobiotics—often drugs. Such polymorphisms, in certain instances, have resulted in grouping individuals as fast metabolizers and slow metabolizers (Rang et al. 1995).

7.7 Increased susceptibility due to socio-economic deprivation

Socially and economically deprived populations can be more at risk of overcrowding, poor nutrition, and poor sanitation, which may increase the prevalence of diseases states such as anaemia, diarrhoea, and infections of the chest and skin. Such socio-economic factors invariably lead to a greater vulnerability to communicable diseases as well as greater vulnerability to toxic insults from chemicals.

These groups may react more strongly to a given exposure, either as a result of increased responsiveness to a specific dose and/or as a result of a larger internal dose of some pollutants than those of a higher socio-economic status exposed to the same concentration.

7.8 Examples of susceptibility and exposure to chemicals

When responding to an incident that involves a potentially harmful chemical, it is important to consider whether there are any susceptible subgroups of the population that may be at greater risk from exposure and adverse health effects compared to the general population. Public health personnel need to be particularly concerned about these groups and to identify them quickly to ensure that they can be removed from the exposure as a priority if they are at an increased risk and treated if they are displaying health effects from the exposure.

7.8.1 Case study of lead exposure

A 3-year-old child was referred to hospital by the general practitioner, who had noticed the child looked pale. A full blood count revealed iron deficiency, microcytic, hypochromic anaemia, and a haemoglobin of 6.6 g/dl. Blood lead levels were found to be 404 µg/l (1.95 µM/l) (a normal result is <100 µg/l). His parents said that he often ate soil from the garden and paint chips from the walls of the house and his usual diet was not thought to be very good.

The child was started on oral iron therapy and the family advised that he should be prevented from eating soil and paint. Community follow-up was arranged through the local health visitors to help improve his diet. One week later his lead level had reduced to 318 µg/l (a sample from his younger sibling at that time was 46 µg/l). Within 2 months his lead level had reduced to 229 µg/l and haemoglobin increased to 11.7 g/dL.

An environmental health officer (EHO) from the local authority visited the house a week after the initial diagnosis and took a water s ample from the kitchen tap, where the results indicated that the lead levels were within permitted bounds at 5 µg/L. A second visit to the house was undertaken by a senior EHO and a consultant in communicable disease control (CCDC) a week later and samples were taken for analysis from the house paint and soil from the garden. The house was built in the 1930s, which meant the most likely source of lead was paint. The parents were strongly advised to make sure that the child did not eat any more paint from the walls.

The lead analysis results were insignificant for most samples, except the paintwork from the stairs, which indicated high lead levels (6.2%), which would pose a problem if eaten over a long period of time. An example of peeling lead paint is shown in Figure 7.2.

The case study illustrates an example of a child receiving high oral exposure to lead-based paint in the home environment and developing symptoms of adverse health effects because of biological sensitivity to lead toxicity, as well as a particular behaviour (in this case pica) causing higher potential for exposure.

7.8.2 Air pollution episodes involving sulphur dioxide

Sulphur dioxide (SO_2) is produced when a material or fuel containing sulphur is burned. Globally, much of the sulphur dioxide in the atmosphere comes from natural sources, but in the UK the predominant sources are power stations burning fossil fuels, principally coal and heavy oils. Widespread domestic use of coal can also lead to high local concentrations of SO_2.

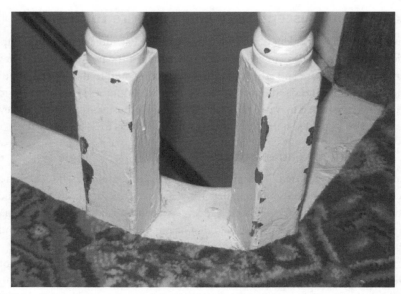

Fig. 7.2 Old paintwork containing high levels of lead that is flaking can lead to oral exposure in children.

According to the UK's Advisory Group on the Medical Aspects of Air Pollution Episodes in 1992 (Department of Health 1992), during episodes of elevated sulphur dioxide concentrations in the air, those suffering from pre-existing respiratory diseases (particularly asthma) may need to take steps to reduce their exposure. The evidence reviewed indicated that although individuals not suffering from respiratory disease should not be affected by the kind of air pollution episodes of elevated concentrations of sulphur dioxide typically found in the UK, asthmatic patients were found to be more sensitive to exposure to sulphur dioxide. Sulphur dioxide pollution is also considered more harmful when particulate and other pollution concentrations are high (UK Air Quality Archive 2007). In parts of the UK, levels of sulphur dioxide can regularly exceed those at which effects of clinical significance, including tightness of the chest, coughing, and wheezing, have been demonstrated in these susceptible individuals, with the effects being acute and reversible, but where medical attention may be needed (Department of Health 1992). Some form of public health intervention may be required, such as an alerting system, so that these susceptible groups can limit their exposure by adapting their behaviour (by, for example, staying indoors).

7.8.3 Health effects of chronic arsenic exposure

Arsenic is widely distributed throughout the Earth's crust. It can be released into the atmosphere by a range of natural processes, such as volcanic activity, or human activities, such as mining, metal smelting, and mobilization into drinking water from geological deposits as a result of drilling wells (World Health Organization 2010). Inorganic arsenic is naturally present at high levels in the groundwater of several countries, including China,

India and Bangladesh, Argentina, Chile, and the USA. In Bangladesh, approximately half of the total population of the country is at risk of drinking arsenic-contaminated water from tube-wells.

Ill-effects as a result of chronic ingestion are most likely to occur as a result of drinking contaminated water. Health effects of long-term exposure include skin changes, e.g. pigmentation and lesions, peripheral neuropathy, liver damage, and circulatory effects. Arsenic has also been classified by the International Agency for Research on Cancer (IARC) as carcinogenic to humans.

The World Health Organization recommends that in areas of contamination, action needs to be taken to reduce arsenic intake by making available drinking water with arsenic concentrations below 10 µg/l. This may be achieved through collecting rainwater for drinking and installing arsenic-removal systems with appropriate disposal and coding handpumps to enable identification of high- and low-arsenic water sources as contaminated water may still be put to other uses, e.g. washing.

7.9 Conclusions

There are variations in the susceptibility of any population exposed to toxic hazards. Special risk assessments are required for vulnerable subgroups such the very young and the elderly. Susceptibility may be revealed by both the dose required to produce effects in vulnerable groups and the time taken for such effects to be noticed. Preventative measures can reduce the risks to susceptible subgroups from toxic exposure to toxic substances.

7.10 Acknowledgement

The authors gratefully acknowledge Dr Charlotte Aus, who prepared an earlier version of this chapter.

7.11 References

COT. (2007) Variability and Uncertainty in the Toxicology of Chemicals in Food, Consumer Products and the Environment. Committee on the Toxicity of Chemicals in Food, Consumer Products and the Environment. Available at: http://www.food.gov.uk/multimedia/pdfs/VUTtoxicityreport.

Department of Health. (1992) Advisory Group on the Medical Aspects of Air Pollution Episodes. Second Report. Sulphur Dioxide, Acid Aerosols and Particulates. HMSO, London.

Eskenazi B, Bradman A, Castorina R. (1999) Exposures of children to organophosphate pesticides and their potential adverse health effects. Env Health Pers 107(s.3):409–419.

Farrow A, Golding J. (1997) Time spent in the home by different family members. Environ Technol 18:605–614.

Health Protection Agency. (2009) A Children's Environment and Health Strategy for the UK. Available at: http://www.hpa.org.uk/web/HPAwebFile/HPAweb_C/1237889522947.

IARC. (1987) Summaries and evaluations: Arsenic and arsenic compounds (Group 1). Lyon, International Agency for Research on Cancer (IARC Monographs on the Evaluation of Carcinogenic Risks to Huamns, Suuplement 7. Available at: http://www.inchem.org/documents/iarc/suppl7/arsenic.html.

Rang HP, Dale MM, Ritter JM. (1995) Pharmacology. 3rd edn. Churchill Livingstone, London.

Risk Assessment and Toxicology Steering Committee. (1999) Risk Assessment Strategies in Relation to Population Subgroups (cr3). Available at: http://ieh.cranfield.ac.uk/ighrc/cr3.pdf

UK Air Quality Archive (2007). Available at: http://www.airquality.co.uk/archive/what_causes.php. Accessed 15 March 2007.

Whitmore R, Immerman F, Camann D, Bond A, Lewis R, Schaum J. (1994) Non-Occupational Exposures to Pesticides for Residents of Two US Cities. *Arch Env Health* **26**:47–59.

World Health Organization. (2010). Exposure to Arsenic: A Major Public Health Concern. Available at: http://www.who.int/ipcs/features/arsenic.pdf.

7.12 Further reading

World Health Organization. (2005) Global update 2005. Particulate matter, ozone, nitrogen dioxide and sulfur dioxide. Chapter 5: determinants of susceptibility in: Air quality guidelines. World Health Organization, Geneva.

Chapter 8

Occupational toxicology

Virginia Murray and Ishani Kar-Purkayastha

Learning outcomes

At the end of this chapter and any recommended reading the student should be able to:

1. understand the importance of occupational toxicology in relation to health protection activities;

2. be aware of important sources of information about toxic agents in the workplace;

3. discuss the methods by which occupational exposure to toxic substances may affect health during manufacture, transport, storage, and use;

4. critically discuss incidents that have resulted from occupational exposures to toxic chemicals, and understand how they are investigated;

5. evaluate the guidelines and protocols that are used to prevent or minimize ill-health due to occupational exposures, and

6. apply acquired knowledge in the analysis and management of hazardous situations.

8.1 Introduction

Occupational toxicology is concerned with the investigation, management, and prevention of diseases arising from chemicals in the workplace. While it is primarily concerned with the health of workers exposed to toxic agents, it recognizes that their families, other household contacts, and the general public may also be affected. There may also be concurrent environmental impacts.

Occupational toxicology is a subset of environmental public health that requires the close co-operation of many professional groups, including occupational physicians, occupational hygienists, environmental health practitioners, government inspectors, health and safety officers, toxicologists, chemists and chemical engineers, design engineers, managers, trade union representatives, information scientists, and the workers themselves (Figure 8.1). Occupational toxicologists provide the other professionals with vital understanding of the nature of toxic agents and hazards, to enable the assessment and management of risks, and appropriate responses to chemical exposures and incidents.

The UK's Health and Safety at Work (etc) Act 1974 (HASAWA) is the primary piece of legislation covering health and safety in the UK. The Act established the Health and Safety

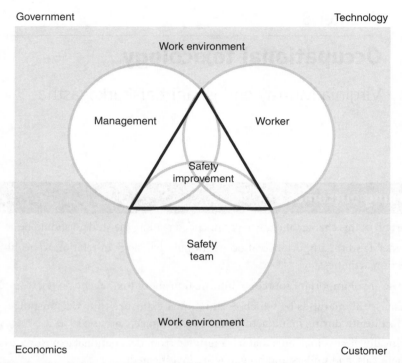

Fig. 8.1 Occupational toxicology is a subset of environmental public health that requires the close co-operation of many professional groups and the workers themselves. Adapted from the University of New South Wales, School of Safety Science, 2008.

Commission (HSC) and its operating arm, the Health and Safety Executive (HSE). In 2008, the HSC and HSE merged, bringing together their powers and functions, and retaining the name Health and Safety Executive. The HASAWA and related legislation, such as the Health and Safety (Offences) Act 2008, is enforced by the HSE or, in certain cases, mainly relating to distribution, retail, leisure, and catering sectors, by local authorities. The Act recognizes the pluralistic approach and places general duties regarding health and safety on all people at work (except domestic servants), including employers, the self-employed, and employees, as well as the HSE itself.

8.2 History of occupational diseases

Occupational toxicology is not new. The Romans recognized that certain occupations were associated with particular diseases. The first such textbook is attributed to Bernardino Ramazzini (1633–1714), who worked as a physician and professor in Padua and Modena, Italy. In 1713 he published *De morbis artificum diatriba* (An account of the diseases of work; Ramazzini 1713), in which he described over 50 occupational disorders, along with an account of working conditions at the time:

- occupational asthma in grain workers;
- pneumoconiosis and other diseases of miners;

- lead poisoning in potters;
- silicosis in stonemasons;
- diseases among metal workers and of gilders and printers;
- workers who cleaned out the city cesspits developed eye infections, which lead to sight loss or total blindness;
- breast cancer occurred more often in nuns than in other women of similar age.

Ramazzini methodically collected data relating to diseases of manual workers in relation to their occupation. In the same way today, when a disease is shown to be more prevalent in a particular group of workers than it is in the general population, it is suggestive of an occupational disease.

8.3 Types of adverse effects

Chemical exposure in the occupational setting can cause a wide range of effects if appropriate controls are not in place. These will depend on various factors, including the exposure route, duration and dose, and the frequency of exposure as well as the individual exposed and any pre-existing diseases or susceptibilities. The effects may be acute or chronic or even delayed, with a long lead time between exposure and disease. This is particularly important with cancer-causing chemicals. Issues relating to fertility and effects on the foetus and the growing child from parental chemical exposure should also be of concern.

In this chapter, two examples of adverse effects from the occupational use of chemicals are provided. The first describes the acute effects of chlorine and the second describes the acute but, more significantly, the chronic effects of vinyl chloride monomer (VCM).

8.3.1 Chlorine: health effects of acute/single exposure

In a properly managed safe system of work, acute exposure to chlorine will not occur. However, should there be an incident in which there is a release the immediate symptoms following inhalation of chlorine include a burning sensation in the eyes and nose, sore throat, cough, chest tightness, headache, fever, wheeze, fast heart rate, and confusion. Sufficient exposure may induce reflex cholinergic bronchoconstriction, with associated signs of coughing, wheezing, and dyspnoea (HPA 2011). Exposure to a sufficiently high dose may result in pulmonary oedema and respiratory failure, the onset of which may be delayed by up to 36 hours. There is some evidence to suggest that exposure to chlorine may be associated with long-term neuropsychological changes (Dilks and Matzenbacher 2003), although further studies are required to confirm this hypothesis. A summary of the acute effects of chlorine exposure by concentration is given in Table 8.1.

8.3.1.1 Delayed effects following an acute exposure

Most studies of survivors of World War I gassing incidents have reported a high incidence of acute respiratory damage and a lower incidence of chronic sequelae following acute exposure (Ayres and Baxter 2004). Similar sequelae have also been reported for individuals following acute exposure to the accidental release of chlorine gas, with the most consistently reported chronic effect being a reduction in the forced expiratory volume (FEV) (IPCS 1999a).

Table 8.1 Summary of acute toxic effects in relation to approximate (air) concentration of chlorine (IPCS 1996)

Concentration		Signs and symptoms
ppm	mg/m³	
1–3	3–10	Mild mucous membrane irritation.
5–15	15–45	Moderate irritation of upper respiratory tract.
30	90	Immediate chest pain, vomiting, coughing.
40–60	115–175	Toxic pneumonitis and pulmonary oedema.
430	1250	Lethal after 30 minutes exposure.
1000	2900	Lethal in minutes.

Concentrations (mg/m³) are approximate conversions from the corresponding ppm value.
Data from IPCS (1996) Chlorine. International Programme on Chemical Safety Poisons Information Monograph PIM 947. Available at http://www.inchem.org/documents/pims/chemical/pim947.htm (accessed 17.08.11)

A relatively recent report relating to accidental exposure to chlorine gas suggests that chronic sequelae following acute exposure may be more frequent than previously anticipated: a follow-up study in July 1999 on 20 individuals (previously exposed in 1995) indicated that 75% had residual lung volumes below 80% of their predicted value and nearly half the subjects tested for airway reactivity to methacholine had a greater than 15% decline in FEV (Schwartz et al. 1990). There is some evidence to suggest that a single, acute exposure to chlorine gas may cause reactive airways dysfunction syndrome (RADS), also known as irritant-induced asthma (Ayres and Baxter 2004; Winder 2001).

8.3.2 Vinyl chloride: exposure and health effects

Vinyl chloride (Figure 8.2), which is produced for industrial use as a chemical intermediate in the manufacture of other compounds, particularly polyvinyl chloride (PVC), is toxic by all routes of exposure. It is metabolized to the active metabolites chloroethylene oxide and chloracetaldehyde, which is responsible for its toxicity. In the absence of proper controls, acute exposure will produce immediate signs and symptoms, such as respiratory irritation, producing coughing, wheezing, and breathlessness following inhalation, and also systemic effects, including headache, ataxia, drowsiness, and coma. In addition, some halogenated hydrocarbons can cause cardiac arrhythmias (IPCS 1999b; NPIS 2004). Ingestion of vinyl chloride may cause sickness, diarrhoea, and stomach pain. Contact of the skin or eyes with vinyl chloride liquid or vapour could cause irritation and dermatitis. Exposure to escaping gas from compressed (liquid) vinyl chloride may cause frostbite (HPA 2008).

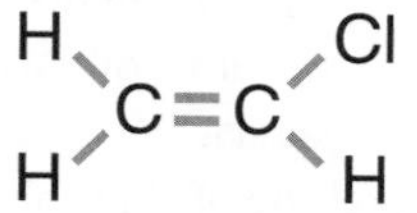

Fig. 8.2 Vinyl chloride monomer.

Where there are inadequate controls, long-term exposure may cause impotence, blood disorders, liver problems (angiosarcoma), and the pathopnemonic disease of acroosteolysis following adult exposure to vinyl chloride. Bone loss in the fingertips due to exposure to VCM has been observed among polyvinyl chloride (PVC) reactor workers (NIOSH 2001). The term 'acroosteolysis' was used to name the condition (the word 'acroosteolysis' is derived from Greek words *akron* = extremity, *osteon* = bone, *lysis*= dissolution) and has been defined as a shortening of the terminal digits.

A Department for Work and Pensions (2005) review concluded that there was consistent evidence that the inhalation of VCM in PVC production workers causes a characteristic clinical triad of osteolysis of the terminal phalanges, scleroderma, and Raynaud's phenomenon, but not all three are invariably present together (Department for Work and Pensions 2005). These effects occurred in workers who had been exposed to levels of VCM very much higher than the current control limits. Surveys of factory workforces have shown that among those exposed to VCM who do not have radiological evidence of osteolysis, the prevalence of Raynaud's phenomenon and scleroderma is greater than in the general population (by a factor of two).

The mechanisms of toxicity for non-cancer VCM effects are not completely elucidated. VCM disease exhibits many characteristics of autoimmune diseases (e.g. Raynaud's phenomenon and scleroderma). B-cell proliferation, hyperimmunoglobulinemia, and complement activation, with increased circulating immune complexes or cryoglobulinemia indicating stimulation of immune response, have been observed.

Postulated mechanisms for the non-cancer effects include:

1. Immunological
   - a reactive vinyl chloride intermediate metabolite, such as 2-chloroethylene oxide or 2-chloroacetaldehyde, binds to a protein such as IgG;
   - altered protein initiates an immune response, with deposition of immune products along vascular endothelium;
   - circulating immune complexes are proposed to precipitate in response to exposure to the cold, and these precipitates are proposed to produce blockage of the small vessels.

2. Resorptive bone changes in the fingers may be due to activation of osteoclast secondary to vascular insufficiency in the fingertips (ATSDR 2006).

However, the International Agency for Research on Cancer has classified vinyl chloride as a known human carcinogen, based on evidence of carcinogenicity in both humans and animals (IARC 1987). It is mutagenic and its carcinogenic action is believed to occur via a genotoxic mechanism. VCM is covered by the Carcinogens Directive, and the current workplace exposure limit of 3 ppm is based on its recognized carcinogenicity rather than non-cancer endpoints.

8.4 Assessing occupational disease and hazardous chemicals

It is important to recognize that occupational diseases are preventable by adopting appropriate control measures, yet they can be responsible for temporary and permanent disablement, discomfort, and distress, as well as lost productivity. The risks extend to co-workers, the worker's family, and the environment. Occupational hygienists stress the importance of *anticipation* and *prevention* before a system of work is introduced.

Diseases can have occupational and non-occupational causes. Occupational causes may be overlooked if the patient presents outside the occupational health sector (Figure 8.3). Occupational illnesses may resemble non-occupational illnesses, and a very long latency period can sometimes exist between exposure and the emergence of signs and symptoms. There are thousands of jobs, chemicals, and diseases, and an association may not be readily apparent. In addition, medical students and most other health professionals are not trained in occupational toxicology.

Occupational disease can be identified by consideration of *health data*, i.e. epidemiological studies, health assessments, the incidence of particular diseases in a workforce, or the appearance of signs and symptoms in individual workers or their families, together with *knowledge of the chemicals* in the workplace, the available data on their toxicity, risk assessment, and monitoring. In most cases, risk assessment will be based on the available toxicology data (largely from experimental studies in animals) together with estimates of exposure.

An investigation into suspected ill-health from workplace exposure to a hazardous chemical will start with an analysis of the system of work, to identify which chemicals are used in which locations by which workers and consideration of the data on their toxicity. The *source-pathway-receptor* model is a useful starting point. The exact activities, times, and durations should be recorded. Existing risk assessment documentation and inventories *should* provide information to identify critical control points, but they must be assessed critically.

Investigations may involve biological/clinical sampling to detect and measure the presence of the toxic agent or its metabolic products in body tissue or excreta—typically blood, urine, or exhalation samples. In some cases it may be necessary for medical examination of the exposed workers and specific organ-function tests. Clearly there are practical and ethical issues here, including consent and confidentiality, not to mention the possibility

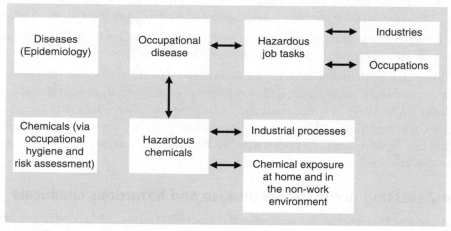

Fig. 8.3 Ways of identifying occupational toxicity-related diseases.

of personal distress, and industrial relations problems. These will need careful handling and good communications.

Environmental sampling may be carried out to provide data for an exposure assessment. This may involve air and dust sampling. In some hazardous situations there may already be continuous monitoring data. The sampling strategy should be appropriate to the pattern of work and activities of individual workers, and their locus and exposure to the particular hazardous chemicals.

Environmental and/or biological sampling data must be complemented by taking the work history, present and past, of the affected individuals, including the type of work and its physical and psychological demands, detailed accounts of working practices, including exposures to physical, chemical, or biological hazards, and the control measures employed (e.g. PPE) should be recorded. This should not be confined to the worker's current work activity and employer, but should if possible cover their entire working lives.

Particular attention should be paid to whether there have been any recent changes in working practices, materials employed, or workplace control mechanisms. Absenteeism, sickness leave, and employee turnover records should be analysed. Analysis and evaluation will lead to recommendations for risk management control measures (see section 8.5 in this chapter).

8.4.1 Multi-exposure to hazardous chemicals

It must be remembered that in the modern workplace it is unlikely that a worker will be exposed to only one hazardous chemical. Multiexposure issues of interactions between substances include:

- **independent**—no cross reaction between the compounds, e.g. carbon monoxide and cadmium;
- **antagonistic**—exposure protects against the production of toxicity, e.g. antidotes;
- **potentiative**—the single compound has no effect unless other is present, e.g. carbon tetrachloride and 2-propanol;
- **additive**—effect is additive in nature, e.g. solvents;
- **synergistic**—effect is multiplicative, e.g. asbestos and smoking.

8.5 Risk management

The exposure of workers to hazardous chemicals must be prevented or adequately controlled. The UK Control of Substances Hazardous to Health Regulations (COSHH) (see section 8.6 below) make risk assessment and risk management mandatory.

A **hierarchy of control measures** is given below. **Elimination** and **substitution** should *always* be considered first, whether as long-term or short-term solutions, before the use of engineering controls. It should be noted that the use of PPE is a final resort after all other controls have been implemented.

- Elimination of hazardous chemical
- Substitution with less hazardous materials or forms of the material (e.g. pellets instead of powder) or processes.

- Minimization of inventories or stocks or amounts of available hazards.
- Engineering controls at source, such as automation or process enclosure.
- Engineering controls to reduce exposure, such as segregation, partial enclosure, mechanical handling, suppression methods, or ventilation.
- Administrative controls, such as safe working procedures, job rotation, good house-keeping.
- Reduction of the number of workers exposed.
- Personnel procedures, such as adequate supervision, information dissemination, and training.
- Health surveillance.
- Personal protective equipment.

COSHH impose special controls over carcinogens. The concept of substitution is encouraged, which is the second most effective measure in the hierarchy of control measures. Table 8.2 provides recommendations for substitution of materials.

8.6 Legal controls and standards

The COSHH made under HASAWA, apply to substances or mixtures of substances classified as dangerous to health under the Chemicals (Hazard Information and Packing for Supply) (CHIP) Regulations. CHIP requires the supplier of a dangerous chemical to identify the dangers associated with the chemical, which is known as 'classification', give information about the hazards to their customers, usually through labelling, and package the chemical safely.

In addition, under the European Union regulations on Registration, Evaluation, Authorisation and restriction of Chemicals (REACH) suppliers are required to provide **safety data sheets** for their products. COSHH require a risk assessment to be carried out and control measures to be implemented to prevent or control exposure. Control measures

Table 8.2 Substitution: some examples

Examples of Chemical Substitution	
Instead of:	**Consider:**
Carbon tetrachloride	1,1,1,-Trichloroethane
Benzene	Toluene, Cyclohexane, Ketones
Lead	Lead-free solders
	Lead-free paints
Organic solvents	Water-based solvents
	Liquid carbon dioxide
Sandstone grinding wheels (silica)	Synthetic grinding wheels such as aluminum oxide

Examples of Chemical Substitution. Accessed 0-662-38542-X; H46-2/04-373E http://www.hc-sc.gc.ca/ewh-semt/occup-travail/whmis-simdut/substitution-eng.php, 2006. Reproduced with the permission of the Minister of Public Works and Government Services Canada, 2012.

may include the monitoring of the exposure of workers and appropriate health surveillance. Workers must be properly trained and supervised, and control measures must be properly maintained and implemented. Occupational exposure limits have been set (see section 8.7 below) and these are found in the HSE publication EH40.

In 2005, existing requirements to follow good practice were brought together by the introduction of eight principles as an update to the Control of Substances Hazardous to Health (Amendment) Regulations 2004 (Box 8.1).

Basic advice on the implementation of the COSHH regulations is also provided on the HSE website COSHH Essentials.

8.7 Occupational exposure limits

8.7.1 Workplace exposure limits

Workplace exposure limits (WEL) have now replaced maximum exposure limits (MELs) and occupational exposure standards (OESs) in the UK. Many of the old MELs and OESs have been converted to WELs, apart from about 100 OESs that have been deleted. There are no WELs for asbestos, lead and other substances that have specific legislative controls.

The list of exposure limits is known as **EH40** and is available from the HSE Direct website. Readers are advised to familiarize themselves with HSE COSHH guidance publications, including EH40 (www.hse.gov.uk).

Box 8.1 Principles of good practice for the control of substances hazardous to health

- Design and operate processes and activities to minimize emission, release, and spread of substances hazardous to health.

- Take into account all relevant routes of exposure—inhalation, skin absorption, and ingestion—when developing control measures.

- Control exposure by measures that are proportionate to the health risk.

- Choose the most effective and reliable control options which minimize the escape and spread of substances hazardous to health.

- Where adequate control of exposure cannot be achieved by other means, provide, in combination with other control measures, suitable personal protective equipment.

- Check and review regularly all elements of control measures for their continuing effectiveness.

- Inform and train all employees on the hazards and risks from the substances with which they work and the use of control measures developed to minimize the risks.

- Ensure that the introduction of control measures does not increase the overall risk to health and safety.

(Control of Substances Hazardous to Health (amendment) Regulations 2004)

All UK WELs are air limit values. They are expressed in both parts per million (ppm) and milligrams per cubic metre of air (mg/m^3) and are given as **long-term exposure limits** (LTELs; 8-hour time-weighted average (TWA) reference period) and **short-term exposure limits** (STELs; 15-minute TWA reference period). The TWA calculation methods are explained in EH40. Some potent substances are only given a STEL.

A 'Comments' column in EH40 gives further advice, for example 'skin' indicates that substance's ability to penetrate human skin.

There are some WELs for multisubstance exposure, prescribing process emissions like welding fumes.

Biological monitoring results may be used as indicators of exposure, although they do not have legal status. **Biological monitoring guidance values** (BMGV) are also provided in EH40.

Employers are now legally obliged to:

- apply the principles of good practice (above) for the control of substances hazardous to health;

- ensure that the WEL is not exceeded; and

- ensure that exposure to substances that can cause occupational asthma, cancer, or damage to genes that can be passed from one generation to another is reduced *as low as is reasonably practicable*.

8.7.2 As low as is reasonably practicable

The duty to control and reduce risks to *as low as is reasonably practicable* (ALARP) has its legal foundations in the case of *Edwards v. The National Coal Board* (1949), which addressed the adequacy of safety precautions in a mine. The Court of Appeal held that:

> "the risk . . . has to be weighed against the measures necessary to eliminate the risk. The greater the risk, no doubt, the less will be the weight to be given to the factor of cost."

The Court decided that 'reasonably practicable' is a narrower term than 'physically possible'. There must be an assessment of the risk on one side, and this must be compared with, on the other side, the 'sacrifice' in terms of the time, trouble, and money necessary for averting the risk. The sacrifice should not be *grossly disproportionate* to the risk. Inherent in the use of the word 'grossly' is a bias on the side of health and safety. Nevertheless, it must be accepted that even when ALARP is adopted there will still be some risk.

Consideration of the balance between risk and cost should be revisited when there is new scientific evidence about the risk (whether higher or lower) or when new control technologies become available.

Complex ALARP decisions involving high risks usually include the consideration of formal cost–benefit analysis (CBA), but ALARP decisions are never based on CBA alone. The inclusion of CBA means that when considering chemicals with no threshold, e.g. genotoxic carcinogens, their use in, say, cosmetics would be prohibited, but industrial exposures, under very strict controls, might still be tolerated.

8.8 Surveillance systems and sources of information

8.8.1 The Health and Occupational Reporting

The Health and Occupational Reporting (THOR) is an example of a UK system for occupational disease surveillance. THOR activity at the Centre of Occupational and Environmental Health, University of Manchester has a range of surveillance programmes. It includes surveillance of work-related and occupational respiratory disease (SWORD), particularly occupational asthma, benign and malignant pleural disease, mesothelioma, lung cancer, and pneumoconiosis surveillance. The most common cause of occupational asthma in the UK consists of the di-isocyanates (used in various industries such as in 'twin-pack' spray painting). Other important asthma hazards include colophony fume (from soldering flux). The SWORD scheme successfully picked up trends such as an increase in asthma associated with exposure to latex, and thus helped in raising awareness and reducing the risks.

8.8.2 International resources in occupational toxicology

The European Community 'REACH' regulation which deals with the Registration, Evaluation, Authorisation and Restriction of Chemical substances (EC 2006) came into force on 1 June 2007. REACH legislation requires manufacturers and importers of chemicals within Europe to submit technical information on the properties of their substances, which will allow their safe handling, and to register the information in a central database run by the European Chemicals Agency (ECHA) in Helsinki.

The American College of Occupational and Environmental Medicine (ACOEM) was founded in 1916. The College periodically issues position papers and committee reports that set practice guidelines for a variety of workplace/environmental settings. These position papers/committee reports cover topics such as spirometry, mould, environmental tobacco smoke, noise-induced hearing loss, multiple chemical sensitivities, workplace drug screening, confidentiality of medical information, depression screening, and reproductive hazards. In their 2005 position paper on toxicology these topics were identified as a core content of occupational and environmental medicine.

8.8.3 Haz-Map

Haz-Map is an occupational toxicology database designed to link jobs to hazardous job tasks which are linked to occupational diseases and their symptoms. It has been published on the website of the National Library of Medicine since 2002. It is a relational database of chemicals, jobs, and diseases. Haz-Map was designed to be a decision-support computer application for occupational safety and health professionals. Its aim is to assist physicians, physician assistants, occupational health nurses, and industrial hygienists in the recognition of diseases caused by toxic chemicals and infectious agents in the workplace.

For more on other toxicology databases such as **TOXNET**, please see Chapter 5.

8.9 References

ATSDR. (2006) Toxicological Profile for Vinyl Chloride. US Department of Health and Human Services, Agency for Toxic Substances Disease Registry, Atlanta, GA.

Ayres J, Baxter P. (2004) Irritant Induced Asthma and RADS. EPAQS short report. World Health Organization, Geneva.

Control of Substances Hazardous to Health (Amendment) Regulations (2004). Statutory Instrument 2004 No. 3386. HMSO, London.

EC. (2006) European Community Regulation on Chemicals and their Safe Use No. 1907/2006. *Official Journal of the European Union* **L396**:2–849.

DWP. (2005) Vinyl Chloride Monomer-Related Diseases. (cm6645) Department for Work and Pensions. HMSO, London.

Dilks LS, Matzenbacher DL. (2003) Residual neuropsychological sequelae of chlorine gas exposure. *Neurotoxicol Teratolol* **25**:391.

Edwards v National Coal Board (1949) All ER 743 (CA). Available at www.safetyphoto.co.uk/sub-site/.../edwards_v_national_coal_board.ht Accessed 20 October 2011.

HPA. (20011) Chlorine. *Compendium of Chemical Hazards*, Version 3. Health Protection Agency, London.

HPA. (2008) Vinyl Chloride. *Compendium of Chemical Hazards*, Version 2. Health Protection Agency, London.

IARC. (1987) Vinyl chloride. International Agency for Research on Cancer—Summaries & Evaluations. Supplement 7, p 373.

IPCS. (1999a) Disinfectants and disinfectant by-products. International Programme On Chemical Safety Monograph. *Environmental Health Criteria* 216.

IPCS. (1999b) Vinyl chloride. International Programme On Chemical Safety Monograph. *Environmental Health Criteria* 215.

NIOSH. (2001) Occupational Dermatoses Program for Physicians: Index of Occupational Dermatoses slides. National Institute for Occupational Safety and Health. Available at: http://www.cdc.gov/niosh/topics/skin/occderm-slides/ocderm18.html. Accessed 28 June 2011.

NPIS. (2004) Vinyl chloride. *TOXBASE®*. National Poisons Information Service. Last updated September 2004. Available at: www.toxbase.org.

Ramazzini B. (1713) *De Morbis Artificum Bernardini Ramazzini Diatriba* [Diseases of Workers: The Latin Text of 1713 Revised]. Wright WC, trans-ed. University of Chicago Press, Chicago, Ill [1940].

Schwartz DA, Smith DD, Lakshminarayan S. (1990) The pulmonary sequelae associated with accidental inhalation of chlorine gas. *Chest* **97**:820–825.

Winder C. (2001) The toxicology of chlorine. *Environ Res* **85**:105–114.

8.10 Further reading

American College of Occupational and Environmental Medicine. Available at: http://www.acoem.org/. Accessed 28 June 2011.

Gardiner K, and Harrington JM. (2005) Occupational Hygiene. Blackwell Publishing, Oxford.

HAZ-MAP. (2011) Occupational Exposure to Hazardous Chemicals, National Library of Medicine. Available at: http://hazmap.nlm.nih.gov/. Accessed 28 June 2011.

Health and Safety Executive. COSHH Essentials. Available at: http://www.coshh-essentials.org.uk/Home.asp. Accessed 28 June 2011.

Health and Safety Executive. (2011) Documentation including COSHH Guidance and EH40. Available at: http://www.hse.gov.uk/legislation/services.htm. Accessed 28 June 2011.

IPCS. (1996) Chlorine. International Programme on Chemical Safety. *Poisons Information Monograph* PIM 947.

Registration, Evaluation, Authorisation and Restriction of Chemical) Information. Available at: http://ec.europa.eu/environment/chemicals/reach/reach_intro.htm. Accessed 28 June 2011.

Stacey NH, and Winder C. (2004) Occupational Toxicology. Taylor and Francis, London.

The Health and Occupational Reporting Network. (2011) University of Manchester. Available at: http://www.medicine.manchester.ac.uk/oeh/research/thor/. Accessed 28 June 2011.

University of New South Wales. School of Safety Science. Available at: http://www.safesci.unsw.edu.au/about/about.html. Accessed 28 June 2011.

Environmental Toxicology

Chapter 9

Air pollution in the United Kingdom

Robert L. Maynard

Learning outcomes

At the end of this chapter and any recommended reading the student should be able to:

1. outline the history of air pollution, and discuss the evolution of concerns about air pollution;

2. explain and discuss the effects of common air pollutants, including ozone, sulphur dioxide, nitrogen dioxide, carbon monoxide, and particulate matter;

3. explain the consequences of organic chemicals, particularly carcinogenic outdoor air pollutants;

4. discuss the problem of indoor air pollution and its relationship with external air quality;

5. understand the setting of air-quality standards;

6. explain the role of international organizations such as the European Union and the WHO in air pollution control, and

7. apply acquired knowledge in the analysis and management of hazardous situations.

9.1 Introduction

What is air pollution? This question is less easy to answer than might be thought: it is generally accepted that the air in busy streets is polluted by emissions from motor vehicles but it is less obvious that secondary pollutants are present in the air in rural areas. Many people associate pollution only with human activity, for example the use of motor vehicles and industrial processes, but so-called natural phenomena also pollute the air. The wind-lift of sea spray leads to the formation of sodium chloride particles and these contribute to the ambient aerosol in coastal districts; the wind lifts sand particles from deserts, leading to deposition far from the source; volcanic activity pours millions of tons of particles and gases into the atmosphere every year. In addition to these sources, there are biological sources: plants produce volatile organic chemicals, which contribute to particle formation in the air, pollen drifts away from plants, the excrement of insects, including house-dust mites, contributes to the indoor aerosol and people carry a cloud, their personal cloud, of particles about with them. So there are many sources of pollution, but in this chapter we shall focus on man-made pollutants and on those known to damage health.

That air pollutants can damage health or, at least, produce unpleasant effects, must have been known since humans first lit fires in caves. Smoke, a mixture of particles and many volatile chemicals, contains irritants of the eyes and nose: acrolein and other alde-hydes are constituents of wood smoke. The use of coal for domestic heating in large cities led to episodes of severe air pollution in the 19th century and the London smog (smog = smoke + fog) became a standard backdrop for writers of the period (Brimblecombe 1987). Cold air lying close to the ground trapped smoke from low chimneys and the Thames valley, especially London, was severely affected in winter. In 1952 a notoriously severe smog episode occurred early in December and at least 4000 people died. At least? Well, the analysis was difficult because of a coincidental epidemic of influenza and perhaps as many as 10,000 deaths were associated with the smog. Concentrations of pollutants rose to what were regarded as unprecedented heights: particles filters became overloaded at about 8 mg/m^3, cinema films could not be shown (the beams from the projectors failed to pierce the smog that had spread indoors), and a performance of an opera in central London was cancelled because the patrons could not see the stage. Such smogs have vanished from London. This is largely a result of the Clean Air Act of 1956, which defined smoke-free zones, provided money for the conversion of domestic fires to the use of smokeless fuel and insisted on tall chimneys for industrial sources of smoke. These measures, at a time when the use of gas and electricity was increasing, did away with London smog. London, today, is a comparatively clean city: the smoke deposits have been removed from the buildings and concentrations of air pollutants are measured in μg/m^3 not mg/m^3. This improvement led some to assume that air pollution no longer has any effects on health: they could not have been more wrong!

At the same time that coal-smoke smog was disappearing in the UK, traffic-generated smog was being studied in Los Angeles (Haagen-Smit 1952). This acidic and irritating mixture of fine particles, nitrogen dioxide, ozone, and related chemicals was a character-istic of a city with heavy levels of traffic (no catalytic converters then and many motor cars had petrol engines of 4–6 litre capacity) and a lot of sunshine. Photochemical reactions driven by sunlight and fuelled by motor vehicle generated pollution produced a new type of smog. This, too, figures in the literature of the period: Raymond Chandler used it as a backdrop to his Philip Marlowe novels, set in Los Angeles in the 1950s. In 1976, record concentrations of ozone were recorded in London and across southern England (Department of Health 1991). Concentrations peaked at about 250 ppb (500 μg/m^3) but, at the time, effects on health were not noted. Later studies suggested an increase in deaths of almost 10%, although it was difficult to separate the possible effects of exposure to ozone from those of temperature.

Mastering this form of pollution has proved to be difficult: fine particles and gases such as nitrogen dioxide are a threat to health in all busy cities today. Progress has been made: emissions from motor vehicles have been dramatically reduced in the last 20 years. The introduction of diesel-powered light vehicles has presented a new problem: diesel engines emit more particles than petrol ones and particle traps are now required on certain classes of diesel vehicles. Low emissions zones, such as that implemented in London, are becoming more common and concentrations of pollutants have fallen. Whether the concentrations of vehicle-generated pollutants are still falling in cities such as London may be doubted: concentrations of both fine particles and nitrogen oxides have been fairly steady for some time. Further efforts will be needed and finding low-cost options is increasingly difficult. At a time when levels of air pollutants are at their lowest for many years in major cities such as London, concern about the effects of air pollutants on health is at its highest. Campaign groups rightly lay emphasis on effects on health and spur governments to greater efforts. Concentrations of fine particles (explained below) in inner London now average about $15 \,\mu g/m^3$ and all but about $1.5 \,\mu g/m^3$ of this is of human (anthropogenic) origin. The majority of the $15 \,\mu g/m^3$ comprises secondary particles (sulphates and nitrates) formed from gaseous emissions not necessarily in London; the contribution from local traffic is only about $2 \,\mu g/m^3$ (Committee on the Medical Effects of Air Pollutants 2010). Further reductions in pollutant concentrations will be costly: the need to weigh costs against benefits is clear.

In addition to traffic and large-scale industry, there are many minor sources of air pollutants. These include bonfires and incinerators. The latter contribute little to the national inventory of pollutants but cause great concern. In terms of effects on health this concern is misplaced: well-managed, modern incinerators emit small amounts of pollutants and, in terms of particles, make only a small contribution even to local ambient concentrations. Concern about local sources of pollution is widespread and is, in part, a result of well-publicized research into the effects of air pollutants on health.

9.2 Methods used to study the effects of air pollutants on health

In broad terms we may think of four methods: epidemiology, experimental studies on volunteers, studies on experimental animals (often referred to by toxicologists as *in vivo* studies), and studies on isolated tissues and cells (*in vitro* studies). To these might be added computer-based, *in silico*, studies. Here we shall discuss only a few of these methods.

9.2.1 Epidemiological studies

Epidemiology is the study of diseases or of the effects of processes and factors harmful to health, at a population level. Epidemiology has been the major contributor to our current understanding of the effects of air pollutants on health. A range of techniques have been applied. These include the following.

Time-series studies examine the relationship between day–to-day changes in concentrations of pollutants and day–to-day changes in the counts of health (or ill-health)-related events such as deaths and admissions to hospital. These studies require very careful control of confounding factors that also vary on a day to day basis. The key confounding factor that varies in this way is ambient temperature. Associations between all the common pollutants (particles, ozone, nitrogen dioxide, sulphur dioxide, and carbon monoxide) and a range of effects, including deaths from cardiovascular and respiratory disease, hospital admissions for heart attacks, and worsening of chronic respiratory conditions and asthma attacks, have been reported. The results of hundreds of such studies have been published and may be grouped as shown in Figure 9.1 (Committee on the Medical Effects of Air Pollutants 2006). This figure deals only with particles (monitored as PM_{10}; see below) and deaths from cardiovascular disease. A consistent effect is seen and meta-analysis shows that a $10\,\mu g/m^3$ increase in PM_{10} is associated with a 0.6% increase in the risk of death from cardiovascular disease (Committee on the Medical Effects of Air Pollutants 2006). This is a small effect. But all the population is exposed to PM_{10} and the effect at a national scale is, inevitably, large.

Cohort studies are quite different from time-series studies. Here defined populations (or, rather, large samples of populations) are followed for long periods and indices of their health (ill-health), such as the risk of dying from cardiovascular disease, are related

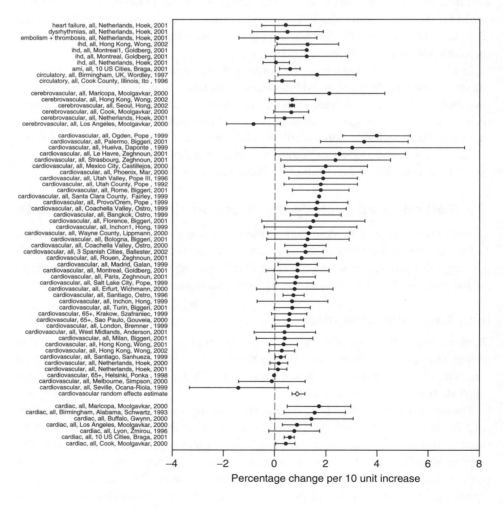

Fig. 9.1 Cardiovascular mortality and PM10. Reproduced from the Committee on the Medical Effects of Air Pollutants (2006) Cardiovascular Disease and Air Pollution. London, COMEAP.

to long-term average concentrations of pollutants. No studies have had a greater impact on thinking than the US Six Cities Study and the American Cancer Society (ACS) Cohort Study (Dockery et al. 1993; Health Effects Institute 2000; Pope et al. 1995, 2002).

These studies, conducted with unexampled care and the closest adjustment for the effects of confounding factors, have shown that long-term exposure to fine particles is associated with an increase in the risk of death from cardiovascular disease and from lung cancer. It is worth noting that the studies show that long-term exposure to $10 \,\mu g/m^3$ of fine particles ($PM_{2.5}$) is associated with a 6% increase in the risk of death from all causes—and a 9% increase in the risk of death from cardio-pulmonary causes. This is a large effect and implies a heavy burden on public health. Adjustment for confounding factors is critically important and, in these studies, factors such as social class, smoking habits, diet, alcohol intake, and education have been found to be important.

Other studies, including panel studies of, generally, small groups of subjects, have been undertaken but it would not be too unfair to say that in comparison with the studies discussed above, their impact has been small.

9.2.2 Chamber studies

Exposing volunteers to pollutants and recording the acute effects on their health, is a well established technique. Heroic, or foolish, exposures to sulphur dioxide were undertaken in the 1950s and 1960s and, more recently, well controlled exposure to diluted diesel exhaust have been reported. These studies allow effects on lung function to be monitored and, unsurprisingly, significant effects have been recorded. The addition of lavage of the airways to these studies has allowed to recovery of cells associated with inflammation: the inflammatory response to diluted diesel exhaust has been found to last longer than effects on lung function. These studies tend to be limited to healthy adult subjects but studies on adults with heart disease have been reported.

9.2.3 *In vivo* studies in animals

These studies have contributed less than might have been expected to our knowledge of the effects of air pollutants on health. In general, much higher concentrations than those shown by epidemiological studies to produce effects of man have been needed to produce well defined effects. This may be due to inter-species differences in sensitivity. Recent use of genetically modified mice (for example the ApoE −/− mouse which is susceptible to atheroma) has shown effects at relevant concentrations Lippmann et al. 2005). Animal work allows effects on organs such as the brain and heart to be investigated in detail.

9.3 Major air pollutants

9.3.1 Particles

More work has recently been done on the effects on health of exposure to ambient particles than on the effects of gaseous pollutants. This research has led to a resurgence of interest in aerosol science, to a surge in work in inhalation toxicology, and to the new field of nano-toxicology. Epidemiological studies have led to a clear understanding of the associations between ambient concentrations of particles and effects on health but little agreement as to the mechanisms underlying those effects has been reached. One theory that is popular at present is that metallic and organic species (especially polycyclic compounds) found in or on ambient particles generate free radicals in the body (see below).

The ambient aerosol comprises a mixture of particles and droplets of varying composition and from varying sources. Particles inhaled via the nose and mouth enter the respiratory tract and may deposit therein. Only particles less than about 10 μm in diameter penetrate beyond the nose and larynx: particles of this size are monitored as PM_{10} and are sometimes, wrongly, referred to as PM_{10s}. PM_{10} is the **mass** of particles of generally less than 10 μm diameter, per cubic metre of air. $PM_{2.5}$ is a subfraction of PM_{10} and is the mass of particles of generally less than 2.5 μm diameter per cubic metre of air. Not all the particles that reach the airways are deposited, the probability or likelihood of their being deposited is controlled by their size and behaviour in the air stream. Larger particles sediment out of the air under the influence of gravity; larger particles fail to follow a diverted air stream at a bifurcation of the airways and therefore deposit at or close to the bifurcations. Smaller particles diffuse in air and deposit in this way. The simple rule is: larger particles deposit mainly in the conducting airways as a result of sedimentation and impaction, and smaller particles deposit mainly in the gas exchange zone, mainly as a result of diffusion. Rather interestingly, of all the particles entering the lung those of about 0.5 μm (500 nm) diameter are least likely to be deposited: they are too small to sediment efficiently and too large to diffuse efficiently. Particles of >10 μm diameter are referred to as coarse particles but confusion has arisen as a result of describing that fraction of the aerosol monitored as PM_{10}–$PM_{2.5}$ as the 'coarse fraction' of PM_{10}.

The ambient aerosol can be described in several ways: by size, by source, by composition. One useful approach is to divide the aerosol into primary and secondary particles. Primary particles are emitted by sources such as motor vehicles; secondary particles are produced by the oxidation of gases, including sulphur dioxide and the nitrogen oxides. Both have effects on health. Primary particles emitted by diesel engines are largely carbon and are only 20–50 nm in diameter. These very small particles aggregate rapidly to form particles of about 0.1 μm (100 nm) diameter. Further reactions may occur and sulphuric acid may condense onto the surfaces of the particles. These processes yield particles of roughly 0.05–2 μm diameter, described as 'accumulation mode' particles. Monitoring the mass concentration of particles as $PM_{2.5}$ reflects this size range.

9.3.2 Effects of ambient particles on health

Particles comprising only soluble material dissolve on being deposited in the airways: ammonium sulphate falls into this category. Dissolution takes place in the fluid that lies on the surface of the cells lining the airways. It is unlikely that inorganic constituents of the particles that dissolve in this way would have any effect on health: the dose would be too small at ambient levels of exposure. Acids that dissolve in the lining fluid might stimulate irritant receptors that lie near the surface of the airway epithelium and cause coughing at high levels of exposure. The point about dose is important. We inhale rather less than 20 m³ of air per day. Let us assume an ambient concentration of particles (PM_{10})

of 100 µg/m^3 (rather high for the UK), then the maximum dose is 2 mg over a period of 24 hours, assuming that all the particles are deposited which will not, in fact, be the case. Two milligrams is a small dose even of sulphuric acid! Buffering in the airways would deal with this without difficulty.

Insoluble particles present different problems. These are rapidly cleared from the conducting airways by the muco-ciliary system and from the gas exchange zone, rather more slowly, by macrophages. In comparison with exposures in dusty trades, exposure to ambient particles is almost trivial. And yet we know from epidemiological studies that exposure to ambient concentrations produces significant effects on health. This mis-match between what we know of the effects of occupational exposure to particles and what we know of the effects of ambient exposure to particles has led to much debate. On the one hand are the doubters who assert that the epidemiological studies reveal associations that may not, in fact, be causal associations; on the other hand are those who accept that the exact mechanism of effect is unknown but who have several attractive hypotheses in play. One such hypothesis is the free radical hypothesis. Those who doubt the causal nature of the association revealed by epidemiology should recall the likely range of response to particles that exists in a population which includes the very young and the very old, the healthy and the very ill, and the highly exposed and minimally exposed.

9.4 Free radical hypothesis

Free radicals are generated continuously by oxidative metabolic processes. Free radicals are highly reactive and dangerous: they can react with lipids and trigger the chain reactions of lipid peroxidation. Inflammatory responses follow, with the synthesis and release of a welter of mediators (Kelly and Mudway 2007) Such effects are guarded against by antioxidants, including reduced glutathione, uric acid, and ascorbic acid. These compounds are secreted into the airway lining fluid. Particles containing metals are thought to be especially active in producing free radicals, for example the Fenton reaction

$$Fe^{++} + H_2O_2 \rightarrow Fe^{+++} + OH \cdot + OH^-$$

has been stressed by some workers. Transition metals other than iron, including copper and nickel, can take part in this reaction. Let us accept that free radicals are produced on inhalation of ambient particles. Unless the defence mechanisms are overwhelmed this should not lead to inflammation. In some individuals with poor production of glutathione due to a genetic defect this might well be the case. A number of studies have linked reduced production of reduced glutathione with cardiovascular responses to inhaled ambient particles (Schwartz et al. 2005). In other individuals with pre-existing disease, sensitivity to further damage might well be raised: this seems to be the case amongst those suffering from diabetes (Stewart et al. 2010).

9.5 The ultrafine hypothesis

The other major hypothesis in the particle field argues that the mass of particles deposited is largely irrelevant but that the number of very small particles (<100 nm diameter) is the controlling factor (Seaton et al. 1995). It was suggested that these very small particles might penetrate the alveolar epithelium and set up an inflammatory reaction in the interstitial tissues of the lung (Seaton et al. 1995).

This in turn might trigger the release of inflammatory factors by the pulmonary capillary endothelium and, in turn, affect levels of clotting factors in the blood. Support for each of these stages has appeared: blood viscosity is related to ambient levels of very small particles, fibrinogen levels increase when levels of ambient particles rise, red cell sequestration in the lung seems to be linked to ambient concentrations of particles (Seaton et al. 1999; Peters et al. 1997; Pekkanen et al. 2000). Could this be the answer? Well, it might be, but there are questions yet to be answered.

One fact, unexpected though it was when it first appeared, that does seem clear is that the major effect of exposure to ambient particles is on the cardiovascular system rather than on the lung. It has been shown that the rate of development of atheromatous lesions is accelerated by exposure to particles, that ultrafine particles can destabilize atheromatous plaques, and that the control of the rhythmicity of heart's beat is affected by particles (Schwartz 2001; Kunzli et al. 2005; Adar et al. 2007). Remarkable findings! Although the exact mechanisms of effect of ambient particles remain unknown and may be very complex indeed, it is accepted that the associations reported by epidemiologists should be regarded as causal.

This conclusion has led to the calculation of the effects (benefits) of reducing concentrations of ambient particles. Such calculations may be based on either time-series studies or on cohort studies. Using the latter, it has been calculated that exposure to 2008 levels of $PM_{2.5}$, in the UK, causes an effect *equivalent to* 29,000 deaths at typical ages in 2008 (Committee on the Medical Effects of Air Pollution 2010). The phrase *equivalent to* is important: it is likely that exposure to particles contributes to many more deaths than 29,000 (this is explained in detail in the recent report by the Committee on the Medical Effects of Air Pollutants (2010)). Reducing concentrations of particles extends life expectancy but cannot, of course, actually prevent deaths: all people die. Such calculations have formed the basis for the cost–benefit analysis that underpins the UK Air Quality Strategy (Department for the Environment, Food and Rural Affairs 2007).

9.6 Gaseous air pollutants

9.6.1 Ozone

Ozone is a classic secondary air pollutant: there are no significant outdoor and few indoor sources of ozone. It is important to distinguish between the ozone of the stratosphere, which protects against UV radiation and which is depleted by halogenated compounds, and the ozone of the troposphere, which affects health. The ozone of the troposphere comes largely from a series of photochemical (light-driven) reactions that depend on three things: light, oxides of nitrogen, and organic compounds. Given this, it is easy to understand why Los Angeles was so affected by photochemical air pollution. Nitrogen oxides (nitrogen dioxide and nitric oxide) are emitted by motor vehicles. Nitric oxide is oxidized to nitrogen dioxide: slowly by oxygen but rapidly by ozone. Ozone concentrations tend to be low near traffic: nitric oxide acts as an 'ozone-sink'. Nitrogen dioxide is broken down by sunlight to nitric oxide and a free, and very reactive, oxygen atom, which reacts with molecular oxygen to produce ozone. The other product of this breakdown reaction, nitric oxide, is oxidized back to the dioxide by reaction with organic peroxy radicals. All this takes some time and occurs as air masses drift away from urban areas, leading, often, to rather higher ozone concentrations in the countryside than in urban areas. Some tropospheric ozone results from incursions from the stratosphere; in the UK this occurs mainly in the spring. Ozone is removed from the air by reaction with plants and the ground: mixing of the air near the ground during the day brings ozone down to ground level and peak concentrations occur in the afternoon. At night, ozone formation ceases and concentrations near the ground fall rapidly.

Ozone causes inflammation of the airways and any effects it has on health must be secondary to this effect as such a reactive gas is unlikely to be absorbed unchanged. Peak tissue absorption occurs at the terminal bronchiole-alveolar duct junction because of the large surface area available and the thin layer of mucus present at this site (Miller et al. 1978). Exposure of animals to high concentrations of ozone leads to severe inflammation with thickening of interalveolar septa and oedema formation. At ambient levels the main effects seen in volunteer studies are an increase in airway resistance to gas flow (reflected by a decrease in the FEV1/FVC ratio), decreased exercise capacity, and pain on deep inspiration. Effects on lung function can be detected on exposure to concentrations as low as 80 ppb ($160 \mu g/m^3$) in subjects exercising in exposure chambers. To produce these effects exposure has to be prolonged to about 6 hours: shorter periods of exposure require higher concentrations to produce the same effects (Horstman et al. 1990). Epidemiological studies, unlike experimental studies with volunteers, have not shown thresholds of effect: effects have been detected at concentrations of only 40 ppb. This may be because sensitive subjects tend not to be studied experimentally, but it is interesting to note that by no means all asthma sufferers are unusually sensitive to ozone. Recent work has suggested that one of the genes that may play a part in the causation of asthma may also confer increased sensitivity to ozone: more work is needed on this. Exposure to concentrations of ozone of over 100 ppb ($200 \mu g/m^3$) may cause eye irritation but whether this is due to ozone per se or to associated photochemical pollutants is uncertain.

The effects on indices of lung function seem to wear off, so to speak, over a few days of exposure: a measure of adaptation seems to occur. Whether this is due to an upgrading of defence mechanisms or to exhaustion of the capacity to respond is unknown (Bromberg and Hazucha 1982). Lavage of the airways after exposure to ozone reveals a brisk inflammatory response with neutrophil leucocytes being prominent in the lavage fluid.

Epidemiological studies show clear associations between ambient concentrations of ozone and a range of indicators of ill-health: deaths from heart attacks and asthma attacks. No association between ambient concentrations of ozone and admissions to hospital for treatment for cardiovascular disease has been reported (Committee on the Medical Effects of Air Pollution 2006). This is odd, given the effect of cardiovascular deaths. The idea that ozone might trigger invariably fatal arrhythmias has occurred to some but this is not certain as yet. Long-term exposure to ozone may be related to the risk of death from respiratory disease but this, too, is not yet unequivocally established (Jerrett et al. 2009). In terms of the effects of short-term exposure to ozone it has been difficult to establish a threshold of effect, i.e. a concentration below which no effects occur. This may be due to a wide range of sensitivity in the population or to the difficulty in establishing an exposure–response rather than a concentration–response, relationship by means of standard epidemiological techniques. This is a common problem in the air pollution field.

9.6.2 Nitrogen dioxide

Nitrogen dioxide is both a primary and a secondary air pollutant: emitted by traffic and formed from nitric oxide, which is also emitted. Time-series epidemiological studies have shown clear associations between ambient concentrations of nitrogen dioxide and a range of effects of the respiratory and cardiovascular systems. In animal studies, high concentrations are needed to produce effects although long-term exposure to concentrations not much greater than occasionally experienced outdoors in the UK can lead to emphysematous changes in the lung. No effects of long-term exposure to outdoor ambient concentrations of nitrogen dioxide seem to have been reported. Studies in volunteers exposed to diluted diesel exhaust containing both high concentrations of particles (largely carbon) and about 300 ppb nitrogen dioxide have shown effects on indices of lung functions and on airway inflammation. Removing the particles greatly reduced the effect.

One of the unusual features of nitrogen dioxide is the wide range of results reported by workers undertaking studies in volunteers (World Health Organization 2006). In normal subjects several mg/m^3 of NO_2 are needed to produce changes in indices of lung function (airway resistance); in those suffering from asthma lower concentrations are effective and there is rather weak evidence for an enhancement of the response to allergens at low concentrations of about 100 ppb (World Health Organization 1987). At all likely ambient concentrations the effects really are rather small. This has led to the suggestion that epidemiological studies have not been able to distinguish between the possible effects of nitrogen dioxide and what are seen, by some, as the better established effects of fine particles. This is a perplexing issue. Vehicles emit both oxides of nitrogen and fine particles; let us assume that ambient concentrations of these pollutants follow each other up and down rather closely, so distinguishing between the effects of these pollutants will be difficult indeed. This has led those who are 'committed to the effects of particles' to downplay the possible effects of nitrogen dioxide. It is, however, fair to say that the current enthusiasm for studies of particles and nanoparticles has largely eclipsed interest in nitrogen dioxide.

Nitrogen dioxide has also been studied as an indoor air pollutant: long-term exposure to the raised concentrations of nitrogen dioxide found in homes provided with gas cookers has been reported to be associated with an increased level of respiratory infection in young children. These studies have been used as the basis for a World Health Organization (WHO) Air Quality Guideline for nitrogen dioxide of 40 µg/m^3 annual average concentration (World Health Organization 2006). This concentration is exceeded at many busy roadsides.

9.6.3 Sulphur dioxide

Sulphur dioxide is an acidic, soluble gas that has effects on the larger airways. High concentrations (irrelevant in terms of ambient air pollution) cause coughing and constriction of the airways in normal subjects (Department of Health 1992). Those who suffer from asthma are often very sensitive to sulphur dioxide and broncho-constriction occurs on exposure to low concentrations. Effects on the airways appear rapidly after exposure begins: this is not the case with ozone. The rapidity of onset of the effects of sulphur dioxide has led to air pollution standards being defined with very short averaging times: 10 or 15 minutes in addition to the more usual averaging time of 24 hours. Despite this, sulphur dioxide is not a major problem as an air pollutant in developed countries today. Sulphate particles, formed from sulphur dioxide, are an important component of ambient secondary particles. This link likely explains the association between long-term average concentrations of sulphur dioxide and effects on health reported from the USA American Cancer Society (ACS) (HEI 2000). Much discussion of the toxicity of sulphate has occurred: it seems clear that pure ammonium sulphate is not toxic in ambient concentrations but may well reflect the functioning of a chain of reactions that does include reactive and toxic intermediates.

9.6.4 Carbon monoxide

Carbon monoxide is the best understood of the classic air pollutants, at least as far as its mechanism of effect is concerned (Maynard 1999). It binds to haemoglobin in precisely the same way as oxygen and thus reduces the oxygen-carrying capacity of the blood. In addition, the oxy-haemoglobin dissociation curve is displaced to the left, making the release of such oxygen as is carried more difficult. Exposure to low concentrations produces headaches and flu-like symptoms; high concentrations kill. Concentrations of carbon monoxide outdoors are generally too low to cause serious effects on health but indoor concentrations can be high and each year many deaths and hospital admissions are caused by accidental exposure to this gas. Damage to the brain may be due to the direct effect of the reduced supply of oxygen but further injury after exposure to carbon monoxide has stopped may also occur. This is an example of re-perfusion injury and is due in part to the formation of oxidative free radicals. Long-term exposure to levels of carbon monoxide that cause only modest symptoms (headaches, tiredness) may be associated with damage to the brain: this is not yet accepted by all experts in the field and more work on this potentially very important effect is needed. Epidemiological studies have shown associations between peak daily concentrations of carbon monoxide and effects on the heart (Samoli et al. 2007). As in the case of nitrogen dioxide, it is difficult to be sure that these effects are due to carbon monoxide per se: they may be due to fine particles.

9.7 Other air pollutants

In addition to the above there is a range of organic compounds, benzene, 1,3-butadiene, polycyclic aromatic hydrocarbon compounds (PAHs), formaldehyde etc., found in ambient air (World Health Organization 1987). A number of these are known carcinogens that act via genotoxic mechanisms. No safe level of exposure can be defined and air quality standards are set at very low concentrations.

9.8 Indoor air pollutants

Much more emphasis has been placed on the study of the effects of outdoor exposure to air pollutants than on those of indoor exposure. This is paradoxical as we all spend more than 80% of our lives indoors and indoor concentrations of pollutants such as nitrogen dioxide and carbon monoxide often exceed those found outdoors. One reason for this disproportionate study of outdoor air pollution is that the means of controlling outdoor levels of air pollutants are more easily adopted by governments. Standards for outdoor concentrations of air pollutants are also more easily enforced than would be standards set for indoor concentrations. The indoor environment is of course connected to the outdoor environment and pollutants generated outdoors infiltrate buildings. Much of our daily exposure to particles generated outdoors must occur indoors. This means that studies which link outdoor concentrations of pollutants with effects on health should not be regarded solely as studies of outdoor exposure.

The indoor environment presents special problems: direct sources of pollutants such as cookers and fires may vent into the limited indoor space. This can lead to high indoor concentrations of pollutants, especially in houses with a low air exchange rate. Modern trends in building design, which reduce the need for space heating by insulation, exacerbate this problem. Some pollutants, including organic species released by carpets and adhesives, reach effective concentrations only indoors; formaldehyde, released from composition boards, is also a special indoor air problem. The dangers of indoor exposure to carbon monoxide have been discussed above. Tobacco smoke is also a special indoor air problem: high concentrations of carbon monoxide and nitrogen dioxide are found in tobacco smoke.

9.9 Air quality standards and the development of strategies to reduce concentrations of air pollutants

It is often assumed that an air quality strategy requires air quality standards; this is not correct. The great advances made in the UK by implementation of the Clean Air Act were achieved in the absence of any air quality standards. What is required is the perception that a problem exists and the political will to solve it. Of course, when concentrations of air pollutants are high it is easy to justify a programme to reduce them; it is much more difficult to justify such a programme when concentrations are low and effects not so apparent. Under such circumstances standards are useful and the WHO's Air Quality Guidelines are useful starting point for setting standards. The guidelines are not standards, per se, but they can and should be adapted for use as standards. Suggestions for how this might be done are set out in the guidelines (WHO 1987). Setting a clear guideline depends on defining a threshold of effect. This cannot be done for genotoxic carcinogens. Modern epidemiological studies do not, perhaps cannot, reveal thresholds of effect of the common, non-carcinogenic, air pollutants. Given this, it will be clear that guidelines are, to a large extent, likely to be arbitrary and to depend on the extent of protection required. The out-dated concept of 'controlling down to the guideline or standard' is slipping away and being replaced by an approach based firmly on the cost–benefit analysis of policy options. As yet this approach has been applied to only a few air pollutants; applying it to all air pollutants is a current challenge.

9.10 International dimensions

For many countries, including the UK, the solution to air pollution problems is impossible without international co-operation. Ozone concentrations in the UK are, in part, dictated by the background hemispheric concentrations of this pollutant. Furthermore the production of volatile organic compounds across Europe affects the photochemical processes that lead to ozone and this too affects the UK. International organizations such as the European Union rightly take a strong interest in air pollution and EC policies are set out in a series of Air Quality Directives. Some specify levels of performances for vehicle engines, others deal with the composition of fuel and some set limit values for air pollutants. These are binding on Member States.

In recent years EC Directive Limit Values have been increasingly based on recommendations from the WHO. These recommendations are summarized in the WHO Air Quality Guidelines. WHO guidelines are set without regard for cost, but cost and feasibility must be taken into account by the EC and dates for achievement of limit values and allowed levels of in excess of these values reflect these considerations.

9.11 References

Adar SD, Gold DR, Coull BA, Schwartz J, Stone PH, Suh H. (2007) Focused exposure to airborne traffic particles and heart rate variability in the elderly. *Epidemiology* **18**:95–103.

Brimblecombe P. (1987) *The Big Smoke*. Methuen, London.

Bromberg, PA, Hazucha MJ (1982) Is 'adaptation' to ozone protective? [Editorial] *Am J Respir Dis* **125**:489–490.

Committee on the Medical Effects of Air Pollutants. (2006) Cardiovascular Disease and Air Pollution. COMEAP, London. Also available at: http://www.comeap.org.uk/documents/reports/html.

Committee on the Medical Effects of Air Pollutants. (2010) The Mortality Effects of Long-Term Exposure to Particulate Air Pollution in the United Kingdom. Health Protection Agency, London. Available at: http://www.comeap.org.uk.

Department for Environment Food and Rural Affairs. (2007) *The Air Quality Strategy for England, Scotland, Wales and Northern Ireland*, Volumes **1** and **2**. Defra, London. Available at: http://www.defra.gov.uk/environment/airquality/strategy/pdf/air-qualitystrategy-vol1.pdf http://www.defra.gov.uk/environment/airquality/strategy/pdf/air-qualitystrategy-vol2.pdf.

Department of Health. (1991) Advisory Group on the Medical Aspects of Air Pollution Episodes. First Report: Ozone. HMSO, London.

Department of Health. (1992) Advisory Group on the Medic al Aspects of air Pollution Episodes. Second Report. Sulphur Dioxide, acid Aerosols and Particulates. HMSO, London.

Dockery DW, Pope CA, Xu X, Spengler JD, Ware JH, Fay ME, Ferris BG, Speizer FE. (1993) An association between air pollution and mortality in six US cities. *N Engl J Med* **329**:1753–1759.

Haagen-Smit AJ. (1952) Chemistry and physiology of Los Angeles smog. *Ind. Eng. Chem* **44**:1342–1346.

Health Effects Institute. (2000) Reanalysis of the Harvard Six Cities Study and the American Cancer Society Study of Particulate Air Pollution and Mortality: A Special Report of the Institute's Particle Epidemiology Reanalysis Project. Health Effects Institute, Cambridge, MA. Available at: http://pubs.healtheffects.org/getfile.php?u=273. Accessed April 2007.

Horstman DH, Folinsbee LJ, Ives PJ, Abdul-Salaam S, McDonell WF (1990) Ozone concentration and pulmonary response relationships for 6.6 hour exposures with five hours of moderate exercise to 0.08, 0.10, and 0.12 ppm. *Am Rev Respir Dis* **142**:1158–1163.

Jerrett M, Burnett RM, Pope CA, Ito K, Thurston G, Krewski G, Krewski D, Shi Y, Calle E, Thun M. (2009) Long-term exposure and mortality. *N Engl J Med* **360**:1085–1095.

Kelly FJ, Mudway I. (2007) Particle-associated extracellular oxidative stress in the lung. In: Donaldson K, Borm K. (eds) *Particle Toxicology*. CRC Press, Boca Raton, op 89–118.

Kunzli N, Jerrett JM, Mack WJ, Beckerman B, LaBree L, Gilliland F, Thomas D, Peters J, Nodis HN. (2005) Ambient air pollution and atherosclerosis in Los Angeles. *Environ Health Perspect* **113**:201–205.

Lippmann M, Hwang JS, Maciejczyk P, Chen LC (2005) PM Source apportionment for short-term cardiac function changes in ApoE -/- mice. *Environ Health Perspect* **113**:1575–1579.

Miller FJ, Menzel DB, Coffin DL. (1978) Similarity between man and laboratory animals in regional pulmonary deposition of ozone. *Environ Res* **17**:84–101.

Pekkanen J, Brunner EJ, Anderson HR, Tiitanen P, Atkinson RW. (2000) Daily concentrations of air pollution and plasma fibrinogen in London. *Occup Environ Med* **57**:818–822.

Peters, A., Doring, A., Wichmann, H.-E. and Koenig, W. (1997) Increased plasma viscosity during an air pollution episode: a link to mortality? *Lancet* **349**:1582–1587.

Pope CA, Thun MJ, Numboodiri MM, Dockery DW, Evans JS, Speizer FE, Heath CW. (1995) Particulate air pollution as a predictor of mortality in a prospective study of US adults. *Am J Respir Crit Care Med* **151**:669–674.

Pope CA, Burnett RT, Thun MJ, Calle EE, Krewski D, Ito K, Thurston GD. (2002) Lung cancer, cardiopulmonary mortality, and long-term exposure to fine particulate air pollution. *JAMA* **287**(9):1132–1141.

Samoli E, Toulomi G, Schwartz J, Anderson HR, Schindler C, Forsberg B, Vigotti MA, Vonk J, Kosnik M, Skorvorsky J, Katsouyanni K. (2007) Short-term effects of carbon monoxide on mortality: an analysis within the APHEA project. *Environ Health Perspect* **115**:1578–1583.

Schwartz J. (2001) Air pollution and blood markers of cardiovascular risk. *Environ Health Perspect* **109**:405–429.

Schwartz J, Park SK, O'Neill MS, Vokonav MS, Sparrow D, Weiss S, Kelsey K. (2005) Glkuthione-S-transferaxe M1, obesity, statins, and autonomic effects of partic.esa. *Am J Respir Crit Care Med* **172**:1529–1533.

Seaton A, MacNee W, Donaldson K, Godden D. (1995) Particulate air pollution and acute health effects. *Lancet* **345**:176–178.

Seaton A, Soutar A, Crawford V, Elton R, McNerlan S, Cherrie J, Watt M, Agius R, Stout R. (1999) Particulate air pollution and the blood. *Thorax* **54**:1027–1032.

Stewart JC, Chaluopa DC, Devlin RB, Frasier LM, Huang L-S, Little EM, Leer SM, Phipps RP, Pietropauli AP, Taubman MB, Utell MJ, Frampton MW. (2010) *Environ Health Perspect* **118**:1692–1698.

World Health Organization. (1987) *Air Quality Guidelines for Europe*. WHO Regional Publications, European Series, No 23. WHO Regional Office for Europe, Copenhagen.

World Health Organization. (2006) Air quality guidelines. Global update 2005. Particulate matter, ozone, nitrogen dioxide and sulfur dioxide. http://www.euro.who.int/InformationSources/Publications/Catalogue/20070323_1.

9.12 Further reading

Department for the Environment, Food and Rural Affairs. (2006) Air pollution in the UK: 2005, London.

Department of Health, Committee on the Medical Effects of Air Pollutants (2006) *Cardiovascular Disease and Air Pollution*. London.

Holgate ST, Samet JM, Koren HS, Maynard RL. (1999) Air pollution and Health. Academic Press, London.

World Health Organization. (2000) Air Quality Guidelines for Europe, 2nd edition. WHO Regional Publications, European Series Number 91. World Health Organization, Geneva.

Chapter 10

Public health risk assessment of contaminated land

Sohel Saikat and James Wilson

Learning outcomes

At the end of this chapter and any recommended reading the student should be able to:

1. describe and discuss the nature of land contamination and the UK's approach to regulation;

2. describe the principles used for assessing land contamination;

3. explain how toxicological and exposure assessment information are used in the UK to assess public health risks posed by land contamination; and

4. apply acquired knowledge to the analysis and management of land contamination cases.

10.1 Introduction

10.1.1 Aims

The aim of this chapter is to provide environmental and public health practitioners with a broad overview of what 'contaminated land' is, how contaminated land is investigated, and how the risks it poses to human health are assessed. Although the chapter is written in the context of UK policy and practice, the principle and approach discussed may be relevant to assessing land contamination in other countries. Contaminated land assessment primarily involves comparing the contaminant concentrations present on a site (especially in soil) to health protection assessment criteria such as the UK Soil Guideline Values. Assessment criteria are generated using toxicological information and exposure assessment models. Therefore, in order for environmental/public health practitioners to contribute to the design or evaluation of a risk assessment strategy or to appreciate the implications of a risk assessment, it is necessary for them to be aware of the rudiments of site investigation procedures, the use of exposure assessment models, and the application of toxicological information. The skills required to undertake contaminated land assessments are clearly varied and may draw on a number of disciplines. Specialist contractors may be commissioned to conduct risk assessments, often on the behalf of regulators. Regulators may

Box 10.1 'Contaminated land' and Part IIA of the Environmental Protection Act (1990)

'Contaminated land' has been defined in the Part IIA of the Environmental Protection Act (1990) as:

> 'any land which appears to the Local Authority in whose area it is situated to be in such a condition, by reason of substances in, on or under the land, that—(a) significant harm is being caused or there is a significant possibility of such harm being caused; or (b) pollution of controlled waters is being, or is likely to be, caused.'

'Harm' is defined as 'death, disease, serious injury, birth defects, and the impairment of reproductive functions. 'Disease' is taken to mean 'an unhealthy condition of the body or a part of it and can include, for example, cancer, liver dysfunction, or extensive skin ailments. Mental dysfunction is only included insofar as it is attributable to the effects of a pollutant on the body of the person concerned.'

in turn seek advice from public health professionals on managing incidents of land contamination.

10.1.2 Definition of 'contaminated land'

The legal definition of 'contaminated land' is given in Part IIA of the Environmental Protection Act (1990). Sites that are undergoing assessment, or might not necessarily fulfil the legal criteria, are generally referred to as 'land affected by contamination' (Box 10.1).

The definition reflects that the presence of chemicals in the ground does not necessarily mean that the land will be classified as contaminated land. The legal definition is to enable the identification and remediation of land where contamination is causing unacceptable risks to human health or the wider environment. The definition is underpinned by the concept of source-pathway-receptor linkage (pollutant linkage), i.e. (i) source of contamination (chemical(s)), (ii) pathway or route (inhalation of dust, ingestion of vegetables grown in contaminated soils) by which the source of contamination can reach the identified receptor, and (iii) the receptor that is likely to be affected (e.g. humans). A pollutant linkage must exist on a given site and the requirements of what constitutes significant harm must be met in line with the statutory guidance which accompanies the legislation.

10.1.3 The nature of land contamination

Land may be contaminated by current and historical activities which cause the release of chemicals. The release may be deliberate or accidental. Although there has been increased control of industrial chemical release and emission, land is still becoming contaminated through common human activities (e.g. land fill, diffuse pollution from agriculture). In the UK, a wide range of industries may be associated with land contamination. Examples include gas/coke works, chemical works, metal works, asbestos works, engineering works, manufacturing plants, oil refineries, textile and dye works, sewage works, timber treatment works, waste recycling works, garages and filling stations, landfills, and electrical

> ## Box 10.2 Extent of land contamination in England and Wales (Environment Agency 2009a)
>
> In the UK there has not been any systematic study to ascertain the geographical extent of land affected by contamination. An estimate by the Environment Agency in 2005 indicated that around 300,000 hectares of land may be contaminated in England and Wales due to industrial activity, which is approximately 2% of the land area of England and Wales.
>
> A total of 781 sites have been determined as 'contaminated land' under Part IIA of the Environmental Protection Act (1990) by the end of March 2007. Of 781 sites, 659 are in England and 122 in Wales. Over 90% of these sites had housing on them when the site was inspected.
>
> Metal, metalloids, and organic compounds were identified as the most common pollutants. The energy and waste industries were the biggest contamination source in England and the deposit of ash was reported as the most common contamination source in Wales in the sites identified as contaminated land.

manufacturing works. In addition to industrial activities, the underlying geology of an area may lead to 'naturally occurring' concentrations of harmful substances which are deemed to be elevated. In the UK, for example, areas in the south-west and the Midlands, contain elevated levels of metals and metalloid in soils linked with mineralization and past mining operations (Box 10.2) (Environment Agency 2009a).

10.2 Risk assessment process

Risk assessment of potentially contaminated area can be a detailed and lengthy process. In the UK, it is undertaken in a tiered assessment structure (Defra/Environment Agency 2004). The tiers are applied to the circumstances of a given site with an increasing level of detail required by the assessor (Figure 10.1). Prior to conducting site investigations, a

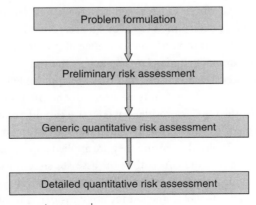

Fig. 10.1 Tiered risk assessment approach.

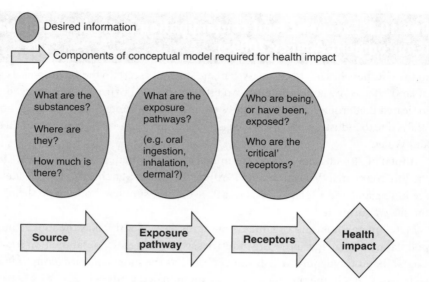

Fig. 10.2 Source-pathway-receptor model.

desk-based study of the land-use history along with its underlying geology is typically con-ducted to identify whether there is a problem due to the presence of hazardous substances. This phase identifies whether or not there is a need for undertaking a systematic risk assessment.

In preliminary risk assessment phase, site reconnaissance activities are undertaken in addi-tion to desk-based studies to ascertain the likely existence of source-pathway-receptor (pollut-ant linkage) linkages on the site and define the exposure scenario (Figure 10.2). Based on the information gathered, a conceptual model of risk for the site is developed. The conceptual model aims to identify the key uncertainties and data gaps, which in turn are used to inform the site investigation design and further stages of risk assessment. If pollutant linkage is identi-fied, the assessment moves into the generic quantitative risk assessment (GQRA) phase.

In the GQRA phase, physical investigation of the ground is conducted which involves collection of environmental samples such as soil, water, and gas. The presence of chemicals and their concentrations is determined by using an accredited laboratory and methods. The quantitative data are used to verify the existence of pollutant linkage and are com-pared with generic assessment criteria (GACs) such as the soil guideline values (SGVs). GACs are typically conservative to ensure that they are applicable to the majority of site conditions. However, GACs should only be used for the purpose for which they are intended. For example, the GAC for residential land use should not be used to assess risk to people working in an office environment. The uncertainties and limitations associated with GACs need to be understood to ensure they are applied appropriately. If the contami-nant concentrations fall above the GACs, then the assessor should use appropriate statis-tical techniques to provide a representative soil concentration value (such as a mean). If the mean value falls below the GAC, the land is not considered to be contaminated and further assessment is not necessary. If the values exceed the GACs, the assessor may consider whether or not further data collection is necessary.

In cases where GQRA assessment indicates that further detailed risk assessment is necessary, the assessor may decide to undertake detailed quantitative risk assessment (DQRA). This phase may involve additional sampling, more detailed assessment of pollutant linkage and exposure scenario, and derivation of site-specific assessment criteria (SSAC). The presence of uncertainty in the toxicology and assumption in the exposure scenario are also evaluated and, where possible, replaced with more site-specific observations and data. The contaminated land exposure assessment (CLEA) model available in the UK to derive the GACs (SGVs) can also be used to derive SSAC for assessing risk from a specific chemical (Environment Agency 2009b). As in the GQRA stage, representative soil concentrations are compared against SSACs and if the values exceed the SSACs, then a risk evaluation can be carried out. If the values do not exceed thef SSACs, the assessor usually decides not to take any further action.

Risk evaluation could consider the likelihood of significant harm, the extent and type of possible effects on the receptor, the risks posed in the context of wider environmental risks, and the socio-economic cost–benefits of regulatory interventions (Defra 2010). If sufficient information is available that suggests that a site fulfils the definition of 'contaminated land', it may be so designated under Part IIA of the Environmental Protection Act (1990). An option appraisal may then be produced which may include a consideration of remedial works that could be undertaken to reduce the risks (Defra/Environment Agency 2004). The aim of remedial work is to break the pollution linkages identified in the conceptual model (such as the removal of the source, breaking exposure pathways, or removal of receptors). If remedial works are undertaken, verification should be carried out to ensure that remedial objectives have been met (for example 'clean' topsoil imported onto a site should be tested to ensure that it really is 'clean').

10.3 Exposure assessment models

Exposure models are necessary to generate assessment criteria such as SGVs, which indicate the concentration of a substance present in soil that may result in a daily intake equal to, or less than, a health criteria value (HCV) (Box 10.3). The exposure pathways present on a given site are identified by constructing a conceptual model indicating potential pollution linkages (Figure 10.2) with degrees of risk associated with them.

In 2009, the Environment Agency released an updated CLEA model (Environment Agency 2009b). The model uses generic assumptions about chemical fate and transport in the environment and a generic conceptual model for site conditions and human behaviour to estimate exposure to contaminants for those living, working, and playing on contaminated sites over long periods. The CLEA model has been used to generate SGVs by comparing the estimated exposure with HCVs.

The CLEA model can be applied for three generic land-use scenarios: residential, allotments, and industrial. The model includes a number of potential exposure pathways (Figure 10.3) and offers flexibility to change/add the pathways and parameters. The approach used is to

Box 10.3 Health criteria values (Environment Agency 2009c)

For substances that exhibit threshold effects, health criteria values (HCVs) take the form of tolerable daily soil intakes (TDSIs), which may be better described as tolerable daily intakes *from* soil. The approach taken for a given substance is to initially identify a tolerable daily intake (TDI), which is expressed as mass of substance per unit mass of body weight per day. This is typically extrapolated from a no observable adverse effect level (NOAEL), often identified from animal experiments. Once this has been identified, a number of uncertainty factors may be applied to account for variability in response resulting from factors such as inter- and intraspecies variation. If a NOAEL is not available for a given substance, the lowest observable adverse effect level (LOAEL) may be adopted with the application of an additional uncertainty factor. Once a TDI has been identified, the mean daily intake (MDI) of substances from sources other than soil is identified (drinking water and food products, for example). The TDSI is equal to the TDI minus the MDI, except in cases where MDI ≥80% TDI. In those cases, the TDSI is equal to 20% of the TDI (in order to ensure that resources are not devoted to inappropriately reducing exposure to substances from soil sources).

For non-threshold substances, HCVs are in the form of 'index doses', which are daily intakes (also expressed as mass of substance per unit mass of receptor body weight per day) that have a corresponding 'minimal' risk of causing adverse health outcomes, typically cancer. Although intakes can be identified which correspond to a minimal risk, there is an additional exhortation that exposure to non-threshold substances should be kept as low as reasonably practicable (ALARP) because no 'safe' level of exposure can be identified. It is also assumed that exposures to non-threshold substances from sources other than soil will also be reduced to levels that are ALARP and as such, intakes of non-threshold substances from sources other than soil are not considered.

Depending on the quantity and quality of toxicology data available, risk assessors can also derive a benchmark dose (BMD) in addition to a NOAEL or LOAEL for an adverse health outcome. This is derived by modelling the dose–response curve and estimating the BMD that causes a predetermined change in response (such as 5–10%). In general, the statistical 95% lower confidence limit of the BMD, called the BMDL, is used in the derivation of HCVs. A large uncertainty factor, such as 10,000, is typically used if the HCV is derived based on a BMDL value.

identify a 'critical receptor' which for a given exposure is likely to receive the greatest dose and therefore potentially be most at risk. For a typical residential site, the critical receptor is taken to be a young female child. The CLEA model can also be used to generate SSACs, where generic exposure parameters are altered to reflect more closely the conditions present on the site of interest.

A number of exposure assessment models have also been developed by other regulatory authorities, such as the Scotland and Northern Ireland Forum for Environmental Research (SNIFFER), Risk-Based Corrective Action (RBCA), and Integrated Exposure Uptake Biokinetic (IEUBK) models. For information on the CLEA exposure model, the Environment Agency's

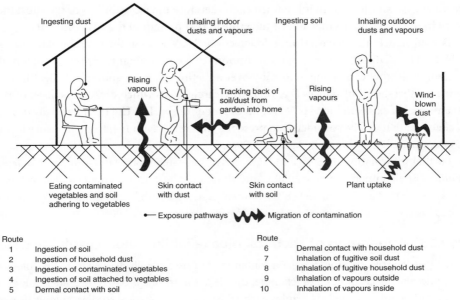

Fig. 10.3 Exposure pathways.

Reprinted with permission from Using science to create a better place: updated technical background to the CLEA model, 2009, pp. 14, Science Report: SC050021/SR3 Environment Agency © Environment Agency 2012.

framework document *Updated technical background to the CLEA model* can be a useful reference (Environment Agency 2009b).

10.4 Toxicological input in risk assessment

10.4.1 Derivation of health criteria value

Toxicological input criteria are central to human health risk assessment in contaminated soil. These are referred to as HCVs in the UK (Box 10.3) and as reference concentrations (RfCs) in the USA. The relationship between SGVs and HCVs is that SGVs are produced using HCVs and the estimates of the amount of substance an individual would take in as a result of exposure to soil. In the context of UK, SGVs provide a link between the concentration of a particular contaminant in the soil and the health risks defined at the HCV under the defined conditions.

HCVs are toxicological benchmarks to an assessor on the level of long-term exposure to individual chemicals in soil that are tolerable or pose a minimal risk (Environment Agency 2009c). They are determined from a review of the evidence from occupational and environmental epidemiological studies, animal studies, and from scientific understanding of the mechanisms of absorption, transport, metabolism, excretion, and toxicity of chemicals within the human body. In the review, consideration has to be given to the toxicological properties of a contaminant/pollutant related to acute as well chronic exposures (including, for example, carcinogenicity, genotoxicity, reproductive toxicity, and teratogenicity). It should be noted that toxicological data are often only available from animal studies and that the form (and therefore bioaccessibility) of the substance used in the experiments may not be the same as that present in the environment.

For substances that have a threshold effect, the HCV is set at the tolerable daily intake (TDI). The TDI is 'an estimate of the amount of a contaminant, expressed on a body weight basis, that can be ingested daily over a lifetime without appreciable health risk'. For non-threshold substances (i.e. genotoxic carcinogens which carry some level of risk at any level of exposure) the HCV is set at the index dose (ID). The ID is 'the daily dose of a chemical that can be considered to present a minimal health risk from exposure to soil contaminants' (Environment Agency 2009c).

Further information on SGV and HCV derivation can be found in *Using Soil Guideline Values* (Environment Agency 2009d) and the framework documents *Updated technical background to the CLEA model* (Environment Agency 2009b) and *Human health toxicological assessment of contaminants in soil* (Environment Agency 2009c).

10.4.2 Consideration of chemical bioavailability/bioaccessibility data

HCVs used in risk assessments of land contamination are generally derived from toxicological or epidemiological studies. For example, the HCV for arsenic is based on epidemiological studies of people exposed via drinking water. In oral toxicological studies, chemicals may be administered via different media, such as drinking water, gavage, and capsules. HCVs tend to assume that a chemical is equally bioavailable in all media. However, this assumption might not be true for soil contaminants because of the binding to soil particles and/or chemical entry inside the soil mineral lattice, which may cause bioavailability to differ between the soil types, chemicals, and chemical forms (Environment Agency 2005; Saikat 2006).

Bioavailability determination requires testing with human volunteers or suitable animal models (*in vivo* models), which may not be ethical to conduct and may also be very costly. In Europe and North America, therefore, academic and regulatory research has been directed into developing *in vitro* methods to measure soil contaminant bioaccessibility, as an indication of bioavailability (Box 10.4). Bioaccessibility methods generally involve laboratory tests that extract metals/metalloids (such as lead and arsenic) from soil by simulating the action of low pH, 37°C and rate of mixing that occurs in the gut (US EPA 2008). However, issues have been identified regarding the validity and robustness of the data produced by such methods and the degree to which they correlate with *in vivo* bioavailability (Saikat 2006; Hagens et al. 2008).

Risk assessment using default estimates of average daily exposure based on a chemical's total concentration in soil may identify many areas of land where contamination may exceed a minimal or tolerable risk level. Therefore the incorporation of site-specific bioavailability or bioaccessibility data into the derivation of SSAC at the DQRA level could make the exposure and risk calculation more realistic to the local situation. In the USA, a validated *in vitro* method for lead has been developed for use in quantitative adjustment of bioavailability data (US EPA 2007, 2008).

Further information on chemical bioaccessibility/bioavailability is available to download free from the Environment Agency website (http://www.environment-agency.gov.uk/landcontamination).

Box 10.4 Concept of chemical bioavailability and bioaccessibility

Bioavailability (or absolute bioavailability) is the fraction of a chemical that is absorbed by the body through the gastrointestinal system, pulmonary system, and/or the skin. It can be expressed as the ratio of the absorbed dose to the intake dose.

$$ABA = \frac{D_s}{D_i}$$

where ABA is the absolute bioavailability of a chemical in dimensionless form, D_s is the absorbed dose in mg/kg body weight per day, and D_i is the intake dose in mg/kg body weight per day. **Relative bioavailability** is the comparison of the extent of absorption between two or more forms of the same chemical (such as lead carbonate versus lead acetate), or the same chemical administered in different media (such as food, soil, water) or at different doses.

Oral bioaccessibility (F_B) is the fraction of a substance that is released from the soil during processes like digestion into solution, making it available for uptake by the body (Environment Agency 2005). Oral bioaccessibility can be expressed as an absolute bioaccessible concentration in soil (e.g. mg/kg) or as a fraction of the total concentration in soil:

$$F_B = \frac{C_{released}}{C_{soil}}$$

where F_B is the oral bioaccessible fraction of a chemical in soil, $C_{released}$ is the amount of chemical released from soil in mg/kg soil, and C_{soil} is the initial total amount of a chemical in soil in mg/kg.

Bioaccessibility is relevant to bioavailability since it represents a step in the overall process of human absorption of a chemical (USEPA 2007; Hagens et al. 2008). Since solubilization is usually required for absorption of a substance across a biological membrane, poorly soluble forms of a chemical with low measured bioaccessibility may also have low bioavailability (USEPA 2007). In certain circumstances, if the solubility of a substance is the controlling factor in overall absorption then bioaccessibility may be a good predictor of bioavailability.

10.5 Health significance of contaminated land

Land contamination may impact on health, the soil quality, and perceptions of the local environment. In the UK, there have not been increased levels of illness observed in people living on 'land affected by contamination'. It may be that health impacts exist but are undetectable with the current epidemiological and analytical methods, and because of small effect sizes or small populations affected, or the effects of confounders (for example, people can be exposed to chemicals from sources separate from land).

In the UK, a project based on published literature was conducted to provide an overview of the different types of risk to human health posed by contaminated land, including an assessment of the uncertainty associated with determining health impacts (FERA 2009). Key findings from this study include:

- There may be a plausible linkage between exposure to land contamination and birth defects, including congenital anomalies and low birth weight.
- There is evidence to both support and refute a link between land contamination and cancer. Overall there is insufficient evidence to demonstrate cause and effect.
- The greatest contributor to the uncertainty is around the toxicological effects of the contaminants, stemming from a lack of adequate data on the capacity of the chemical to cause disease.

Further details of this project are available on the Defra website (http://sciencesearch. defra.gov.uk/Document.aspx?Document=SP1002_8879_SD5.pdf).

10.6 Conclusion

Assessing the health risks posed by land contamination is a complex process, requiring an understanding of site investigation, exposure modelling, and the use of toxicological information. Environmental/public health practitioners should be familiar with the rudiments of risk assessment, some of which are discussed here. Soil sampling and analysis should provide a reliable, representative indication of contaminant concentrations to which receptors may be exposed via pathways. These data may then be compared to assessment criteria generated using assumptions appropriate for the land use of a given site and authoritative toxicological information. Quantitative risk assessment is a powerful tool used in health protection. However, resource limitations and uncertainties associated with exposure and effect (along with differences between individuals' perceptions of risk) will result in the need for informed judgements to be made when remedial options (or other interventions) are being considered.

10.7 References

Defra. (2010) Consultation: changes to the contaminated land regime under Part2A of the Environmental Protection Act 1990. Department of Environmental, Food and Rural Affairs (Defra), London, UK. Available at: http://archive.defra.gov.uk/corporate/consult/contaminated-land/index.htm.

Defra/Environment Agency. (2004) Model Procedures for the Management of Land Contamination. Environment Agency, Bristol, UK. http://publications.environment-agency.gov.uk/pdf/SCHO0804BIBR-e-e.pdf.

Environment Agency. (2005) Environment Agency's Science Update on the use of Bioaccessibility Testing in Risk Assessment of Land Contamination. Environment Agency, Bristol, UK. Available at: http://www.environment-agency.gov.uk/commondata/acrobat/science_update_1284046.pdf.

Environment Agency. (2009a) Dealing with contaminated land in England and Wales: a review of progress from 2000–2007 with Part 2A of the Environmental Protection Act. Environment Agency, Bristol, UK. Available at: http://publications.environment-agency.gov.uk/PDF/GEHO0109BPHA-E-E.pdf.

Environment Agency. (2009b) *Updated technical background to the CLEA model.* Environment Agency, Bristol, UK. Science Report SC050021/SR3. Environment Agency, Bristol. Available at: http://www.environment-agency.gov.uk/clea.

Environment Agency. (2009c) *Human health toxicological assessment of contaminants in soil.* Science Report SC050021/SR2. Environment Agency, Bristol, UK. Available at: http://www.environment-agency.gov.uk/clea.

Environment Agency. (2009d) *Using Soil Guideline Values.* Science Report SC050021/SGV introduction. Environment Agency, Bristol, UK. Available at: http://www.environment-agency.gov.uk/clea.

FERA. (2009) Potential health effects of contaminants in soil, Defra. Department for Environment, Food and Rural Affairs (Defra), London, UK. Available at: http://sciencesearch.defra.gov.uk/Document.aspx?Document=SP1002_8879_SD5.pdf.

Hagens WI, Lijzen JPA, Sips AJAM, Oomen AA. (2008) The bioaccessibility and relative bioavailability of lead from soils for fasted and fed conditions, Letter Report 711701080. National Institute for Public Health and the Environment, Bilthoven, The Netherlands.

Saikat S. (2006) Bioavailability/bioaccessibility testing in risk assessment of land contamination – a short review. Chemical Hazards and Poisons Report 6, 44-45, Health Protection Agency, London, UK.

US EPA. (2007) Estimation of Relative Bioavailability of Lead in Soil and Soil-Like Materials Using In Vivo and In Vitro Methods. OSWER 9285.7–77. United States Environmental Protection Agency, Washington, DC, USA. Available at: http://www.epa.gov/superfund/health/contaminants/bioavailability.

US EPA. (2008) Standard Operating Procedure for an In Vitro Bioaccessibility Assay for Lead in Soil, EPA 9200.1–86. United States Environmental Protection Agency, Washington, DC, USA. Available at: http://www.epa.gov/superfund/health/contaminants/bioavailability.

10.8 Useful internet links

Chartered Institution of Environmental Health http://www.cieh.org/knowledge/environmental_protection/contaminated_land.

Contaminated Land: Applications in Real Environments http://www.claire.co.uk.

Defra http://www.defra.gov.uk/environment/land/contaminated/index.htm.

Environment Agency http://www.environmentagency.gov.uk/subjects/landquality/113813/?version=1&lang=_e.

Health Protection Agency http://www.hpa.org.uk.

United Kingdom Accreditation Service (UKAS) http://www.ukas.com/about_accreditation/.

Chapter 11

Management of incidents affecting drinking water quality

Gary Lau

Learning outcomes

At the end of this chapter and any recommended reading the student should be able to:

1. explain the processes and guidelines for the provision of safe public water supply in England and Wales;

2. evaluate the roles of the Drinking Water Inspectorate (DWI), local authorities, and the water utilities;

3. explain the importance of good analytical support and toxicological advice, plus inter-agency assistance and effective communications in the event of the chemical contamination of public water supplies;

4. critically discuss examples of chemical water contamination incidents and evaluate the manner in which investigations were carried out, and

5. apply acquired knowledge in the analysis and management of hazardous situations.

11.1 Introduction

This chapter outlines the arrangements for public water supply in England and Wales, and the role of the DWI in enforcing regulatory requirements. The management of incidents affecting drinking water quality is described using examples to highlight some of the issues associated with minimizing harm to the population. Analytical support, health risks and toxicological advice, inter-agency assistance, and communication are considered.

The need for effective and rapid communications between all relevant bodies in the event of a chemical contamination incident affecting public water supplies and the ready availability of an assessment of potential health risks and provision of toxicological advice are highlighted.

11.2 The Drinking Water Inspectorate

11.2.1 Background

The DWI was formed on 2 January 1990 following the privatization of the water industry. It provides independent reassurance that public water supplies in England and Wales are safe and acceptable to consumers.

11.2.2 Public water supplies

A public water supply is one which is provided for the purposes of drinking, washing, cooking and food production by a statutorily appointed water company. From December 2005, non-domestic consumers who use at least 50 m³ of water a year were able to purchase water from either their existing company or from a licensed water supplier.

11.2.3 Private water supplies

Water that is not supplied by a statutorily appointed water company is called private water. Local authorities are responsible under the Water Industry Act 1991 for checking the safety and sufficiency of water supplies in their area, including private water supplies. The DWI provides expert technical advice to local authorities but has no regulatory role. Private water supplies make up less than 2% of the total water supply in England and Wales, and most such supplies are in rural and remote parts of the country.

11.2.4 Regulatory framework

The Water Industry Act 1991 sets out the regulatory framework and defines the powers and duties under which the DWI operates as well as the responsibilities of water companies. Under the Act, the Secretary of State for Environment, Food and Rural Affairs and the National Assembly for Wales are responsible for regulating the quality of public water supplies. These two authorities appoint the Chief Inspector of Drinking Water to act on their behalf to enforce water quality standards and, where appropriate, initiate prosecutions. The Water Act 2003 (Section 57) provides for the appointment of the Chief Inspector of Drinking Water and amends the Water Industry Act to allow for the appointment of inspectors.

11.2.5 Wholesome water

By law (Section 68 of the Water Industry Act 1991) water companies must supply water that is wholesome at the time of supply. Wholesomeness is defined by reference to drinking water standards and other requirements set out in the Water Supply (Water Quality) Regulations 2000 (2010 in Wales) (the Regulations). Many of these regulations derive from the 1998 European Drinking Water Directive (Council Directive 1998), which came fully into force on 25 December 2003. Until December 2003, the standards contained within the Water Supply (Water Quality) Regulations 1989 applied.

The standards are directly linked to the World Health Organization (WHO) guideline values for drinking water quality, which are intended to protect public health as well as ensuring that water supplies are aesthetically acceptable to consumers. Under the EC Directive, standards will be subject to revision in the light of new knowledge. The new Regulations contain some new and revised standards; others that are no longer appropriate have been withdrawn. Although the Directive focuses on those parameters of importance to human health, others are included which relate to the control of water treatment processes and the aesthetic quality of drinking water. The Directive allows member states to set additional or tighter national standards to preserve the already good quality of drinking water and to prevent future deterioration.

11.2.6 Testing and reporting

Water companies are required to collect and test samples of the water leaving water treatment and service reservoirs and from randomly selected consumers' properties. The tests to be carried out and the frequency of testing are detailed in the Regulations and the Water Supply Regulations (2010). The DWI checks independently that the testing is carried out to the highest standards and that appropriate quality control checks are in place to assure the integrity of the analytical information produced. Water companies have a duty to make the results of their testing available to consumers and the DWI also publishes summary information on individual companies both in an annual report and on its website.

11.2.7 Water safety

The Regulations also make some provisions for drinking water safety. There are specific requirements concerning *Cryptosporidium*, there is a requirement to adequately treat and disinfect water supplies, and there are controls over chemicals and materials of construction that drinking water supplies might come into contact with.

11.3 Water quality incidents

11.3.1 Incident notification

When events occur that might impact on the quality or sufficiency of the water supplied, water companies are required to notify such events to the DWI under the terms set out in the Water Industry (Supplier's Information) Direction 2009 (DWI 2009a). This duty is enforceable under Section 202 of the Water Industry Act 1991.

The Direction requires water companies to inform the DWI of all events that have affected, or are likely to affect, drinking water quality or sufficiency of supplies where, as a result, there may be a risk to consumers' health (Box 11.1). When notified of such events the DWI assesses the water company's provisional information to determine whether the event is an incident. If the event is deemed to be an incident a full report from the company may also be required.

11.3.2 What should be notified?

The wording of the current Direction and its predecessors deliberately leaves it to water companies to decide what to notify. This is because an event that appears significant to a small company could appear to be less so to a larger company. Furthermore the trigger for consumer contacts may be very different between a rural area and a highly populated inner city area. However, the DWI has issued guidance on the type of events that it considers should be notifiable (DWI 2009b). The guidance also gives information on the investigation process by which the DWI investigates incidents.

11.3.3 Incident investigation

The DWI assesses the information provided by water companies to determine whether the event meets the criteria of an incident, as defined by the DWI (Box 11.2).

Box 11.1 Notification requirements of the Water Industry (Supplier's Information) Direction 2009

Water companies are required to notify the Inspectorate of:

- the occurrence of any event which, because of its effect or likely effect on the quality or sufficiency of water supplied by the supplier, gives rise, or is likely to give rise, to a significant risk to the health of persons to whom the water is supplied (including any event notified by the supplier to a local authority, the Health Protection Agency, or local health board under regulation 35 of the Water Supply (Water Quality) Regulations 2000.

- any other matter relating to the supply of water that:
  - in the opinion of the supplier, is of national significance; or
  - has attracted or, in the opinion of the supplier, is likely to attract significant local or national publicity; or
  - has caused or, in the opinion of the supplier, is likely to cause significant concern to persons to whom water is supplied.

- any reports of disease that might be associated with water supplied by the supplier.

Most incidents are relatively minor, but all are assessed thoroughly (Box 11.3) and may result in recommendations to the company concerned on the actions needed to minimize the risk of future failures. Where the lessons to be learnt might benefit other companies, generic guidance may be issued to the industry. Consideration is given to whether during the incident the company contravened any of the wholesomeness standards set out in the Regulations. The DWI also considers whether the company contravened any other enforceable regulatory duty. If contraventions occurred, the DWI then decides whether the breaches were trivial or likely to recur and whether enforcement action under Section 18 of the Water Industry Act 1991 is required.

Box 11.2 Definition of an incident

An incident can be defined as (DWI 2003):

- a non-trivial or unexpected breach of Part II of the Water Supply (Water Quality) Regulations 1989, as amended; or
- a breach of Part IV of the 1989 Regulations; or
- an unusual deterioration in water quality; or
- a significant risk to the health of consumers; or
- a significant number of consumers perceiving adverse water quality changes; or
- significant local or national media interest on a water quality issue that could result in consumer concern.

Box 11.3 Key components of the Inspectorate's assessment of incidents

During an incident, the DWI assesses (DWI 2011):

- what caused the problem and whether or not it was avoidable;
- what the company did in response and how it handled the incident;
- what lessons can be learned to prevent similar incidents in the future;
- if there were any breaches of enforceable regulations; and
- whether an offence has been committed.

These criteria apply only to public water supplies. As mentioned above, the responsibility for monitoring private water supplies rests with local authorities.

11.3.4 Unfit water

The Regulations define water as wholesome if its quality meets the standards contained in the Regulations. Water which breaches those standards is considered to be unwholesome. Depending on the circumstances, the DWI may have to consider whether water unfit for human consumption was supplied during the incident. If there is sufficient evidence to show that water unfit for human consumption was supplied (Box 11.4), that the Company did not exercise all due diligence to prevent the incident from occurring, and if it is in the public interest, then prosecution under Section 70 of the Water Industry Act may be considered.

Section 70 of the Act makes it a criminal act for a water company to supply water that is unfit for human consumption. In 1994, the DWI developed a policy that it would consider prosecution of a water company for an alleged offence under section 70 of the Water Industry Act 1991 of supplying water unfit for human consumption.

It will be obvious that a prosecution of a water company for supplying unfit water involves considerable effort in obtaining sufficient and robust evidence that meets the exacting requirements demanded to support a charge in a criminal court.

The definition of 'unfit' was clarified in 2000 when, after a legal challenge, it was concluded (Jones 2000) that either:

'. . . the water if drunk would be likely to, or when drunk did in fact, cause injury to the consumer; or the water, by reason of its appearance and/or smell, was of such a quality that it would cause a reasonable consumer of firm character to refuse to drink it or use it in the preparation of food.'

Although the DWI may bring a prosecution if it believes that a water company supplied unfit water, it is for the courts to decide whether or not an offence has been committed and, if a company is found guilty of supplying water unfit, what the level of fine should be (up to a maximum of £20,000 per count).

For those incidents that do not justify full court proceedings the DWI may issue a caution which the court could take into account in any future offences.

Box 11.4 Evidential and other requirements before considering prosecution of a company for supplying unfit water

In order to prosecute a water company for an incident, the Inspectorate must consider (DWI 2010b):

a) Evidence to demonstrate that:

    (i)   illness or other health effects were experienced by at least two consumers using the water supplied;

    (ii) the quality of the water supplied was such that at least two consumers rejected it for drinking or cooking or food production on aesthetic grounds;

    (iii) the analytical results showed the presence of organisms or substances at a concentration at which illness or other health effects may be expected, even when none were manifest in the community at the time;

b) the 'relevant person' does not have a defence that it took all reasonable steps and exercised all due diligence for securing that:

    (i)   the water was fit for human consumption on leaving its pipes, or

    (ii) the water supplied was not used for human consumption;

c) such a prosecution is regarded as being in the public interest.

11.3.5 Outcomes of investigations

There are several typical outcomes of an incident assessment by an inspector (DWI 2011):

- a letter sent to the company, copied to other relevant parties;
- a letter sent to the company, copied to other relevant parties, making recommendations for action which the company must take to address deficiencies revealed by the incident;
- enforcement action initiated against the company: a legal process to ensure the company takes all the necessary action to prevent further breaches of either a regulatory duty or a drinking water standard (other relevant parties are informed), and
- initiation of prosecution proceedings against the company or the issue of a formal caution for a criminal offence (other relevant parties are informed).

11.3.6 Number of water-related chemical incidents reported to the DWI

Between 1990 and 2001 there was a steady year-on-year increase in the number of notifications received from water companies. This was attributed to the industry becoming more familiar with the process and the type of events that should be notified. In recent years some 60–70% of notifications have been classified as non-incidents. Occasionally the DWI is made aware of a water quality problem by a third party. For example, a health authority may inform the DWI of an increase in the number of reported cases of cryptosporidiosis at the same time as it informs the water company.

Table 11.1 Number of notifications made to DWI between 1995 and 2005

Year	Number of notifications	Number of incidents	Number resulting in prosecutions or cautions
1995	157	83	3
1996	176	76	3
1997	197	95	16
1998	300	120	17
1999	388	166	10
2000	429	139	4
2001	459	138	0
2002	398	130	1
2003	353	99	1
2004	304	89	2
2005	391	92	2

Table 11.1 shows the number of notifications received between 1995 and 2005. It also shows the number that were classified as incidents and the number of cases taken forward for prosecution or for which a caution was issued.

In earlier years, many of the incidents related to bacteriological failures or problems at water treatment works. In 1997, 33% of incidents related to the supply of discoloured water. This increased to more than 60% in 1998, which was attributed to the condition of the distribution systems and the associated remediation work being carried out. The DWI considered that many of these incidents were avoidable. Since 1998 the number of discoloured water incidents has gradually decreased as companies have responded with improved planning and better operational management.

11.4 Examples of chemical water contamination incidents

11.4.1 Example 1

A consumer reported a petrol-like taste in the water supply, which continued for some 30 days. Analytical results confirmed that the value for odour exceeded the standard. A neighbour reported a benzene-like taste in the water supply.

The presence of dissolved hydrocarbons up to a concentration of 31 μg/l was subsequently confirmed. The local authority and health authority were advised and the latter sought toxicological advice. Bottled water was supplied to consumers in the seven properties affected. Investigations by the company revealed no obvious source of the contamination. The company decided to replace the medium-density polyethylene (MDPE) communication pipe and during excavations discovered a layer of bituminous material some 0.5 m thick close to one of the affected properties just under pavement level. This had an odour similar to that found in the consumers' supply and was subsequently shown to contain toluene, kerosene, and diesel hydrocarbons.

11.4.2 Example 2

A consumer reported a taste in the water supply. Three affected properties were supplied with bottled water and the consumers were advised not to use the water. The water company sampled on day two and confirmed the presence of organic chemicals, including 2-(methylthio)benzothiazole at concentrations up to 0.5 μg/l and unidentified hydrocarbons at concentrations up to 10 μg/l.

Toxicological advice related to health risks and toxicology was limited. No specific toxicological information was available for the compounds in question and data were only available for related compounds.

11.4.3 Example 3

The manager at a water treatment works was informed that concentrations of isoproturon, a herbicide, had been detected by online organic monitoring equipment at concentrations up to 4.3 μg/l in the raw water source supplying the treatment works. Isoproturon was found in the treated water leaving the works at concentrations of up to 1.3 μg/l. The water company increased the dose of powdered activated carbon to absorb the isoproturon. Subsequent samples taken from the associated service reservoirs and some consumers' properties contained up to 1.5 μg/l isoproturon, in excess of the standard but less than the WHO guideline value.

11.4.4 Example 4

An unknown quantity of chlorpyriphos was discharged into a river, 6 km upstream of the abstraction point supplying a water company's water treatment works. Invertebrate deaths occurred in the river. The company was notified some eight days later and immediately arranged for the analysis of the sample taken the previous day for chlorpyriphos. It also arranged for further samples of the raw water to be taken. Chlorpyriphos was found at a concentration of 0.325 μg/l in the raw water, although none was found in the treated water leaving the works. No samples were taken of water in supply.

11.4.5 Example 5

An incident in Wem, Worcestershire, started at about 07:50 on Friday 15 April 1994 when the water company began to receive customer complaints of an unusual taste and odour in the public water supply to Worcester. It was evident that these were consistent with a problem at Barbourne Water Treatment Works on the River Severn, where the works operator confirmed that there was an odour and taste in the final water. The company isolated the treatment works, where treatment comprised conventional clarification, filtration, and disinfection. Unlike some works, there were no facilities for dosing activated carbon.

By later in the morning the number of complaints had risen to 60 and the decision was made, in collaboration with the Consultant in Communicable Disease Control (CCDC), Worcestershire Health Authority, to advise customers in the Worcester area not to drink the water. The health risk assessment was made even more difficult by the inconsistency in describing the odour, e.g. sweet, sewage, paint stripper etc. At 12:30 a meeting took place of the Worcester Health Emergency Incident Team (HEIT).

A crisis management team was convened at Severn Trent Water and worked in close association with the Worcester HEIT. The first press statement issued by the HEIT advised customers that an organic chemical had entered the water supply system and first indications were that this did not pose any serious threat to health. Until further information became available, the public were advised not to drink the water or to use it in food preparation.

Early on the Saturday, there was a report of a strong solvent smell entering Wem Sewage Works in Shropshire. The identity of one of two chemicals present was confirmed as 2-ethyl-4-methyl-1,3-dioxolane (2EMD). The second chemical was identified 13 days later as 2-ethyl-5,5-dimethyl-1,3-dioxane (2EDD). Both chemicals were at sub ppb levels (i.e. very low concentrations) in the potable water supply.

The Crisis Management Team met with the Regional Director of Public Health, West Midlands Regional Health Authority. He agreed that the water might taste and smell unpleasant for the next couple of days, but that there was no threat to public health.

It has always been known that certain chemical compounds can cause a highly detectable odour even in trace quantities and the potential impact on potable water systems was thought to be negligible. It was not possible to identify the compound 2EDD by conventional analysis.

Chemical products passing from river sources through water treatment are traditionally removed as part of the process. The organic compounds involved in this incident were not broken down through coagulation, filtration, and chlorination. Absorption through carbon treatment can be effective. There was no advanced carbon treatment at the works as Barbourne Water Treatment Works was due to be shut down.

The public health advice given verbally and early to Severn Trent was that people should be advised not to consume the water. This was confirmed when the HEIT met at lunchtime on the Friday. Potentially vulnerable groups such as nursing homes, the Worcester Royal Infirmary, nurseries, play groups, schools, and residential homes were all alerted through pre-arranged cascade systems, as were all food producers. GPs were contacted through a telephone cascade system.

The two chemicals contaminating the tap water were found at concentrations of less than 1 ppb. Medical toxicologists from the National Poisons Centre and the Department of Health advised that these chemicals at the very low concentrations found were not hazardous to health. A press statement was issued, assuring the public that the water was safe to drink, although taste and smell problems may still occur in some areas.

Severn Trent Water was prosecuted for the above incident for 'supplying water not fit for consumption' despite the fact that there was no risk to health and complimentary comments from the Judge on the effectiveness of the emergency response. There were a number of recommendations from the independent report which were aimed at the water industry as a whole.

Other examples have been presented and discussed at two conferences, the proceedings of which have been published (Gray and Thompson 2004, 2006).

11.5 Conclusion

Over recent years a number of incidents of chemical contamination of water have been reported in England and Wales. Fortunately, few have resulted in significant adverse health effects. However, experience in responding to these events has shown that to provide effective support to the public and consumers, close links between public health organizations, water companies, the regulators, and other related bodies are essential elements for a successful response. This chapter has addressed some of the common features between the perspectives of medical toxicology, public health, and drinking water quality regulation. From this collaboration it is possible to identify learning needs.

It has been said that the water industry needs to consider planning, preparation, and performance when considering the impact of incidents affecting drinking water quality (Jackson 2004). Planning requires the need to think the unthinkable and plan to deal with it. Preparation must ensure the provision of analytical facilities and appropriate expertise to interpret the results of such analyses. It also requires the ability to assess any impact on public health and to have available safe alternative supplies of drinking water. There is a need to cope with the unexpected and at the same time maintain public confidence. Learning points must be identified after each incident (or emergency) and incorporated into any emergency response plan.

11.6 Acknowledgement

The editors gratefully acknowledge the work of John Gray for this chapter in the first edition.

11.7 References

Council Directive. (1998) *Council Directive 98/83/EC of 3 November 1998 on the quality of water intended for human consumption.*

DWI. (2003) *Part 3—Inspectorate objectives and key results.* DWI, London. Available at: http://dwi.defra. gov.uk/about/annual-report/2003/chapters_a_to_k.pdf. Accessed 9 January 2012.

DWI. (2009a) *Guidance on the Notification of Events.* DWI, London. Available at: http://dwi.defra.gov. uk/stakeholders/guidance-and-codes-of-practice/notification%20of%20events.pdf. Accessed 9 January 2012.

DWI. (2009b) *Water Industry (Supplier's Information) Direction 2009.* DWI, London. Available at: http://www.dwi.gov.uk/stakeholders/information-letters/2009/06_2009annexA.pdf. Accessed 9 January 2012.

DWI. (2010) *Guidance on the regulatory responsibilities of new (inset) appointees in relation to public water supplies.* DWI, London. Available at: http://www.dwi.gov.uk/stakeholders/guidance-and-codes-of-practice/inset.pdf. Accessed 11 January 2012.

DWI. (2011) *Events and prosecutions.* Available at: http://www.dwi.gov.uk/press-media/incidents-and-prosecutions/index.htm (updated 7 July 2011). Accessed 9 January 2012.

Gray J, Thompson KC (eds). (2004) *Water contamination emergencies: can we cope?* Royal Society of Chemistry, Cambridge.

Gray J, Thompson KC (eds). (2006) *Water contamination emergencies: enhancing our response.* Royal Society of Chemistry, Cambridge.

Jackson C. (2004) Problems, perceptions and perfection—the role of the drinking water inspectorate in water quality incidents and emergencies. In: Thompson, KC, Gray J (eds). *Water contamination emergencies: can we cope?* Royal Society of Chemistry, Cambridge, pp 38–43.

Jones N. (2000) *Judgment.* Leeds Crown Court, 28 July 2000.

Water Act 2003. (c.37). HMSO, London.

Water Industry Act 1991. (c.56). HMSO, London.

Water Supply (Water Quality) Regulations 1989. SI 1989/1147. HMSO, London.

Water Supply (Water Quality) Regulations 1989. SI 1989/1147. HMSO, London.

Water Supply Regulations 2010. SI 2010/991. HMSO, London.

11.8 Further reading

Dawson A, West P (eds). (1993) *Drinking water supplies: a microbiological perspective.* HMSO, London.

Twort AC, Ratnayaka DD, Brandt MJ (eds). (2000) Water supply, 5th edn. Arnold, London.

World Health Organization, (2010) *Guidelines for drinking-water quality.* 4th ed. Gutenberg, Malta.

Chapter 12

Food additives and contaminants

Diane Benford

Learning outcomes

At the end of this chapter and any recommended reading the student should be able to:

1. explain the principles of toxicological risk assessment as applied to food additives and contaminants;

2. discuss its use in assessing consumer safety, and in setting regulatory limits for chemicals in food, and

3. apply acquired knowledge in the analysis and management of hazardous situations.

12.1 Chemicals in food

Food is a complex mixture of chemicals, the vast bulk of which are naturally part of the food. Some are contaminants that are present inadvertently, as a result of environmental pollution, microbial metabolism, cooking, or food processing (referred to as process contaminants) (see Box 12.1). Others are purposefully used or added during food production and processing, including food additives (see Box 12.2), pesticides, and residues of veterinary medicines.

All of these chemicals have the potential to be harmful if ingested in excessive amounts, and the primary aim of the food toxicologist is to determine how much can be consumed without *appreciable* risk to health. This terminology is used in recognition of the fact that it is never possible to guarantee absolute safety but based on the available evidence any risk is likely to be extremely small. The main difference between these categories of chemicals is that those with an intentional use are subject to regulatory approval processes, and will have a manufacturer or 'sponsor' who is responsible for generating the data to support the risk assessment. Therefore the database of regulatory toxicology studies is normally more complete for additives. In contrast, there may be more mechanistic studies, and sometimes epidemiological studies, available for contaminants than for additives.

12.2 Risk assessment of food chemicals

The general principles of risk assessment were described in Section 1 of this book. In the first instance, the risk assessment for food chemicals is conducted by scientific advisory

Box 12.1 Examples of chemical food contaminants

Environmental pollutants, e.g.

- dioxins and dioxin-like polychlorinated biphenyls
- polycyclic aromatic hydrocarbons
- heavy metals, such as lead and cadmium.

Natural toxicants, e.g.

- aflatoxins
- shellfish biotoxins.

Process contaminants, e.g.

- acrylamide
- heterocyclic amines
- polycyclic aromatic hydrocarbons.

committees, which allows separation of the independent assessment of the science from the societal and political influences that need to be taken into account in risk management. The major independent scientific advisory committees that have assessed the safety of food additives and contaminants are:

- UK Committee on Toxicity of Chemicals in Food Consumer Products and the Environment (COT) and its sister committees on Mutagenicity (COM) and Carcinogenicity (COC);
- EU Scientific Committee on Food (SCF) (until 2002);
- European Food Safety Authority (EFSA) (since 2002);
- Joint FAO/WHO Expert Committee on Food Additives and Contaminants (JECFA).

The approach taken to risk assessment (or safety assessment) of food chemicals with threshold effects is summarized in Figure 12.1. In brief, the highest dose that has no observed adverse effect in a study of the most sensitive relevant toxic endpoint is

Box 12.2 Food additives

Food additives have a technological function in food. Important subcategories are:

- colours
- flavour enhancers and flavourings
- preservatives
- sweeteners
- antioxidants
- emulsifiers, stabilizers, gelling agents, and thickeners.

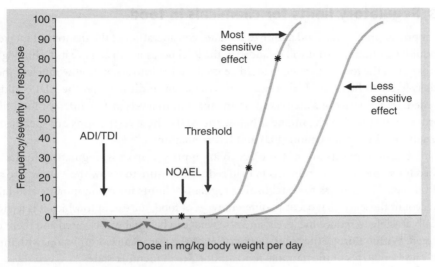

Fig. 12.1 Derivation of an acceptable or tolerable daily intake.

identified (the NOAEL). The NOAEL is divided by uncertainty factors (or safety factors) to allow for interspecies differences if the NOAEL is derived from a study in laboratory animals, and for interindividual variability in the human population. The aim is to protect the most susceptible subgroups, if that is possible. A combined uncertainty factor of 100 is often used, but a larger factor may be used if key data are missing, and a smaller factor may be used if specific data are available relating to effects in humans. Dividing the NOAEL by the uncertainty factor results in establishment of a health-based guidance value referred to as the acceptable daily intake (ADI) or tolerable daily intake (TDI). The term 'acceptable' is used for food additives since they are subject to regulatory approval. The term 'tolerable' is used for contaminants and the health-based guidance value may be related to weekly or monthly intake for contaminants that have the potential to accumulate in the body. In addition the term 'provisional' is conventionally used by JECFA. The ADI and TDI are normally expressed in relation to body weight (e.g. mg/kg bodyweight per day) in order to allow for individuals of different body size, especially children. Regardless of the terminology used, these health-based guidance values are considered to be amounts that can be consumed over an entire lifetime without appreciable risk to health (Box 12.3).

Box 12.3 Health-based guidance values

Additives:

◆ acceptable daily intake (ADI).

Contaminants

◆ tolerable daily intake (TDI)

◆ provisional tolerable weekly intake (PTWI).

12.3 Regulatory limits for chemicals in food

The approval process for food additives includes consideration of the theoretical intake of the additive assuming that it will be added at the level necessary to achieve its technological purpose in all the foods in which it could be used, taking into account how much of those foods is likely to be eaten. If this exposure assessment indicates that the ADI could be exceeded, then restrictions are placed on the maximum levels or the different food uses, in order to ensure that the intake is below the ADI. These restrictions are specified in international, European Union (EU) and UK regulations.

Whilst contaminants are not subject to an approval process, regulatory limits are applied for some key contaminants to help reduce exposure to below the TDI, where one could be set. The process for establishing regulatory limits for contaminants also takes into account the levels that occur in different types of food, the extent to which it is technologically feasible to reduce the levels, and also what can be reliably measured and therefore enforced. Within Europe the regulations are set by the European Commission, with input from representatives of the national food authorities in member states.

Because of the different ways that regulatory limits are set, a food exceeding the regulatory limit for a particular additive or contaminant will not inevitably result in intakes above the ADI or TDI.

12.4 Implications of exceeding the ADI or TDI

When foods are found to exceed regulatory limits for additives or contaminants, or when assessing levels of unregulated contaminants, it is important to first assess the anticipated intake for average and high-level consumers of the foods containing the additive or contaminant. Consideration of children's food consumption is generally important because young children have a higher caloric requirement, expressed in relation to body weight. If the estimates of total dietary exposure for different subgroups are below the ADI/TDI, then there is not considered to be a health risk. If, the ADI/TDI is exceeded by some subgroups, then it is necessary to consider if the available toxicological information allows further conclusions to be drawn. The ADI/TDI is not a threshold of toxicity, and for a substance that does not have acute effects, occasionally exceeding the ADI/TDI is unlikely to be harmful. The greater the degree by which it is exceeded, and the longer the period of potential exceedance, the more likely it becomes that adverse effects will occur. In such situations, action may be taken to withdraw the affected food from sale, and if appropriate, specific advice may be given to subgroups at particular risk.

12.5 Recent health concerns related to food additives and contaminants

12.5.1 Aspartame

Aspartame is an intense artificial sweetener that is widely used in beverages and processed foods. Some people have concerns that aspartame could be the cause of a wide range of human illnesses, largely based on unsubstantiated information available on the internet.

In fact, the available evidence on aspartame has been reviewed on many occasions (see EFSA (2011) for an overview of the evaluations) over the past two to three decades. It is metabolized in the gastrointestinal tract into two amino acids (aspartic acid and phenylalanine) and methanol, all of which are present naturally in many foods and in the human body. Ingestion of aspartame at the level of the ADI does not result in elevation of these components within the blood. EFSA (2006) concluded that intakes of aspartame at the ADI do not lead to toxicologically relevant systemic exposure and confirmed that there was no reason to revise the previously established ADI. Estimates of intakes, even for high-level consumers, are well below the ADI. Since 2006, EFSA has reviewed a number of scientific studies on aspartame and concluded that they did not influence the previous conclusions (EFSA 2011).

12.5.2 Sudan dyes

Sudan dyes have never been approved as food colours in the UK. Although not tested to current standards, the available information indicates that they are genotoxic and carcinogenic. Therefore the expert opinion is that it is not possible to propose a TDI and exposures should be reduced to as low as reasonably practicable. In 2003 it was discovered that Sudan dyes were being used illegally to increase the market value of some spices, such as chilli powder, and legislation was introduced to require testing of chilli and chilli products imported into the EU (EC 2003). Since then there have been a number of occasions in which Sudan dye adulterated foods have been found on the UK market. At the levels detected the cancer risk is likely to be extremely small, but it is an unnecessary risk that can be avoided if action is taken to prevent these dyes from being added to food.

12.5.3 Acrylamide

Acrylamide has been used as an industrial chemical since the mid-1950s, but its presence in food was only discovered in 2002 (FAO/WHO 2006). There has been extensive international effort to investigate how acrylamide forms in food and how formation could be reduced, and also to develop and refine risk assessment for dietary exposure to acrylamide. Acrylamide is known to be neurotoxic in humans as a result of occupational and accidental exposure. Studies in animals have shown that it can cause reproductive effects and that it is genotoxic and carcinogenic. It is not known whether dietary exposure to acrylamide could cause cancer in humans, but based on the evidence from the animal studies, it is considered possible. Research conducted since 2006 has confirmed the earlier conclusion that estimates of dietary exposure to acrylamide indicate a health concern (FAO/WHO 2011). As with the Sudan dyes, the expert opinion is that it is not possible to propose a TDI and intakes should be reduced to as low as reasonably practicable. However, because acrylamide is present in a wide variety of cooked foods, it is not possible to have a healthy balanced diet that avoids acrylamide. It is also likely that it has been in our food for generations.

Research is underway to investigate how acrylamide formation can be reduced without incurring other food risks, but so far this has had limited impact on levels of acrylamide in food and total dietary exposure. The Food Standards Agency advises that people should not change their diets because of concern about acrylamide, but should follow the healthy eating guidelines that help to protect against some cancers as well other chronic diseases.

12.5.4 Contaminants in fish

Fish is an important source of nutrients, and most people in the UK eat less than is recommended for health benefits. However, fish also contain contaminants that can be a health concern. There are two main issues: methylmercury accumulates in large predator fish, regardless of whether they are oily or non-oily, and persistent organic pollutants, such as dioxins, have the potential to accumulate in oily fish. Fish is the major source of exposure to methylmercury. Dioxins and related compounds are widely present in other foods, although levels have decreased significantly over the past three decades.

The Food Standards Agency asked an expert group of nutritionists and toxicologists to advise on the benefits and risks associated with fish consumption (SACN/COT 2004) in order to give cohesive advice to consumers. Methylmercury is neurotoxic and the most sensitive effect is impaired neurodevelopmental as a result of pre-natal exposure. Dioxins have a wide range of health effects, the most sensitive of which was considered to be on development of the male reproductive system as a result of pre-natal exposure. The expert group advised that the tolerable intakes set to protect against accumulation of methylmercury and dioxins in a woman's body to levels that could have adverse effects on the foetus should also be applied to susceptible subgroups.

However, as seen in Figure 12.1, if the most sensitive effect relates to exposure during pregnancy, the TDI could be over-precautionary for people who are not pregnant. Therefore the COT set additional guidelines, based on the next most sensitive effect, to be applied for men and for women who were not or would not become pregnant, for the range of fish consumption at which there would be nutritional benefits without undue risks from the contaminants. Combined with information on the levels of contaminants present in different types of fish and other dietary sources of dioxin-like compounds, this opinion forms the basis of Food Standards Agency advice to consumers.

12.6 References

EC. (2003) Commission decision 2003/460/EC of 20 June 2003 on emergency measures regarding hot chilli and hot chilli products. *Official Journal of the European Union.* L 154/114.

EFSA. (2006) Opinion of the Scientific Panel on Food Additives, Flavourings, Processing Aids and Materials in Contact with Food (AFC) on a request from the Commission related to a new long-term carcinogenicity study on aspartame. Adopted on 3 May 2006. Available at: http://www.efsa.europa.eu/EFSA/efsa_locale-1178620753812_1178620765743.htm.

EFSA. (2011) EFSA Statement on the scientific evaluation of two studies related to the safety of artificial sweeteners. EFSA Journal 9(2):2089. doi:10.2903/j.efsa.2011.2089. Available at: www.efsa.europa.eu/efsajournal.

FAO/WHO. (2006) Safety evaluation of certain food additives. *Food Additive Series No 56.* World Health Organization, Geneva. Available at: http://whqlibdoc.who.int/publications/2006/9241660554_eng.pdf.

FAO/WHO. (2011) Safety evaluation of certain contaminants in food. Food Additive Series No 63. World Health Organization, Geneva. Available at: http://whqlibdoc.who.int/publications/2011/9789241660631_eng.pdf.

SACN/COT. (2004) Scientific Advisory Committee on Nutrition Reports. Available at: http://www.sacn.gov.uk/reports/#. Accessed February 2008.

12.7 Further reading

IPCS. (2009) Environmental Health Criteria 240. Principles and methods for the risk assessment of chemicals in food. http://www.who.int/foodsafety/chem/principles/en/index1.html.

12.8 Useful internet links

COT opinions: http://www.food.gov.uk/science/ouradvisors/toxicity/.

EFSA opinions: http://www.efsa.europa.eu/en/science.html.

Food Standards Agency website: http://www.food.gov.uk.

JECFA procedures and opinions: http://www.who.int/ipcs/food/jecfa/en/and http://www.inchem.org/.

SCF opinions: http://ec.europa.eu/food/fs/sc/scf/outcome_en.html.

Section 4

A Review of Some Toxic Agents

Chapter 13

Carbon monoxide poisoning

Lakshman Karalliedde and Catherine Keshishian

Learning outcomes

At the end of this chapter and recommended reading the student should be able to:

1. explain the manner in which carbon monoxide causes toxicity;

2. describe and discuss common sources of carbon monoxide poisoning and the population groups that are considered vulnerable;

3. describe and differentiate between acute and chronic carbon monoxide poisoning;

4. discuss the long-term effects following acute and chronic poisoning;

5. provide basic information for treatment, and

6. apply acquired knowledge in the analysis and management of hazardous situations.

13.1 Introduction

Carbon monoxide (CO) is a colourless, odourless, tasteless, non-irritant gas which when inhaled in excessive amounts can cause death or serious ill-health. CO poisoning is an important cause of ill-health and accidental death in the UK, causing an estimated 50 fatalities and 200 hospital admissions a year, with many more cases going unreported or unrecognized (Department of Health 2010). Intentional self-harm with CO resulted in 174 deaths in England and Wales in 2005 (ONS 2007). CO is also a toxic component of smoke from fires, with 44 deaths reported (ONS 2007).

Poisoning due to low-level concentrations of CO can result in chronic symptoms of flu-like illness and cognitive impairment continues to be a significant health problem. Many cases of chronic illness go undiagnosed and there are no reliable prevalence data to indicate the magnitude of the problem.

13.2 Sources of carbon monoxide

When there is insufficient oxygen for organic compounds to burn efficiently, there is production of CO. If there is enough oxygen for complete combustion, carbon dioxide (CO_2) is formed.

The most common source of CO poisoning in the home is from faulty or improperly installed heating or cooking appliances, where either insufficient oxygen leads to the production of CO or CO is not properly removed, such as a defect in a flue or ventilation system. A common misconception is that CO is only generated by such faulty gas appliances, whereas many incidents involve wood-, oil-, or charcoal-burning appliances, or even inappropriate use of well-functioning appliances, e.g. using over-large cooking utensils that prevent oxygen from reaching the flame. Data from the UK show that non-gas fuels are a considerable source of unintentional, non-fire related deaths, and that more deaths occur in winter where use of heating appliances is more common (de Juniac et al. presented at the 23rd Annual Conference of the International Society of Environmental Epidemiology, Barcelona, 2011). Following the four major hurricanes in the USA during 2004, electric power failures meant that many people used gasoline-powered generators designed for outdoor use inside, for warmth and cooking or to dry out flooded properties. The end result was 167 people seeking treatment for CO poisoning in 10 hospitals and six deaths attributed to CO toxicity (MMWR 2005).

Automobile exhaust fumes are a major source of ambient CO, for which air quality guideline levels exist (see Table 13.1). In enclosed spaces such as garages, CO concentrations from motor vehicle engines kept running can rise rapidly to lethal concentrations, causing many accidental deaths. Poor ventilation between living spaces and garages, and exposure to traffic fumes can also give rise to significant exposure to CO. Occupational groups such as traffic wardens and car park attendants are therefore at risk of CO exposure.

Tobacco smoke is an important source of CO exposure, and smokers have a higher baseline CO level than non-smokers (see section 13.3.1.2).

A relatively uncommon source of CO poisoning is from the paint stripper methylene chloride, which can enter the body by inhalation, ingestion, or through the skin. Methylene chloride is metabolized by the human liver to CO. In such instances, because of the continued metabolic production of CO in the body, the time taken for the haemoglobin to

Table 13.1 Standards or guideline values for carbon monoxide exposure

Guideline/objective*	Concentration of CO (ppm)	Concentration of CO (mg/m³)	Duration
Indoor Air Quality Guideline (WHO 2010)	7	7	24 hours
	10	10	8 hours
	30	35	1 hour
	90	100	15 minutes
Air Quality Guideline (WHO 2000)	10	10	8 hours
	25	30	1 hour
	50	60	30 minutes
	90	100	15 minutes
Workplace Exposure Limit (HSE 2005)	30	35	8 hours
	200	232	15 minutes

*NB: Not all are legally enforceable standards in the UK.

free itself from CO may be as long as 12 hours (i.e. twice the time taken following cessation of CO exposure by inhalation from other sources).

Small amounts of CO are also produced endogenously in the human body by the degradation of haem proteins by the enzyme haem oxygenase. The amount of CO produced naturally within the body can be affected by disease status, with oxidative stress and inflammatory processes leading to higher levels of CO (Owens 2010).

13.3 Toxicology of carbon monoxide in the body

Carbon monoxide gas enters the body by inhalation and readily crosses from the lung into the bloodstream. CO is eventually removed from the body through expiration, with a small amount being oxidized to CO_2. Carbon monoxide can be toxic to the body in a number of ways, depicted in Figure 13.1.

13.3.1 Binding of carbon monoxide to haemoglobin

Haemoglobin, found in red blood cells, carries oxygen to all cells in the body for the cells to be metabolically active and survive. CO has an affinity for haemoglobin that is 200–250 times more than that of oxygen, thus in the presence of CO haemoglobin competes and preferentially binds to CO, forming carboxyhaemoglobin (COHb). CO remains bound to haemoglobin for a longer period than oxygen, accumulating in blood and preventing oxygen from reaching binding sites.

Haemoglobin has four oxygen binding sites. If CO is bound to one, it strengthens the bond between oxygen and haemoglobin at the other sites, meaning that any oxygen that is being carried is less available for use by tissues. This is known as a shift in the oxygen–haemoglobin dissociation curve to the left.

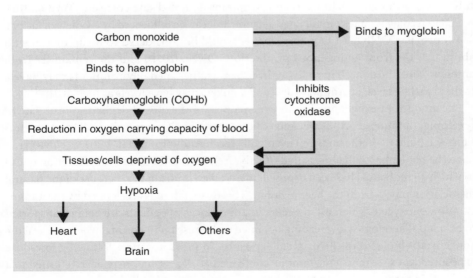

Fig. 13.1 Actions of carbon monoxide in the body.

These actions deprive cells, including those of the heart, muscle, brain, and nervous system, of their usual supply of oxygen, referred to as hypoxia, which prevents them from functioning normally.

This binding is reversible, and once exposure has ceased oxygen competes with CO for binding sites and the CO is expelled. Usually, 50% of the haemoglobin dissociates from CO in 4–6 hours when an individual is breathing air; this is known as the half-life. Following inhalation of 100% oxygen, CO dissociates much faster, with 50% of the haemoglobin being freed to carry oxygen in about 1 hour (a half-life of 1 hour). Oxygen therapy therefore can and will be life-saving. Oxygen can also be given at above atmospheric pressure (hyperbaric oxygen therapy); the increase in oxygen dissolving in plasma under hyperbaric conditions may be helpful in accelerating the dissociation of CO from haemoglobin. However, there is debate about the added value of providing hyperbaric oxygen (Buckley et al. 2011).

13.3.1.1 Measuring carboxyhaemoglobin

COHb is the most common biomarker available to confirm exposure to CO and is most often measured by taking venous blood samples, which are analysed in a laboratory. Non-invasive methods of measuring CO exposure have recently been developed. Breath analysers measure the concentration of CO in the expired air (air breathed out); however, the method usually relies on patients being fit enough to take deep breaths and exhale hard. COHb saturation in the blood can also be measured using a spectrophotometer, also known as a pulse co-oximeter, which is slipped over the finger to provide readings. These instruments are useful screening tools for use in the field, such as by paramedics or smoking cessation clinics, but are not as reliable as measurements taken directly from blood.

13.3.1.2 Interpreting carboxyhaemoglobin concentrations

It is well known that COHb levels and symptoms do not always correlate (WHO 2010). A COHb reading requires careful interpretation as it can be influenced by a variety of factors.

A 'normal' COHb level in a non-smoker would be considered to be up to 2%, with about 0.3–1% from endogenous production (Owens 2010) and the remainder from ambient contributions. Those living in urban, traffic-filled environments may have a higher baseline level, at around 3–4%, and smokers may have levels as high as 10–15%.

The amount of exogenous CO to which a person is exposed depends on the rate of breathing, duration of exposure, and concentration of CO in the air. COHb concentrations will build up in the body but eventually reach equilibrium (HPA 2011). However, it has to be remembered that measured COHb rarely reveals the actual concentration of CO to which an individual has been exposed unless taken immediately, because of the natural dissociation of CO from the haemoglobin. This dissociation is accelerated by the administration of oxygen, which often occurs in ambulances as patients are being transported to hospital. Therefore, a low reading obtained on admission to hospital will not reveal the concentration of CO of the original exposure. In most instances following low-dose exposure, exposure to CO may not be confirmed at all as values may have returned to a level within the normal range by the time they are measured in hospital.

13.3.2 Binding of carbon monoxide to myoglobin

Myoglobin is the oxygen-binding protein in muscle and is similar to haemoglobin in the blood. It too has an increased affinity for CO when compared to oxygen, forming carboxymyoglobin, but the difference is only 60-fold. However, the lack of adequate oxygen supplies to the muscle results in fatigue or decreased exercise tolerance and early onset of tiredness. About 15% of the CO that enters the body binds to myoglobin (Coburn 1970).

13.3.3 Other toxic effects of carbon monoxide

During CO exposure, cells are deprived of their normal oxygen supply due to reduced oxyhaemoglobin levels, but cells are also unable to utilize the oxygen that they do receive due to CO interfering with the activity of enzymes such as cytochrome oxidase, and other mechanisms that are involved in the utilization of oxygen by the cells.

CO is also directly toxic and several other symptoms, signs, and biochemical changes following acute CO exposures have been reported, although they have not been substantiated by studies in humans. Some studies suggest that the re-oxygenation process may affect the central nervous system and that the production of oxygen radicals may damage cells (Ernst and Zibrak 1998).

13.4 Health effects of acute and chronic carbon monoxide poisoning

Adverse health effects associated with CO are related to the concentration of COHb in the blood (Tables 13.2 and 13.3) and the duration of exposure. There are two well-defined forms of CO poisoning. Acute poisonings are usually due to exposure to high

Table 13.2 Human health effects following exposure to carbon monoxide

Blood carboxyhaemoglobin levels (%)	Observed health effects
<2	No significant health effects
2.5–4.0	Decreased short-term maximal exercise duration in young healthy men
2.7–5.1	Decreased exercise duration due to increased chest pain (angina) in patients with ischaemic heart disease
2.0–20.0	Equivocal effects on visual perception, audition, motor, and sensorimotor performance, vigilance, and other measures of neurobehavioural performance
4.0–33.0	Decreased maximal oxygen consumption with short-term strenuous exercise in young healthy men
20–30	Throbbing headache
30–50	Dizziness, nausea, weakness, collapse
>50	Unconsciousness and death

Adapted from the Department of the Environment, Transport and the Regions (1998) and the Department of Health (2004).

Table 13.3 Threshold toxicity values for exposure to carbon monoxide by inhalation

Concentration of CO in air (ppm)	Concentration of CO in air (mg/m³)	Exposure duration	Symptoms
~100	~115	Indefinite	Slight headache, flushing of skin
200–300	230–345	5–6 hours	Headache
400–600	460–690	4–5 hours	Severe headache, weakness, dizziness, nausea, vomiting
1100–1500	1265–1840	4–5 hours	Increased pulse and breathing rate, syncope, coma, intermittent seizures
5000–10,000	5750–11,500	1–2 minutes	Weak pulse, depressed respiration/respiratory failure, death

Reproduced from Carbon Monoxide Incident Management, HPA 2010, http://www.hpa.org.uk/web/HPAwebFile/ HPAweb_C/1194947341118, with data from IPCS 1996 Poisons Information Monograph http://www.inchem.org/ documents/pims/chemical/pim947.htm

concentrations of CO for short durations (minutes or hours). Chronic poisonings occur when exposure takes place at lower but nevertheless toxic concentrations of CO over more prolonged periods, such as days, weeks, or even years. Both types have non-specific symptoms that mimic other common diseases, such as influenza or food poisoning, which may lead to mis-diagnosis (Department of Health 2010).

13.4.1 Acute carbon monoxide poisoning

13.4.1.1 Immediate effects

With acute, high-level exposure to CO, headache, nausea, and vomiting are early symptoms and there may be rapid progression to dizziness, confusion, shortness of breath, blurred vision, loss of consciousness, fits, and death.

Following acute exposures, patients are likely to seek immediate medical assistance. However, disease progression may be so rapid that confusion and un-coordination may be severe enough to prevent the patient from dialling 999 or asking for help. Death is likely if the person is not immediately evacuated or removed from the source of exposure and treated with high concentrations of oxygen.

Acute poisoning may be severe enough to cause brain damage and damage to the heart muscle. Irregular heart rhythms (arrhythmias) are commonly seen, as are signs and symptoms of heart attacks. In 2005, Satran et al. reported that permanent damage to heart muscle (myocardial injury) is common in patients hospitalized following moderate to severe CO poisoning (Satran et al. 2005). The group showed that enzymes that confirmed injury to heart muscle were raised and that there were abnormal changes in the electrocardiogram. They also showed that those who sustained damage to heart muscle died earlier than those who did not.

Many CO poisoned patients have symptoms and signs of abnormal brain function such as impaired memory, tendency to abnormal involuntary movements, gait abnormalities, and some disturbances of vision. Twenty-four hours after acute severe exposure to CO, where there has been loss of consciousness, CT scanning may show changes indicative of brain damage. Damage to the basal ganglia is a characteristic of CO-induced brain damage.

Neurological symptoms such as headache, lethargy, irritability, and Parkinsonism may be delayed for 2–240 days post exposure, although the mechanisms for this are not well understood (Ernst and Zabrik 1998).

13.4.1.2 Long-term effects

Following recovery from acute exposure, many patients suffer from a wide range of residual ill-health.

a. The exposure itself may have been so emotionally traumatic that symptoms of post-traumatic stress disorder may occur.

b. The patient may suffer from the effects of brain damage due to the lack of adequate oxygen to the brain cells during the period of severe poisoning. These symptoms may range from personality changes to memory loss to deterioration of mental acuity or mental sharpness.

c. The patient may suffer damage to heart muscle, which may result in changes in the electrocardiogram associated with an elevation of enzymes, indicative of injury to heart muscle (Sartran et al. 2005). For example, plasma levels of a structural protein found in the myocardium, troponin, may increase. This damage to the heart muscle would make an individual more vulnerable to subsequent ischaemic episodes and also pre-disposed to clinical states such as heart failure.

d. Damage to muscle cells due to a lack of oxygen during exposure may lead to a break-down of muscle fibres and release of myoglobin, which can damage the kidneys and cause renal failure.

13.4.2 Chronic carbon monoxide poisoning

13.4.2.1 Immediate effects

Chronic CO toxicity occurs when there has been long-term exposure (months or even years) to low but toxic doses of CO. This usually occurs in homes and more rarely at workplaces or in cars. It is therefore usual for more than one person to have been exposed to the toxic environment and for other household members, including pets, to present with similar symptoms. Symptoms often improve once the patient is away from their home for a period of time and may worsen over weekends and during the winter months when more time is spent indoors, resulting in prolonged exposures.

With such exposures, death is most unlikely and patients usually seek assistance from GPs, often on a very regular basis. It is very difficult to make a diagnosis without a high index of awareness of the nature of ill-health associated with such exposures as the signs and symptoms are very non-specific.

Patients tend to attend the surgeries of GPs with recurrent flu-like illnesses, sore throats, coughs, impaired memory, and confusion. It is unfortunate that most of these patients are diagnosed as suffering from minor ailments or from depression, anxiety, or another psychiatric illness. In the vast majority of cases, the identification of the cause of ill-health as exposure to CO is only made or confirmed following the detection of a faulty appliance at the home or another source of exposure. As discussed in section 13.3.1, the short half-life of COHb makes biological confirmation difficult if exposure was to low levels and time has passed since exposure ceased.

13.4.2.2 Long-term effects

The main problem with exposure to low but toxic concentrations of CO is that diagnosis is often delayed and as a result patients have suffered considerable emotional, mental and physical disability. Patients may have suffered from months or years of poor memory, impaired concentration, poor effort tolerance, apathy, and lethargy. They may have a sense of frustration as they have not been diagnosed for a long period despite repeated medical consultations and treatment schedules.

Following cessation of exposure, these patients require considerable encouragement to resume their normal lives. A substantial degree of recovery can be expected within about three years of cessation of exposure provided no further exposure takes place. Patients may benefit from cognitive behavioural therapy to overcome their deficits. However, some may not show significant recovery and may fail to lead the lives they led prior to toxic exposure. This can be especially important for children, who may have performed poorly at school due to impaired concentration and mental ability.

In recognition of the importance of chronic CO poisoning and its toxicological differences to acute poisoning, the World Health Organization in 2010 published a guideline value for chronic (24-hour mean) exposure to CO in the indoor environment (WHO 2010; Table 13.1).

13.5 Vulnerable population groups

13.5.1 Extremes of age

Children are considered more sensitive to the effects of CO than adults because of their higher metabolism and lower body weight, and they may become symptomatic at levels as much as 10% below evaluated levels. In older patients, particularly those with decreased blood supply to the heart muscle (ischaemic heart disease), symptoms of restricted blood supply to the heart (angina pectoris) may develop at much lower concentrations than in healthy young adults (Karalliedde, 2006).

13.5.2 Pregnancy

Carbon monoxide readily crosses the placenta. Maternal poisoning is known to cause severe neurological deficits in the child after birth and the foetus has to be considered to be particularly vulnerable. Maternal exposure may also cause still birth (Van Hoesen et al. 1989). Foetal haemoglobin has a higher affinity to CO than that of adult haemoglobin, and the elimination of CO is also slower from foetal circulation. It is therefore important to remember that measured maternal COHb levels will not accurately reflect foetal COHb levels (Copel et al. 1982) and may be up to 10–15% higher in the foetus (Longo 1977), which can have significant implications for treating the exposed expectant mother. Treatment with hyperbaric oxygen is considered by some following CO exposure during pregnancy.

13.5.3 Those with pre-existing systemic disease

People with cardiovascular disease, including coronary heart disease, angina, and anaemia, are at significant risk of CO poisoning as the level of oxygen that they can carry to major organs is already decreased (Karalliedde 2006). Some diseases increase endogenous CO production, raising baseline COHb levels, with the potential to leave patients unable to cope with additional exogenous CO exposure, leading to risk of toxicity (Owens 2010).

See Chapter 7 for more on susceptible populations.

13.6 Treatment and incident response

13.6.1 Treatment

1. Immediate removal from source of exposure.
2. Administer 100% oxygen.
3. Treat convulsions if present.
4. Monitor basic physiological parameters: pulse rate, blood pressure, arterial oxygen concentration, electrocardiograph.
5. Measure carboxyhaemoglobin concentration.
6. Consider treatment with hyperbaric oxygen.

For detailed information on treatment for CO poisoning refer to *Toxbase*, the clinical toxicology database of the UK National Poisons Information Service (www.toxbase.org).

13.6.2 Incident response

Both acute and chronic CO poisoning can be difficult to identify for two reasons. Firstly CO poisoning causes non-specific symptoms, potentially leading to it being overlooked as a diagnosis. Secondly, due to the relatively short half-life of COHb and the removal of ambient CO through ventilation, exposure to CO cannot always be confirmed clinically or environmentally. It is therefore important that measurements are taken as soon as possible. Fire services in the UK have CO detection equipment to measure ambient air samples. Specialist ambulance staff, known as hazardous area response teams (HART), carry non-invasive monitors to test patients where symptoms suggest CO poisoning. However, because of the factors mentioned above, lack of biological or environmental confirmation of CO does not exclude a diagnosis of CO toxicity, and health protection staff should consider all the aspects and context of the situation.

Immediately upon notification of a CO poisoning case, consideration should be given to others who may be affected at present or who may be exposed in the future. CO is a small molecule which mixes freely with air and can therefore travel between floorboards, through cracks in walls, and via shared chimneys and flues to neighbouring rooms and properties. If emergency services are present, they will usually have assessed and, if necessary, evacuated surrounding premises. Other people who may have been exposed should be encouraged to seek medical treatment.

Fire service personnel will remain on scene until the area is immediately safe (i.e. CO levels are below acute risk guideline values) and responsibility has been handed over, for example to a building manager, National Grid gas emergency service, or local authority. It may be necessary for health protection staff to work with these agencies to ensure that all appropriate actions are taken to identify the source and either disable or remove it before the area is re-opened to the public. Low-level CO incidents with no emergency phase may be particularly difficult to manage and resolve. Guidance on managing CO incidents is available on the HPA website (www.hpa.org.uk/chemicals/co).

Health professionals should encourage residents to have all fuel-burning appliances tested by qualified engineers annually and install CO alarms.

13.7 Conclusions

Carbon monoxide poisoning remains a major public health concern. It is a major contributor to urban air pollution, and many hundreds of millions of people around the globe are further chronically exposed to CO indoors (WHO 2010). The primary toxic mechanism of CO is its ability to bind to haemoglobin, preventing body tissues from accessing oxygen.

In high-level exposures, this can lead to death. In low-dose exposures, diagnosis is difficult and can be often missed by doctors because of low clinician awareness and because symptoms can mimic other common diseases.

Acutely exposed patients require urgent treatment with oxygen after immediate removal from the source of exposure to prevent neurological and cardiac sequelae. During pregnancy, the use of hyperbaric oxygen by some authorities is rationalized due to the increased vulnerability of the foetus to lower concentrations of CO in comparison to normal healthy adults.

Long-term low but toxic exposure may lead to protracted ill-health, primarily because diagnosis is delayed until the source of exposure has been confirmed. These patients may require prolonged care and encouragement for years following cessation of exposure. As children are more vulnerable to CO exposure than adults, symptoms may initially manifest in the school environment where there may be lack of concentration, mental acuity, and disinterest in extra-curricular activities.

CO is dangerous because it is undetectable by the human senses, leaving the individual unaware in most cases that he or she is being poisoned. Public awareness as well as regular educational activities for healthcare professionals to raise awareness of this silent killer are essential. The public should be urged to install CO alarms routinely, as with smoke alarms. To minimize the hazard, fuel-burning appliances should be annually checked by a qualified engineer, such as Gas Safe Register, the Solid Fuel Association, or the Oil Firing Technical Association, and chimneys should be regularly swept.

13.8 References

Buckley NA, Juurlink DN, Isbister G, Bennett MH, Lavonas EJ. (2011) Hyperbaric oxygen for carbon monoxide poisoning. *Cochrane Database Syst Rev* **13**;4:CD002041.
Coburn RF. (1970) The carbon monoxide body stores. *Ann N Y Acad Sci* **174**:11–22.

Copel JA, Bowen F, Bolognese RJ. (1982) Carbon monoxide intoxication in early pregnancy. *Obstet Gynecol* **59**:26S–28S.

Department of the Environment, Transport and the Regions. (1998) Indoor Air Quality in the Home (2): Carbon monoxide. Institute of Environmental Health, Leicester.

Department of Health. (2004) Guidance of the effects of health of indoor air pollutants. Committee on the Medical Effects of Air Pollutants. Available at: http://comeap.org.uk/documents/reports/85-indoor-air-pollutants.html.

Department of Health. (2010) Carbon monoxide poisoning: Needless deaths, unnecessary injury. *Letter from the Chief Medical Officer and Chief Nursing Officer.* Department of Health, London, PL/CMO/2010/02, PL/CNO/2010/02.

Ernst A, Zibrak JD. (1998) Carbon monoxide poisoning. *New Engl J Med* **339**:1603–1608.

HSE. (2005) Workplace exposure limits. Health and Safety Executive EH40/2005. HMSO, Norwich.

HPA. (2011) HPA Compendium of Chemical Hazards: Carbon monoxide. Health Protection Agency, v3. Available at: www.hpa.org.uk/chemicals/compendium.

Karalliedde L. (2006) Carbon monoxide poisoning *Int J Clin Prac* **60**(12):1523–1524.

Longo LD. (1977) The biological effects of carbon monoxide on the pregnant woman, fetus, and newborn infant. *Am J Obstet Gynecol* **129**:69–103.

MEDITEXT® Medical Management (2010). Carbon monoxide. In: Klasco RK (ed), TOMES® System. Thomson Micromedex, Greenwood Village, Colorado. Accessed August 2010.

MMWR. (2005) Carbon Monoxide Poisoning from Hurricane-Associated Use of Portable Generators—Florida, 2004. *Morbid Mort Week Rep* **54**(28):697–700.

ONS. (2007) Mortality statistics: Injury and poisoning. Review of the Registrar General on deaths attributed to injury and poisoning in England and Wales, 2005. Office for National Statistics, London.

Owens EO. (2010) Endogenous carbon monoxide production in disease. *Clin Biochem* **43**(15):1183–1188.

Satran D, Henry CR, Adkinson C, Nicholson CI, Bracha Y, Henry TD. (2005) Cardiovascular manifestations of moderate to severe carbon monoxide poisoning. *J Am Coll Cardiol* **45**(9):1513–1516.

Van Hoesen KB, Camporesi EM, Moon RE et al. (1989) Should hyperbaric oxygen be used to treat the pregnant patient for acute carbon monoxide poisoning? A case report and literature review. *J Am Med Assn* **261**:1039–1043.

WHO. (2000) Air Quality Guidelines for Europe. WHO Regional Publications, European Series, No. 91, 2nd edn. World Health Organization Regional Office for Europe, Copenhagen.

WHO. (2010) Carbon monoxide. WHO guidelines for indoor air quality: selected pollutants. 1st edn. World Health Organization European Centre for Environment and Health, Bonn.

13.9 Further reading

Flomenbaum NE, Howland MA, Goldfrank LR, Lewin NA, Hoffman RS, Nelson LS. (eds) (2006) *Goldfrank's Toxicologic Emergencies.* 8th edn. McGraw-Hill, New York.

IPCS. (1999) Carbon monoxide. *Environmental Health Criteria* 213. International Programme on Chemical Safety, World Health Organization, Geneva.

Jones A, Karalliedde L. (2006) Carbon Monoxide Poisoning. In: Boon, N.A., Colledge, N.R., Walker, B.R., and Hunter, J.A. (eds), *Davidson's Principles and Practice of Medicine.* 20th edn. Churchill Livingstone, London.

WHO. (2000) Air Quality Guidelines for Europe. WHO Regional Publications, European Series, No. 91, 2nd edn. World Health Organization Regional Office for Europe, Copenhagen.

WHO. (2010) Carbon monoxide. WHO guidelines for indoor air quality: selected pollutants. 1st edn. World Health Organization European Centre for Environment and Health, Bonn.

Chapter 14

Toxicity of heavy metals and trace elements

Lakshman Karalliedde and Nicholas Brooke

Learning outcomes

At the end of this chapter and any recommended reading the student should be able to:

1. Understand the terms 'trace element' and 'heavy metal';

2. Explain, with reference to case studies, the source and health effects of some trace elements, e.g. lead, zinc, mercury, arsenic, thallium, aluminium, and chromium, and

3. Apply acquired knowledge in the analysis and management of hazardous situations.

14.1 Introduction

14.1.1 Heavy metals

'Heavy metals' is a somewhat ambiguous term used to describe chemical elements that have metallic or metalloid properties with a specific gravity that is around five times or more than the specific gravity of water. Specific gravity is a measure of density, which compares a given amount of a solid substance to an equal amount of water. The specific gravity of water is 1 at 4°C (39°F). Some well-known toxic metallic elements with a specific gravity that is five or more times that of water are arsenic (5.7), cadmium (8.65), iron (7.9), lead (11.34), and mercury (13.546) (Lide 1992).

There are approximately 23 heavy metals that are important or relevant to health protection and toxicology. Small amounts of some of these heavy metals are necessary for normal body function and good health, and are known as 'trace elements' (see below), e.g. iron, copper, and cobalt. Trace elements are present in the environment and in our diet. However, they can be toxic at higher doses. Other metals such as lead and mercury have no beneficial effects on health and are toxic at low dose levels. Some heavy metals have the potential to cause disorders of function of many body organs, including the nervous system, cardiovascular system, kidneys, liver, and lung. In addition, allergies may also occur (e.g. to nickel). There are data to indicate that long-term (chronic) exposures to some heavy metals, e.g. arsenic and hexavalent chromium, cause cancer (CIS 1999).

The heavy metals of particular concern to public health are antimony, arsenic, bismuth, cadmium, cerium, chromium, cobalt, copper, gallium, gold, iron, lead, manganese, mercury, nickel, platinum, silver, tellurium, thallium, tin, uranium, vanadium, and zinc (Glanze 1996).

14.1.2 Trace elements

In the toxicological/biological sciences, trace elements are generally considered to be those elements, including some heavy metals, which are essential to health in trace amounts, or where there is some evidence to support claims that they have some benefit to health. These are described as 'essential' or 'probably essential' and are often commercially available in multivitamin products or other food supplements. The Expert Group on Vitamins and Minerals (EVM) lists the following as trace elements: boron, chromium, cobalt, copper, germanium (now withdrawn as a supplement due to toxicity), iodine, manganese, molybdenum, nickel, selenium, tin, vanadium, and zinc (EVM 2003).

14.2 Heavy metal toxicity

In general, heavy metal toxicity is rare in clinical practice. However, when it does occur, diagnosis may be delayed, compounding the clinical effects with delayed or inappropriate treatment and resulting in serious ill-health (Ferner 2001).

Symptoms of acute heavy metal toxicity may be more easily recognized if there is a sufficient degree of suspicion and awareness of potential sources of exposure. Following acute toxic exposures, symptoms usually appear rapidly, thus diagnosis and treatment are often prompt (Ferner 2001). However, symptoms of chronic toxicity can be vague, so the establishment of a cause and effect relationship becomes difficult and symptoms may be misdiagnosed as those of a non-toxicological illness. The symptoms of chronic toxicity, e.g. impairment of brain function (cognitive dysfunction), learning difficulties, nervousness, insomnia, lethargy, and general malaise, also tend to vary in intensity with time. Heavy metal toxicity usually needs to be confirmed by appropriate laboratory investigations (e.g. via blood or urine analysis), therefore there are often delays in diagnosis and in the implementation of appropriate therapy following chronic exposures.

In order for an individual to be exposed to a substance there has to be a pathway linking the source to the person, known as the source-pathway-receptor model (see Section 2.3), therefore the presence of a heavy metal in the environment does not always result in exposure. Exposure is influenced by the concentration of the metal in the environment and its form (e.g. inorganic vs organic). Important exposure pathways that need to be considered are inhalation, skin contact, and ingestion via food or water.

People may be exposed to heavy metals through their everyday applications. In medicine, heavy metals can be used in diagnostic medical applications, such as the direct injection of radioactive isotopes of gallium during radiological procedures, and chromium used in intravenous feeding (parenteral nutrition) (Roberts 1999). Occupational exposure can result from heavy metal use in industrial applications such as in the manufacture of pesticides, batteries, alloys, electroplated metal parts, textile dyes, and steel (CIS 1999). Many products containing these chemicals are also found in our homes and improve our quality of life when properly used.

Heavy metals may enter the human body through food, water, or air, or by absorption through the skin. Ingestion is the most common route of exposure in children (Roberts 1999). Pica is the term used to describe individuals, particularly children, with an eating disorder characterized by the consumption of non-foodstuffs. Small children may ingest potentially toxic quantities of heavy metals from hand-to-mouth activity involving contaminated soil, by actually eating objects that are not food, such as dirt, and through sucking and gnawing on paintwork, such as on windowsills. Toys contaminated with heavy metals pose a particular risk to children when the metals are deliberately or accidentally introduced during the manufacturing process. These can then leach out of toys when children handle, suck, or swallow them. This has resulted in the highly publicized recall in 2007 of lead-painted toys manufactured in China and more recently in the withdrawal of children's jewellery containing cadmium (Becker et al. 2010).

People may be exposed in manufacturing, pharmaceutical, industrial, and residential settings; industrial exposure is a common source of exposure for adults. Less common routes of exposure are during radiological procedures, from inappropriate dosing during intravenous (parenteral) nutrition or from a commonly used instrument that is damaged or broken, such as a clinical thermometer (Smith et al. 1997). Heavy metals have been used as agents for both suicide and homicide.

Individuals may also be exposed to heavy metals via traditional medicines. Ayruvedirc medicines are extremely popular within South Asian populations and can be split into two major groups: herbal only and Rasa Shastra. Rasa Shastra involves the deliberate combination of herbs with heavy metals for therapeutic reasons. One study identified that one-fifth of ayurvedic medicines bought via the internet following manufacture in the USA and India contained lead, mercury, or arsenic at concentrations higher then regulatory limits (Saper et al. 2008). There is further discussion on the toxicity of heavy metals found in traditional medicines in Chapter 16.

Acute toxicity is more likely to occur in the workplace as a result of inhalation or skin contact from dust, fumes, or vapours. However, lower levels of contamination may occur in industrial and residential settings, particularly in older properties with lead paint or old lead plumbing.

As with any other potentially toxic agent in an occupational or public exposure context, a risk assessment is necessary if exposure to heavy metals and trace elements is likely to occur. The main difference with risk assessment of trace elements compared with other toxic agents is the need to consider the minimum amounts that may be necessary for health, in addition to the levels that may be toxic.

Toxic heavy metals with no beneficial effect should be considered as any other toxic substance and, where possible, tolerable daily intakes should be identified, or in the case of genotoxic compounds for which we assume no threshold, exposure should be kept as low as reasonably practicable (see Box 14.1). This is also true for lead, for which the general assumption is that there is no threshold dose for the adverse effects of lead on the developing

Box 14.1 The concept of 'as low as reasonably practicable'

As low as reasonably practicable

In the case of genotoxic compounds for which we assume no threshold, exposures must be kept ALARP, i.e. 'as low as reasonably practicable'. The concept of ALARP involves the consideration of the risks and benefits of the exposure, and so this could mean that some exposures to the chemical may not be permitted at all. For example, such compounds would not be used in household products, cosmetics, food additives, and similar products which are frequently used. However, industrial use could be allowed under strictly controlled conditions.

nervous system, which may result from an intake in the developing foetus during pregnancy, during infancy or during early childhood.

Once absorbed into the body heavy metals may partition between the blood, soft tissue, liver, kidney, bone, and teeth, although this varies dependent on the properties of the metal under consideration. Elimination of heavy metals from the body may take months or even years. For example, absorbed lead has an elimination half-life of 27 years from bone and is excreted primarily in urine.

Numerous chelating agents exist that are able to bind to and enhance the rate of excretion of heavy metals from the body following acute and chronic poisoning. Table 14.1 lists those chelating agents currently recommended to be kept by emergency departments in the UK for heavy metal poisoning (College of Emergency Medicine 2008).

The following sections contain a brief introduction to the toxicity of some of the more common heavy metals.

14.3 Lead

Lead is not required as a trace element in the body. The harmful effects of lead have been recognized for centuries and have even been reported as a contributing factor in the downfall of the Roman Empire. Metallic lead is used in storage batteries, cables, and electronic equipment. Inorganic lead salts are used in the production of pesticides, paint, ceramics, glass, plastic, and rubber products.

Lead does not have any specific historical medicinal usage, although it has been an ingredient in cosmetic products (and is still illegally used in skin-lightening products).

Lead is present in both inorganic and organic forms. Lead has an affinity for bone and acts by replacing calcium. It is deposited in growing bone and will accumulate with repeated exposures. Ingested lead is absorbed more readily by children, which makes children more sensitive to the toxic effects of lead than adults: in children, 40% of ingested lead is absorbed, whereas only 5–15% is absorbed by adults (HPA 2007). Approximately 50–90% of inhaled lead enters the blood. Children under 3 years are especially vulnerable because they both absorb lead more effectively than adults and usually have greater exposures

Table 14.1 Chelating agents currently recommended for storage by emergency departments for heavy metal poisoning

Antidote	Indication
Desferrioxamine	Iron
Prussian Blue	Thallium
Sodium calcium edetate	Heavy metals (particularly lead)
Succimer (DMSA)	Heavy metals (particularly lead and arsenic)
Unithiol (DMPS)	Heavy metals (particularly mercury)
Penicillamine	Copper

Data from College of College of Emergency Medicine, Guideline on Antidote Availability for Emergency Departments (May 2008) www.collemergencymed.ac.uk/asp/document.asp?ID=4685

because of their exploratory behaviour and frequent hand-to-mouth activity. As the developing nervous system in children is much more vulnerable to damage than the nervous system in adults, pregnant women are also a high-risk group. Lead follows similar metabolic pathways to calcium in the body, so can pass through the placenta, and infants can also be exposed during lactation.

The toxicology of lead is summarized in the Health Protection Agency (HPA) Compendia of Chemical Hazards Series (HPA 2007); the summary of the health effects is given below.

14.3.1 Toxicity of lead

Lead is classically a chronic or cumulative toxic substance. Few adverse health effects are observed following an acute exposure at low dose levels. Acute effects including gastrointestinal disturbances (loss of appetite, nausea, vomiting, abdominal pain), neurological effects (encephalopathy, malaise, drowsiness), hepatic and renal damage, and hypertension have been reported.

Chronic lead exposure may cause anaemia, basophilic stippling (presence of many bluestaining granules within red blood cells), and decreased haemoglobin synthesis. Neurological effects may also be observed such as fatigue, sleep disturbance, headache, irritability, lethargy, slurred speech, convulsions, muscle weakness, ataxia, tremors, and paralysis.

Epidemiological studies in children have shown an inverse relationship between blood lead concentrations above 10 μg/dl and intelligence quotient (IQ). There is some evidence that even lower exposures are also harmful, and it is therefore assumed that there is no completely harmless level of exposure to lead.

Nephropathy (kidney disease) and renal tubule dysfunction (dysfunction in the tubules of the filtering units—nephrons—in the kidney) may arise following chronic lead exposure. Hepatic damage has been reported in a few cases only, following occupational exposure to lead. Gastrointestinal disturbances such as nausea, vomiting, anorexia, constipation, and abdominal cramps have also been observed in workers.

Chronic exposure to lead may cause adverse effects on both male and female reproductive functions. Females may experience spontaneous abortion, stillbirths, or low birth weight following occupational exposure before or during pregnancy. Males may experience reduced libido and/or have low semen volumes and sperm counts along with a decrease in sperm motility.

Occupational exposure to lead has been reported to cause an increase in sister chromatid exchange and chromosomal aberrations, with worker blood concentrations of 80 µg/dL. However, such increases were not observed in environmentally exposed children with blood concentrations between 30 µg/dL and 63 µg/dL.

Based on epidemiological and experimental data, the Working Group of the International Agency for Research on Cancer concluded that inorganic lead compounds are probably carcinogenic to humans (Group 2A) (IARC 2006).

14.3.2 Regulation of lead

The high toxicity of lead has been recognized for many years and has led to a raft of regulation to reduce exposures wherever reasonably practical over the past two decades. The elimination of lead in petrol has been of critical importance, although there are concerns about the resultant increased use of benzene, a recognized carcinogen, to sustain high octane ratings, however legislation (in 2000) reduced the maximum amount of benzene in petrol to 1%.

Lead is banned in cosmetics manufactured or marketed in the EU (and the UK). However, cosmetics are sometimes brought into the UK from abroad for personal use or bought via the internet, so should not be ruled out as a possible source of exposure. Lead has recently been found in kohl, a widely used traditional cosmetic mainly worn around the eyes.

Legislation controlling the marketing and use of lead in paint in the UK came into force in 1992 with the Environmental Protection (Controls on Injurious Substances) Regulations. However, voluntary agreements between the Paintmakers' Association (now called the British Coatings Federation) and the UK government initially came into being in 1963 (revised in 1974). Under this accord, paints which contained more than 1% lead in dry film had to be labelled with a warning that they were not to be used on surfaces accessible to children. In practice, however, the UK paint industry had begun to replace its use of white lead (lead carbonate/lead sulphate) in the 1950s with alternatives, such as titanium dioxide, that are technically superior and also considered less hazardous. In the 1960s, lead-drying agents also began to be phased out, along with coloured lead pigments in decorative paints, so that ordinary paints in the UK were virtually lead-free from the 1960s. Some very limited uses of lead did continue, such as in thin primer paints on some prefabricated domestic wooden windows up to the 1980s, and in products intended for professional use. The Lawther Working Party for the then Department of Health and Social Security estimated in its 1980 report that lead-based paints accounted for less than 3% of the current market.

The occupational use of lead is strictly governed by the Control of Lead at Work Regulations 2002 and the Health and Safety at Work (etc.) Act 1974.

The use of lead water supply pipes is no longer permitted in new dwellings or in repairs to old systems. In areas with a plumbosolvent public water supply (water that is able to dissolve lead) grants are available from local authorities for the removal of old pipe-work, although these are usually means-tested and therefore of limited impact.

In addition, lead solder may still legally be used in central heating supply pipes and there has been at least one incidence where this has inadvertently been used in pipes for a drinking water supply.

As a result of these efforts, blood-lead levels in the UK have fallen dramatically in recent decades and surveys indicate that the great majority of UK children are now well below the target level for blood-lead of 10 µg/dl, set by the International Miami Declaration on Children's Environmental Health, which the UK signed in May 1997.

It is reasonable to expect further reductions in blood-lead levels, as older legislation continues to have an effect and newer actions, such as lowering limits for lead in drinking water, are introduced. However, it is important to note that the 10 µg/dl level does not denote a concentration at which lead poisoning begins, rather it is a target to minimize the possibility of harm to populations at risk. Indeed recent evidence suggests that some intellectual impairment may occur at levels below 10 µg/dl. The underlying assumption is that no exposure to lead is completely harmless and the aim is therefore to reduce exposure wherever reasonably practicable.

The Housing Act 2004 introduced a new system for rating the 'fitness' of housing. The system is used by local authority environmental health practitioners to secure the remediation of hazards, including domestic lead exposure, such as from old paintwork and lead water pipes. However, the removal of lead paintwork can itself present hazards— from paint dust and vapours from the use of paint-stripping hot-air guns. Advice on safe removal is given in a DEFRA advice sheet (DEFRA 2005).

14.4 Zinc

Zinc salts are used in soldering, cement additives, horticultural chemicals, and dry cells. Zinc phosphide is used as a rodenticide and zinc is also found in numerous topical skin preparations as zinc oxide.

Zinc is a good example of an essential trace element. It was reviewed by the EVM in their report *Safe Upper Levels for Vitamins and Minerals* (EVM 2003).

Meat and cereals are good sources of zinc in the diet. The Committee on Medical Aspects of Food Nutrition and Policy (COMA) determined a reference nutrient intake (RNI) for zinc. An RNI is the amount of nutrient that is enough or more than enough for most (usually at least 97%) people in a group; if the average intake in this group is at the RNI then the risk of deficiency in the group is very small. The RNI for zinc is 5.5–9.5 mg/ day for men and 4.0–7.0 mg/day for women (COMA 1991).

Zinc is essential as it is a constituent of more than 200 enzymes and is necessary for cell division. Zinc deficiency is associated with a range of adverse effects, including poor pre-natal development, mental retardation, impaired conduction of nerve impulses, reproductive failure, dermatitis (inflammatory disorders of the skin), hair loss, diarrhoea, loss of appetite (anorexia), anaemia, susceptibility to infection, delayed wound healing, and macular degeneration (change in the eye which affects vision).

14.4.1 Toxicity of zinc

Symptoms of acute toxicity caused by over-exposure to zinc include abdominal pain, nausea and vomiting, lethargy, anaemia, and dizziness.

Prolonged use of high doses of zinc can result in secondary deficiency of copper, which gives rise to a wide range of effects. These include hypocupraemia (reduced copper content in the blood) and impaired iron mobilization.

Changes in the blood also occur due to deficiencies in copper, including anaemia, leucopaenia (decreased white cells in the blood), neutropaenia (a decrease in neutrophils—a specific type of white blood cell), increased plasma cholesterol, and increased low-density lipoprotein to high-density lipoprotein (LDL:HDL) cholesterol ratio. The increase in LDL:HDL ratio is considered harmful as low density lipoproteins are associated with heart attacks, whereas high density lipoproteins are considered protective against heart attacks.

Other toxic effects associated with zinc-related copper deficiency include decreased erythrocyte superoxide dismutase activity, decreased cytochrome C oxidase activity, decreased glucose clearance (decreased removal of glucose in the blood by the kidneys), decreased methionine, decreased leucine enkephalins, abnormal cardiac function, and impairment of the pancreatic enzymes amylase and lipase.

Acute toxicity occurs in humans after oral doses of 200 mg of zinc or more. The most sensitive indicator of zinc toxicity is the reduction in copper absorption, measured through effects on the copper-dependent enzyme erythrocyte superoxide dismutase. Repeated daily exposure to 50 mg for several weeks results in effects on this enzyme and a reduction in haematocrit (the blood test which measures the ratio of volume of cells to volume of plasma) and serum ferritin levels. Doses greater than 100 mg per day have resulted in an altered ratio of LDL:HDL cholesterol. This may be why excess zinc is considered atherogenic, i.e. able to cause the formation of lipid deposits within the lumen of arteries.

The EVM recommend a safe upper level for daily consumption of 25 mg zinc/day for supplemental zinc (EVM 2003).

Inhalation of zinc compounds may result in local irritation of the nose and throat, causing shortness of breath (dyspnoea), cough, chest pain, headache, nausea, and vomiting. Chronic exposure may cause changes in the lung tissues, fibrosis of the lung, or inflammation of lungs (pneumonitis).

14.4.1.1 Metal fume fever

Under occupational exposure conditions, inhalation of zinc compounds (mainly zinc oxide fumes) can result in a condition referred to as 'metal fume fever'. Metal fume fever's unique symptoms have been described in welders/metal workers since the early 19th century. It is an acute, self-limited syndrome characterized by a delayed onset (4–12 hours) after exposure to welding fumes. Symptoms tend to resolve spontaneously in 24–48 hours and treatment is generally supportive and non-interventional. The precise underlying disorders are not known with certainty, and metal fume fever can occur either following the first exposure to metal fumes or after repeated exposures. There is a tendency for attacks to be worse at the beginning of the working week—hence the popular name Monday Morning Fever (Greenberg et al. 2003).

The clinical features of metal fume fever are irritation of the nasal passages, cough, abnormal sounds in the lungs (known as rales) when breathing is heard through a stethoscope, reduced lung volumes, increased rate of breathing (hyperpnoea), and an alteration in the ability of gases to diffuse across the lung to the blood (as detected by a carbon monoxide diffusing capacity test), headache, altered taste, fever, weakness, sweating, pains in legs and chest, and an increase in white blood cells (leukocytosis).

Although metal fume fever occurs in occupationally exposed workers, it is essentially an acute reversible disorder that is unlikely to occur under chronic exposure conditions. The workplace exposure limit for zinc chloride fumes is 1 mg/m^3 over an 8-hour period (HSE 2005).

14.5 Mercury

Mercury has in the past been used as an ingredient in diuretics, antibacterial agents, antiseptic skin ointments, laxatives, and hair-conditioning agents, and was used in dentistry for many centuries. Mercurous (calomel) salts were also historically used as a purgative. Mercuric salts (e.g. mercuric chloride) were used as disinfectants and because of their high solubility and acute toxicity have been used as homicidal agents.

14.5.1 Forms of mercury

14.5.1.1 Organic mercury

Organomercury compounds such as methyl mercury are a particular environmental concern because of their formation through the methylation of inorganic mercury by microorganisms in aqueous environments. Methyl mercury is accumulated in the aquatic food chain and the mercury concentrations in shellfish or predatory fish (e.g. shark, swordfish) are of particular concern to public health (see Section 3.4 on food contaminants). Organic mercury is readily absorbed through the gastrointestinal system into the systemic circulation and readily crosses the blood–brain barrier; it is concentrated in the brain as well as the kidney, liver, hair, and skin. Organic mercury also readily crosses the placenta.

Organic mercury compounds may have significant volatility and may be readily absorbed by inhalation and through the skin as well as orally.

14.5.1.2 Inorganic mercury

When ingested, inorganic mercury salts can be absorbed from the gastrointestinal tract. However, they are poorly lipid-soluble and only around 10% of an ingested dose would be absorbed. Once absorbed, inorganic mercury is concentrated in the kidneys. Inorganic mercury compounds do not in general pose a significant risk by the inhalation route as they are not encountered in a respirable form. However, there have been recent reports of the use of mercury-containing skin-lightening creams containing significant quantities of mercury being associated with the development of nephrotic syndrome (Choudhury 2011).

14.5.1.3 Elemental mercury

Elemental mercury, as present in mercury thermometers, is not absorbed through the intact gastrointestinal tract to any significant extent, nor through the skin. However, elemental mercury vapour is readily absorbed by inhalation. Mercury can pose a health risk from exposure to modest amounts, such those found in thermometers if spills are not cleaned up effectively.

The toxicology of inorganic and elemental mercury is summarized in the HPA Compendia of Chemical Hazards Series (HPA 2007); the summary of the health effects is given below.

14.5.2 Toxicity of mercury

Mercury poisoning may often be misdiagnosed as the symptoms are non-specific and insidious in nature. The gastrointestinal system, the nervous system, and the kidneys are the most common organ systems affected.

Following an acute exposure to elemental mercury vapour via inhalation, respiratory effects such as cough, dyspnoea (shortness of breath), chest tightness, bronchitis, and decreased pulmonary (lung) function may occur. Cognitive, personality, sensory, or motor disturbances may also arise, including tremor, irritability, hallucinations, muscle weakness, and headaches. Because of the accumulation of mercury in the kidneys, acute renal failure indicated by proteinuria (passage of proteins in the urine), haematuria (passage of blood in the urine), and oliguria (passage of reduced amounts or volumes of urine) is commonly reported. Acute inhalation of elemental mercury may also cause gastrointestinal effects such as stomatitis (inflammation of the mouth), abdominal pain, vomiting, diarrhoea, and ulceration of the oral mucosa, as well as cardiovascular effects such as hypertension (high blood pressure) and tachycardia (increase in heart or pulse rate).

Inorganic mercury compounds are highly irritating to the gastrointestinal tract and an acute ingestion may cause a metallic taste, abdominal pain, vomiting, diarrhoea, and necrosis of the intestinal mucosa, possibly leading to circulatory collapse and death. Ulceration of the mouth, lips, tongue, and gastrointestinal tract may also occur. If patients survive damage to the gastrointestinal tract, acute renal failure may occur within 24 hours of ingestion. Hypertension and tachycardia have also been reported following ingestion of inorganic mercury compounds.

Acute dermal exposure to elemental mercury vapour can cause erythematous (reddish) and pruritic (itchy) skin rashes, reddening and peeling of skin on palms of feet and hands associated with acrodynia, and contact with soluble inorganic mercury compounds may cause irritation, vesiculation, and contact dermatitis.

Chronic exposure to elemental mercury vapour via inhalation may cause neurotoxicity, resulting in decreased psychomotor skills (skills requiring co-ordinated thinking and muscle activity) and neuropsychological symptoms including fatigue, tremor, headaches, depression, irritability, and hallucinations. Nephrotoxicity (toxicity to the kidney) leading to proteinuria and increased urinary enzyme excretion was observed following occupational exposure to elemental mercury, as well as stomatitis (inflammation of the mouth), sore gums, and ulceration of the oral mucosa.

Chronic ingestion of inorganic mercury compounds may cause irritability, weakness, insomnia (inability to fall asleep), muscle twitching, swollen gums, excess salivation, anorexia, and abdominal pain.

There is little convincing evidence that exposure to mercury causes chromosomal damage or other mutagenic effects. The IARC have classified elemental mercury and inorganic mercury compounds as category 3 carcinogens, i.e. not classifiable as to its carcinogenicity to humans (IARC 1997a).

Conflicting evidence regarding the incidence of spontaneous abortion following inorganic mercury exposure has been presented. Some studies have reported a higher incidence of reproductive failures (spontaneous abortions, still births, congenital malformations) and irregular, painful, and haemorrhagic menstrual disorders in occupationally exposed women compared to unexposed women.

14.5.2.1 Toxicity of mercury dental amalgams

The toxicity of mercury from dental amalgams is a contentious issue. The views of the Committee on Toxicity of Chemicals in Food, Consumer Products and the Environment (COT) were first sought on this issue in 1986. At that time, the Committee recognized that some mercury may be released from completed dental restorations but was of the opinion that the use of dental amalgam is free from risk of systemic toxicity and that only a very few cases of hypersensitivity may occur (COT 1986).

The Committee, when asked for further advice in 1997, particularly regarding any nephrotoxic or neurotoxic effects arising from dental amalgams, came to the following conclusions:

- Their former conclusions regarding lack of systemic toxicity and only very few cases of hypersensitivity should remain unchanged.

- Nephrotoxicity (toxicity to the kidney) was not associated with exposure of healthy subjects to mercury amalgam from dental restorations. Also, the Committee considered that neurotoxicity (toxicity to the nervous system) caused by exposure to mercury vapour was a matter of greater concern in the occupational setting than in dental patients.

- There was no available evidence to indicate that the placement or removal of dental amalgam fillings during pregnancy was harmful. The Committee was of the opinion, however, that the toxicological and epidemiological data were inadequate to assess fully the likelihood of harm occurring in such circumstances. Until appropriate data were available, they concurred with the view that it may be prudent to avoid, where clinically reasonable, the placement or removal of amalgam fillings during pregnancy.

- Further research in a number of areas was recommended (COT 1997).

- Further studies have come to similar conclusions and in May 2008 a Scientific Committee of the European Commission addressed the safety concerns for the public and professionals regarding the use of mercury-containing dental amalgams. It was concluded that dental amalgams are effective and safe, both for patients and staff, and noted that alternative materials are not without clinical limitations and toxicological hazards (EC 2008).

14.6 Arsenic

Arsenic is the heavy metal (or metalloid, as it has properties of both metals and non-metals) that has been arguably responsible for the largest number of individuals adversely affected by an environmental chemical. Chronic arsenic poisoning from naturally occurring arsenic in drinking water has been a threat to approximately 70 million people in Bangladesh and 45 million in West Bengal. Similar health hazards have been reported to exist in Nepal, Thailand, Taiwan, China, Mexico, and some other countries in South America. The World Health Organization (WHO) guideline value for arsenic content in drinking water is 10 μg/l.

Historically, arsenic compounds were commonly used as medications for various disorders such as syphilis, acne, malaria, and anaemia. In addition, arsenic has been used as a poison since the 15th century and was considered the 'perfect poison' because it is odourless, tasteless, and resembles sugar. Fowler's solution of 1% potassium arsenite was used for over 150 years for the treatment of various ailments, including psoriasis, rheumatism, asthma, cholera, and syphilis. Arsenicals are still used in the treatment of African trypanosomiasis (sleeping sickness) and in the treatment of rare forms of leukaemia. Some arsenic compounds may also be found in Chinese and Indian traditional medicines and rarely in some herbal preparations.

Arsenic exists in both organic and inorganic forms. The organo-arsenicals are mainly found in marine organisms or as metabolites in the detoxification pathway in mammals. The Food Standards Agency estimate that the average daily intake of arsenic is 65 μg in the UK, mostly from fish, and that the bulk of this is in the form of organo-arsenicals (DEFRA and EA 2002). Organo-arsenicals are less toxic than the inorganic compounds and are not considered further in this review.

Soluble inorganic arsenic compounds are well-absorbed following ingestion. Arsenic binds to specific groups of chemicals which are essential for enzyme function, e.g. sulphydryl groups, and thus the activity of many enzymes in the body is inhibited. Hence, very few organs escape the toxic effects of arsenic. Arsenic also replaces inorganic phosphorus in enzymes and thus prevents certain metabolic reactions (e.g. it inhibits oxidative phosphorylation).

The toxicology of inorganic arsenic compounds is summarized in the HPA Compendia of Chemical Hazards Series (HPA 2007); the summary of the health effects is given below.

14.6.1 Toxicity of inorganic arsenic compounds

Single doses of inorganic arsenic may be highly toxic by ingestion and inhalation (70–180 mg orally are widely cited as being fatal). However, survival has been reported following ingestion of 20,000–50,000 mg in adults and 14.6 mg/kg in a child. Trivalent arsenic is, in general, more toxic than pentavalent arsenic.

Inorganic arsenic is a known human carcinogen which acts via a genotoxic mechanism. It is assumed, therefore, that there is no threshold for such effects and that risk management measures should ensure that exposures are prevented whenever possible or otherwise kept as low as reasonably practicable (see Box 14.1 for more on the concept of ALARP). There is sufficient evidence that chronic exposure to inorganic arsenic in drinking water causes non-melanoma skin cancers and an increased risk of bladder and lung cancers in humans.

The effects of inorganic arsenic on the peripheral blood vessels are well documented. Long-term ingestion of contaminated drinking water may lead to Raynaud's phenomenon and acrocyanosis with progression to endarteritis obliterans and gangrene of the lower extremities (black foot disease). An increased incidence of cardiovascular disease has also been noted. Anaemia and leucopaenia may occur together with other disturbances of haem synthesis.

Chronic exposure to inorganic arsenic compounds may lead to peripheral and central neurotoxicity. Early events may include paraesthesia (pins and needles) followed by muscle weakness. Both motor and sensory peripheral neurones are affected. Characteristic dermal lesions after chronic oral or inhalation exposure may include hyperpigmentation and hyperkeratosis.

Other toxic effects associated with chronic exposure to inorganic arsenic include liver damage, cardiovascular disease, and diabetes mellitus.

There are limited data from epidemiology to suggest that inorganic arsenic may be a human developmental toxicant, but it is not possible to draw any definitive conclusions. Administration of high doses may cause death or foetal malformations in laboratory animals. Inorganic arsenic may cause irritation of the mucous membranes, leading to conjunctivitis and pharyngitis and rhinitis after inhalation. Skin irritation and allergic contact dermatitis may occur after exposure to inorganic arsenic compounds.

14.7 Thallium

Thallium is used in small quantities industrially in the production of special glasses used in the electrical and electronics industry. In the past it was used as a rodenticide and for medical purposes. Thallium compounds have also been used in suicides and homicides.

Thallium compounds are highly toxic if inhaled, ingested, or absorbed through the skin (IPCS 1996). Following ingestion, the onset of gastrointestinal symptoms may occur after 12–48 hours. These include nausea, vomiting, metallic taste in the mouth, hypersalivation, and retrosternal and abdominal pain. Systemic features occur 2–5 days post exposure, the main effects being, in addition to gastroenteritis, a polyneuropathy characterized by numbness around lips, paraesthesia of fingers and toes becoming severe and spreading to arms and legs, and paralysis eventually affecting all muscles. Hair loss (alopecia) occurs at 10–15 days. Death is usually from cardio-respiratory failure and often occurs 10–12 days post exposure, although with very high doses death may occur within 24 hours. In some cases it may take symptoms 2–3 weeks to reach their maximum severity. If recovery occurs following thallium poisoning it is likely to be slow.

The neurological effects of thallium are believed to be due to impairment of the action of the Na/K pump (the mechanism by which exchange of the ions sodium and potassium occurs in cells), since the affinity of thallium for the enzyme sodium/potassium ATPase is 9–10 times that potassium.

The characteristic effects of thallium poisoning are often considered the triad gastroenteritis, polyneuropathy, and alopecia, but in some cases gastroenteritis and alopecia are not observed (IPCS 1996).

14.8 Aluminium

Aluminium is the third most prevalent element and the most abundant metal in the earth's crust. Aluminium in the diet is therefore ubiquitous, with very small amounts in food and water, the permitted WHO drinking water standard being 0.2 mg/l. The main intakes other than diet are from the use of aluminium-based antacids (grams consumed) and to a lesser extent from aluminium compounds in toothpastes.

Soluble forms of aluminium (e.g. aluminium chloride, aluminium fluoride, aluminium oxide, aluminium sulphate, and aluminium citrate) are potentially more toxic than insoluble forms (e.g. aluminium hydroxide, which is used as an antacid).

Aluminium compounds are poorly absorbed orally and have low acute toxicity by this route. There is some evidence of neurotoxicity following repeated oral exposure in animals, particularly when given by injection. Osteomalacia (softening of the bones) has also been produced at high exposure levels. Studies in animals and other experimental systems indicate that aluminium compounds do not have any significant mutagenic or carcinogenic effects or effects on the reproductive system.

It has been suggested that aluminium ingestion may be a risk factor for the development of Alzheimer's disease and impaired cognitive function in the elderly. A large number of studies have investigated this concern (IPCS 1997). However, consideration of all the data from mechanistic studies and from epidemiology suggests that aluminium exposure does not cause Alzheimer's disease or non-specific impaired cognitive function (IPCS 1997).

Patients with chronic renal failure necessitating dialysis (a process which artificially replaces the failing kidney's functions to remove waste, salt, and fluid) for many months are at risk from the toxic effects of aluminium. This may manifest as dialysis encephalopathy or a form of osteomalacia or microcytic anaemia (anaemia associated with red blood cells smaller than normal). These effects can be prevented by ensuring that the dialysis fluid contains less than 30 µg of aluminium per litre or by using deionized water.

14.8.1 Lowermoor incident

Possibly the best-known environmental toxic episode associated with aluminium in the UK was the Lowermoor incident. In July 1988, 20 tonnes of aluminium sulphate solution was discharged into the incorrect tank at the Lowermoor water treatment works in North Cornwall. The total amount of aluminium added in the incident was 850 kg. Aluminium sulphate is used in the water treatment process as a flocculant to bind suspended solid matter and dissolved organic acids in the raw water before filtration, so some aluminium is usually present in drinking water. The maximum permitted level is 0.2 mg/l. However, following the Lowermoor incident, levels up to 109 mg/l were recorded in the water supply system by the water authority and levels up to 720 mg/l were reported in samples taken by private individuals.

The acidity of the contaminated water was sufficient to cause corrosion of metallic plumbing materials, storage tanks, and other fittings, leading to the release of increased amounts of copper, zinc, iron, and, in some cases, lead into the water supply. Flushing of the mains distribution system to remove the contaminated water resulted in the disturbance of old mains sediments containing iron and manganese oxides and, in some cases, possibly lead and lead salts, which resulted in higher than usual amounts of these chemicals in the water at the tap.

A number of acute effects were reported after the incident by individuals who drank the contaminated water. These included mouth ulceration, skin irritation, and gastrointestinal effects such as diarrhoea and abdominal pain. The gastrointestinal effects are almost certainly attributable to the contaminated water, which was reported as tasting very unpleasant. Although the recorded pH values of the water after the incident were not low enough to cause the cases of skin irritation reported, it may be that high concentrations of sulphate and metal salts rendered the water more irritant than would be anticipated from its pH alone.

A number of chronic symptoms have also been reported by people affected by the incident, including impaired memory, joint pains and/or swelling, tiredness/lethargy, and problems with coordination and concentration. A number of expert groups have been convened by the government over the years to investigate whether chronic effects such as these are likely to have resulted from exposure to the contaminants released during the incident. Full details are given in the draft report of the Committee on Toxicity of Chemicals in Food Consumer Products and the Environment's Subgroup Report on the Lowermoor incident (COT 2005).

Studies to date have concluded that there is no evidence that a harmful accumulation of aluminium has occurred within the exposed population, nor that the prevalence of ill-health (e.g. cancer incidence) among those exposed to the contaminated water is greater than normal.

14.9 Chromium

Chromium was reviewed by the EVM in their report *Safe Upper levels for Vitamins and Minerals* (EVM 2003).

Chromium is a trace element that can exist in a number of oxidation states, the trivalent and the hexavalent being the most important biologically. The trivalent form (chromium III) is ubiquitous in nature whilst hexavalent (chromium VI) compounds are man-made and do not occur naturally. Chromium in foodstuffs and as food supplements is in the trivalent form, with the highest levels in processed meats and whole-grain products.

Committee on Medical Aspects of Food and Nutrition Policy (COMA) has not set RNIs for chromium, but has suggested that an adequate level of intake of trivalent chromium lies above 0.025 mg/day for adults and between 0.0001 and 0.001 mg/kg/day for children and adolescents. COMA also noted that no adverse effects were observed at intakes of trivalent chromium of 1000—2000 mg per day (COMA 1991).

Trivalent chromium has been shown to potentiate insulin action and thereby affect carbohydrate, lipid, and protein metabolism.

Although referred to as an essential trace element in humans, deficiency has only been observed in patients on long-term parenteral nutrition (feeding by the intravenous route). The symptoms of chromium deficiency observed were impaired glucose tolerance and glucose utilization, weight loss, neuropathy, elevated plasma fatty acids, and abnormalities of oxygen and nitrogen metabolism.

In contrast to trivalent chromium, hexavalent chromium has no beneficial effects. It is much more toxic than the trivalent compound and is a mutagen and a carcinogen (see below).

Trivalent chromium compounds are poorly absorbed orally (0.5–2.0%) and absorbed material does not enter blood cells but binds to plasma proteins such as transferrin and is transported to the liver. In contrast, hexavalent chromium does penetrate red blood cells, where it is reduced by glutathione to trivalent chromium, which binds to haemoglobin. Excess hexavalent chromium is taken up into the kidneys, spleen, liver, lungs, and bone.

There is only limited data on the toxicity of trivalent chromium compounds following ingestion, although this appears to be low because of the poor absorption. The EVM felt unable to derive a safe upper level for trivalent chromium. However, based on one repeated-dose study in the rat where no effects were seen at 15 mg/kg body weight per day, they did for guidance purposes suggest a value of 0.15 mg/kg body weight per day (EVM 2003). No recommendations were possible for hexavalent chromium and as this has both mutagenic and carcinogenic properties it is not possible to derive a safe exposure level.

The toxicology of chromium compounds is summarized in the HPA Compendia of Chemical Hazards Series (HPA 2007); the summary of the health effects is given below.

14.9.1 Toxicity of chromium compounds

The toxicity of chromium depends on the oxidation state, hexavalent chromium being more toxic than the trivalent form. In addition, hexavalent chromium is the more readily absorbed by both inhalation and oral routes.

The respiratory tract is the primary target for inhaled chromium following acute exposure, although effects on the kidney, gastrointestinal tract, and liver have also been reported.

Acute ingestion of high doses of hexavalent chromium compounds, the exact quantity of which is not usually known in accident scenarios, results in acute, potentially fatal, effects in the respiratory, cardiovascular, gastrointestinal, hepatic, renal, and neurological systems.

Due to the corrosive nature of some hexavalent chromium compounds, dermal exposure can lead to skin ulcers. At high doses, systemic toxicity leading to effects on the renal, haematological and cardiovascular systems, and death has been reported.

Studies of the effects of chronic occupational exposure to chromium compounds have proven difficult due to co-exposures to other toxic substances in the relevant working environments. Occupational exposure to some inhaled hexavalent chromium mists may cause nasal septal ulceration and perforation, respiratory irritation and inflammation, dyspnoea, cyanosis, and gastrointestinal, hepatic, renal, and haematological effects and lung cancer. Chronic exposure to hexavalent chromium compounds can also cause allergic responses (e.g. asthma and allergic dermatitis) in sensitized individuals. Chronic exposure to trivalent chromium resulted in weight loss, anaemia, liver dysfunction, and renal failure.

Hexavalent chromium compounds are positive in the majority of *in vitro* mutagenicity tests reported and may cause chromosomal aberrations and sister chromatid exchanges in humans. The mechanism of genotoxicity has been proposed to be a result of sequential reduction of hexavalent chromium within the cells to trivalent chromium and the binding of trivalent chromium to macromolecules, including DNA.

Trivalent chromium is not considered to be mutagenic in most cellular systems and there is no firm evidence that *in vivo* it is mutagenic to humans or experimental animals. Studies have not shown chromium (III) to be carcinogenic.

Hexavalent chromate ions are transported into cells, whereas trivalent chromium compounds are more poorly absorbed into cells, this may account for the differences in genotoxicity.

Hexavalent chromium has been classified as a Group 1 known human carcinogen by the inhalation route of exposure and chromium metal and trivalent chromium compounds are not classifiable as to their carcinogenicity to humans (Group 3) due to inadequate evidence in humans (IARC 1997b).

Potassium dichromate may be toxic to the reproductive system and the developing foetus. There is insufficient evidence to suggest that trivalent chromium compounds are reproductive or developmental toxicants.

14.10 Copper

Copper was reviewed by the EVM in their report *Safe Upper levels for Vitamins and Minerals* (EVM 2003).

Copper is an essential trace element, being involved in the function of certain enzymes, such as cytochrome C oxidase, amino acid oxidase, superoxide dismutase and monoamine oxidase. Because of the heat and electrical conductivity of copper, as well as its resistance to corrosion, ductility, and malleability, it has many industrial applications and is widely used in electrical wiring, switches, electroplating, plumbing pipes, coins, metal alloys, and fireworks. Copper sulphate is used as a fungicide, an algaecide, and in some fertilizers.

COMA has set a RNI for copper of 1.2 mg/day (COMA 1991). Food is the major source of copper intake, with particularly high concentrations found in nuts (8 mg/kg), shellfish, and offal (40 mg/kg).

The absorption of copper is kept under tight homeostatic control in the body to prevent accumulation of excessive amounts. Where dietary levels are high, absorption is reduced and, in particular, biliary excretion is increased. Copper toxicity only occurs when these defences are overwhelmed.

14.10.1 Toxicity of copper compounds

Acute copper toxicity is rare in humans but can occur from contamination of food or drink (e.g. from leaching into drinking water from pipes) and very rarely intoxication has followed ingestion of large amounts of coins. The emetic properties (induction of vomiting) and unpleasant taste of copper salts mitigate against frequent accidental or deliberate ingestion. Signs of acute toxicity include salivation, epigastric pain, nausea, vomiting, and diarrhoea. Intakes in the range 25–75 mg have been quoted as sufficient to induce vomiting but individual susceptibility varies and lower intakes may produce effects if taken on an empty stomach. Intakes of above about 100 g of copper sulphate produce intravascular haemolysis (breakdown of red blood cells), acute hepatic failure, acute tubular renal failure, shock, coma, and death.

Other clinical features of acute copper toxicity observed include anaemia, neutropaenia, and bone abnormalities. Less frequent signs and symptoms include hypopigmentation of the hair, hypertonia (increased tone of muscles), impaired growth, increased susceptibility to infection, abnormalities in metabolism of glucose and cholesterol, and cardiovascular changes. Copper exposure via inhalation has also been linked to the development of metal fume fever (see section 14.4).

There are insufficient data in humans to assess the chronic toxicity of copper and only limited data in animals. Studies in human volunteers suggest that daily doses of 7.5–10 mg of copper in food or supplements are not associated with adverse effects. In animals, there is marked species variability, with copper salts being relatively well tolerated in pigs and rats, but in sheep, copper toxicosis develops at low dietary intakes.

Copper compounds are believed not to have any significant mutagenic or carcinogenic properties. Reproductive effects have been reported in laboratory animals but these findings were not consistent.

The EVM used a well-conducted subchronic toxicity study in the rat to derive a safe upper limit of exposure. In this study the NOAEL was 16 mg/kg body weight per day. Higher dose levels resulted in damage to the fore-stomach, kidney, and liver. This was divided by an uncertainty factor of 100 to give the safe upper exposure level. The recommended safe upper exposure level was set at 0.16 mg/kg body weight per day (EVM 2003).

14.11 Acknowledgement

The authors gratefully acknowledge input for this chapter from a previous edition from Dr Robin Fielder.

14.12 References

Becker M, Edwards S, Massey RI. (2010) Toxic chemicals in toys and children's products: limitations of current responses and recommendations for government and industry. *Environ Sci Technol.* **44**(21):7986–7991.

Choudhury K, Morris J, Harrison H, O'Moore E. (2011) Use of skin lightening creams. Dangers from mercury. *British Medical Journal*, 342:d1327.

CIS. (1999) Metals. In: *Basics of Chemical Safety.* International Occupational Safety and Health Information Centre (CIS), International Labour Organization, Geneva. Available at: www.ilo.org.

College of Emergency Medicine. (2008) Guideline on Antidote Availability for Emergency Departments. Guy's and St Thomas' poison unit, Royal College of Surgeons of England, British Association for Emergency Medicine, London. Available at: http://www.emergencymed.org.uk.

COMA. (1991) Committee on Medical Aspects of Food and Nutrition Policy: Dietary Reference Values for Food Energy and Nutrients for the UK. HMSO, London.

COT. (1986) Statement on Dental Amalgam prepared for the Committee on Dental and Surgical Materials. Committee on Toxicity of Chemicals in Food, Consumer Products and the Environment, London.

COT. (1997) Statement on the toxicity of dental amalgam. Committee on Toxicity of Chemicals in Food, Consumer Products and the Environment. Available at: http://www.food.gov.uk/multimedia/pdfs/committee/cotstatementdentalamalgam1997.

COT. (2005) Subgroup Report on the Lowermoor Water Pollution Incident. Lowermoore Subgroup, Committee on Toxicity of Chemicals in Food, Consumer Products and the Environment. Available at: http://cot.food.gov.uk/cotwg/lowermoorsub/.

DEFRA. (2005) Restoration methods and safe working. Advice on lead in old paint—Advice Sheet 3, last updated 16 August 2005. Department for Environment and Rural Affairs, London. Available at: http://www.defra.gov.uk/environment/chemicals/lead/.

DEFRA and EA. (2002) TOX1 Arsenic. *Contaminants in soil: collation of toxicological data and intake values for humans.* Department for Environment, Food and Rural Affairs and the Environment Agency, London. Available at: http://www.environment-agency.gov.uk/commondata/acrobat/tox1_arsenic_675423.pdf.

European Commission: Scientific Committee on Emerging and Newly Identified Health Risks. (2008) The Safety of Dental Amalgam and Alternative Dental Restoration Materials for Patients and Users. Available at: http://ec.europa.eu/health/ph_risk/committees/04_scenihr/docs/scenihr_o_016.pdf.

EVM. (2003) Safe Upper levels for Vitamins and Minerals. Expert Group on Vitamins and Minerals (EVM). Available at: http://www.food.gov.uk/multimedia/pdfs/vitmin2003.pdf.

Ferner DJ. (2001) Toxicity, heavy metals. *eMed J* **2**(5): 1.

Glanze WD. (1996) Mosby Medical Encyclopedia. rev. edn. Signet, New York.

Greenberg MI, Hamilton RJ, Phillips SD, McCluskey GJ. (2003) Occupational, industrial and environmental toxicology. 2nd edn. Mosby, Pennsylvania.

HPA. (2007) *Compendium of Chemical Hazards series.* Available at: http://www.hpa.org.uk/chemicals/compendium/.

HSE. (2005) *EH40/2005 Workplace exposure limits.* Health and Safety Executive, HMSO, London.

IARC. (1997a) Beryllium, Cadmium, Mercury, and Exposures in the Glass Manufacturing Industry. *IARC Monographs* Volume 58. International Agency for Research on Cancer, Lille.

IARC. (1997b) Chromium, Nickel and Welding. *IARC Monographs* Volume 49. International Agency for Research on Cancer, Lille.

IARC. (2006) Inorganic and Organic Lead Compounds. *IARC Monographs* Volume 87. International Agency for Research on Cancer, Lille.

IPCS. (1996) Thallium. *Environmental Health Criteria* No 182. International Programme on Chemical Safety, World Health Organization, Geneva. Available at: www.inchem.org/pages/ehc.

IPCS. (1997) Aluminium. *Environmental Health Criteria* No 194. International Programme on Chemical Safety, World Health Organization, Geneva. Available at: www.inchem.org/pages/ehc.

Lide DR. (ed.) (1992) Handbook of Chemistry and Physics. 73rd edn. CRC Press, Boca Raton.

Roberts JR. (1999) Metal toxicity in children. In: *Training Manual on Pediatric Environmental Health: Putting It into Practice.* Children's Environmental Health Network, Emeryville. Available at www.cehn.org.

Saper RB, Phillips RS, Sehgal A, Khouri N, Davis RB, Paquin J, Thuppil V. (2008) Lead, mercury, and arsenic in US- and Indian-manufactured Ayurvedic medicines sold via the Internet. *J Am Med Assn* **300**(8):915–23.

Smith SR, Jaffe DM, Skinner MA. (1997) Case report of metallic mercury injury. *Pediatr Emer Care* **13**(2):114–116.

Chapter 15

The toxicology of pesticides

Timothy C. Marrs and Lakshman Karalliedde

Learning outcomes

At the end of this chapter and any recommended reading the student should be able to:

1. define and classify pesticides, and explain the common terminology of the toxicology of pesticides;

2. define and classify insecticides, describe the various types and the main toxic effects of each type, e.g. organochlorines, organophosphorus compounds, pyrethrins, and synthetic pyrethroids;

3. discuss insecticides of biological origin other than pyrethrins and nicotine;

4. define and classify fungicides, describe the various types and the main toxic effects of each type;

5. define and classify herbicides, describe the various types and the main toxic effects of each type;

6. define and classify rodenticides and molluscicides and discuss their main toxic effects, and

7. apply acquired knowledge in the analysis and management of hazardous situations.

15.1 Introduction

A precise definition of a pesticide is difficult. A dictionary definition would be an agent used to kill unwanted living organisms. In legislation, the definition may be different. In the European Union (EU), those that are used to kill unwanted living organisms on crops are called plant protection products and those used for other purposes are called biocides and the two groups are regulated separately. Furthermore, some compounds that regulate plant growth are also regulated as plant protection products. Substances similar or the same as those used on plants are regulated as veterinary drugs in the EU when used on animals. These include substances used to kill parasites on farm animals such as sheep dips (used to control sheep scab and fly-strike) and flea killers for dogs and cats. Some compounds are even used in human medicine (e.g. for head lice); these are controlled as human medicines. In common parlance all these agents may be called pesticides and this chapter makes no distinction between them.

The organisms against which the pesticides are used are referred to as target species and any other living organism as the non-target. The art of producing successful pesticides is toxicological specificity for killing the target and not non-target organisms. Thus an insecticidal plant protection product should not damage plants. A pet flea treatment should not harm domestic pets.

15.2 Use of pesticides

The main use of pesticides is in agriculture and this gives the opportunity for exposure of consumers via food and importantly of farmers and farm workers. Nearly 50% of the world labour force is employed in agriculture (Lichfield, 2005) and during the past five decades there has been a massive increase in utilization of pesticides and fertilizers to enhance crop protection and production, food quality, and food preservation. Pesticides are also employed for public health purposes and for domestic use. The role of insecticides in the control of vector-borne diseases should not be underestimated. Malaria, the best-known vector-borne disease, affects more than 500 million people in 90 countries causing 1.1–2.7 million deaths a year, mostly among children under 5 years of age (UN Millennium Project 2005). Diarrhoeal diseases (vectors being the common house fly) account for 17% of deaths among children under 5 years worldwide or nearly two million deaths per year (UNICEF 2007). Other important vector-borne diseases include yellow fever and dengue. Insecticides have contributed to the elimination of some vector-borne diseases in Africa (such as River Blindness).

Small amounts of pesticides are used in horticulture and in the UK those used by private individuals are particularly tightly controlled.

15.3 Toxicity of pesticides

Pesticide are, like antibiotics and disinfectants, intended to be toxic to their target organisms and are deliberately spread into the environment. Pesticides have a variable but generally limited species selectivity. Many insecticides target the insect nervous system and these may also target the mammalian nervous system, whereas other insecticides target structures peculiar to insects (see below) and these are often of very low mammalian toxicity as are some herbicides, e.g. glyphosate. Pesticide toxicity depends on the compound family and is generally greater for older compounds. In humans, pesticides may be responsible for acute poisonings as well as for long-term health effects, including cancer and adverse effects on reproduction. Because of the potential of pesticides to produce toxicity, in most countries a specific and complex legislation prescribes a thorough risk assessment process for pesticides prior to their entrance to the market (pre-marketing risk assessment). The risk assessment is carried out for possible food exposure and for occupational exposure to pesticides in agriculture. Occupational exposure may be important for product distributors, mixers and loaders, applicators, bystanders, and rural workers re-entering the fields shortly after treatment. For non-food crops, e.g. cotton, where plant protection products are used to preserve the quality of the cotton and prevent damage, the main concern is operator exposure. Post-marketing surveillance of pesticide residues is undertaken for those pesticides used on food crops. The systems of regulation of plant protection products, biocides, and veterinary and human medicines differ in detail but the general principles are similar. However, the EU, which previously used a purely risk-based regulatory system for plant protection products, now uses a risk- and hazard-based system.

15.4 Risk assessment and management

Assessing and managing the occupational health risks posed by the use of pesticides in agriculture is a complex but essential task for occupational health specialists and toxicologists. In the EU, the USA, and elsewhere, the risk assessment process will generate reference doses, such as the acceptable daily intake (ADI), for food consumers, and the acceptable operator exposure level (AOEL), for workers. These figures are based on the toxicological data (usually from animal studies performed before the pesticide is marketed). The toxicological studies will include 90-day repeated dose and lifetime studies in experimental animals as well as studies of reproduction and developmental toxicity. If field trials using the pesticide on crops in the proposed way suggest that either the ADI or AOEL will be exceeded, it may be possible to alter the conditions of use to remedy the situation. This will be done by, for example, altering the conditions of use or, for workers, mandating the use of individual protective equipment. Guidelines for safe storage and disposal are being addressed regularly to improve operator and environmental safety. Attempts are made to determine optimal regimens of treatment for poisoned patients and effective antidotes. In many countries, despite the economic and social importance of agriculture, the health protection of agricultural workforce has been overlooked for too many years, causing a heavy load of avoidable diseases, human sufferance, and economic losses. Particularly in the developing countries, where agricultural work is one of the predominant jobs available, a sustainable model of development calls for more attention to occupational risks in agriculture. The experience of many countries has shown that prevention of health risk caused by pesticides is technically feasible and economically rewarding for the individuals and the whole community. Proper risk assessment and management of pesticide use is an essential component of this preventative approach.

There are considerable difficulties in obtaining accurate data on worker ill-health attributable to pesticides from developing countries. It is generally accepted that such ill-health is likely to be frequent. The WHO estimated in 2006 that pesticides, insecticides in particular, have caused 3.5–5 million acute poisonings per year, which were associated with 250,000 deaths. In contrast, the rate of occupational acute pesticide poisonings in agricultural workers in developed countries is 1–4% of the several million cases of occupational injuries and ill-health in agricultural workers worldwide (Litchfield 2005). Arguably, Sri Lanka amongst the so-called developing countries has been the location for a considerable degree of information associated with pesticide ill-health. Although there are no national data for the incidence of self-poisoning in Sri Lanka, two recent studies reported annual incidences of 315 and 363 per 100,000 acts of self-poisoning in rural Sri Lanka. Since more than half of self-poisoning is due to ingestion of pesticides, the incidence is likely to be around 150–200 per 100,000 per year. The major official source of information on health statistics is the Annual Health Bulletin of Sri Lanka, which reports hospital admissions.

Although this source should be viewed with caution due to errors of reporting, it can provide some information on trends on deaths and patient admissions. Until the end of the 1980s, pesticide poisoning was not listed among the 10 leading causes of hospital deaths in any Sri Lankan district. This changed markedly over the next decade, pesticide poisoning becoming the sixth most common cause of hospital deaths in Sri Lanka, whereas in certain districts it was listed as the leading cause of hospital deaths. Interestingly, this increase is not likely to be due to a simple increase in the incidence of poisoning but due to ingestion of less-toxic, more slowly acting pesticides in the 1990s, which allowed patients to reach hospital before dying. The actual number of deaths peaked in the late 1980s and has fallen by more than 50% over the past 13 years (Figure 15.1). Pesticide self-poisoning currently remains the 10th most common cause of hospital death in Sri Lanka. A review of 37,125 death certificates issued over the 20 years from 1967 in a single semi-agricultural district revealed an increasing number of deaths by self-poisoning (from 11.8 per 1000 deaths in 1967 to 43.0 in 1987). The majority of pesticide poisoning deaths are in men between the economically productive ages of 20 and 60 years.

It has been shown that the easy availability of highly toxic pesticides is an important contributor to the high case fatality from pesticide poisoning seen in Sri Lanka. Restriction of pesticides has been in operation from the 1970s in Sri Lanka. In the early 1990s, import of WHO Class I organophosphorus compounds was initially restricted and then totally banned in 1995. In 1998 endosulfan, an organochlorine associated with status epilepticus and high frequency of mortality, was banned in Sri Lanka. Restriction of these compounds was associated with a reduction in the incidence of deaths from self-poisoning with pesticides, without any effect on agricultural output. The pesticide registrar of Sri Lanka has

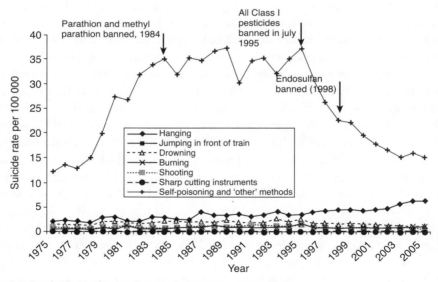

Fig. 15.1 Method-specific suicide rates in Sri Lanka, 1975–2005.

Reproduced from Gunnell et al. (2007), The impact of pesticide regulations on suicide in Sri Lanka, *Int. J. Epidemiol.* **36**(6): 1235–1242 with permission from Oxford University Press.

recently taken steps to ban the import of dimethoate and fenthion—the organophosphorus pesticides believed to be responsible for a large proportion of pesticide poisoning deaths. Further, import of paraquat formulations at concentrations above 6.7% was banned in mid-2008, and import of paraquat will be banned in 3 years. These changes are expected to substantially reduce the number of poisoning deaths in Sri Lanka. Future projects will target interventions at a community level, screening for suicide risk and empowering people with coping skills.

15.5 Suicide

Suicide by intentional ingestion of pesticides is a continuing tragedy in developing countries. In rural China, pesticides account for over 60% of suicides. The rates for Trinidad and Malaysia are 68% and 90%, respectively (Gunnell and Eddleston 2003; WHO 2006).

15.6 Nomenclature of pesticides

Pesticides have chemical names and national common names (for example British Standards Institute [BSI] and American National Standards Institute [ANSI]). Pesticides also have international common names bestowed by the International Organization for Standardization (ISO). ISO names are allocated in a number of languages, including English and French, and it is important to note that the English language ISO name is not always the same as the BSI or ANSI common name. A number of pesticides are used in human or veterinary medicine. As such they have international non-proprietary names (INNs). In some cases these differ from the ISO pesticide names, examples being trichlorfon, an insecticide which has trichlorfon as the ISO pesticide name and which is the same as metrifonate (INN), used in tropical medicine. Another example is the fungicide imazalil (ISO), which has the INN enilconazole when used as a human pharmaceutical.

15.7 Classification of pesticides

Pesticides may be classified on the basis of their use as follows:

- insecticides/acaricides
- fungicides
- herbicides
- rodenticides
- molluscicides.

15.7.1 Insecticides/acaricides

Insecticides comprise a large group of pesticides, which are often active against other arthropods, such as mites (acaricides). They may be divided on the basis of their chemical structure and mode of action as follows:

- organochlorine compounds, e.g. DDT
- anticholinesterase agents, e.g. organophosphorus compounds, carbamates

- pyrethrins and synthetic pyrethroids
- nicotine and neonicotinoid compounds
- insecticides that target structures/systems unique to insects
- other insecticides.

15.7.1.1 Organochlorine compounds

Organochlorine compounds such as DDT (dichloro-diphenyl-trichloroethane) and the 'drins'—aldrin, dieldrin, and endrin—and related insecticides such as lindane (γ-hexachlorocyclohexane) and endosulfan primarily cause toxicity to the nervous system. This is due to these insecticides interfering with the function of sodium channels (see appendix for more details), which are needed to function normally for transmission of nerve impulses and for normal activity of the nervous system. Some are also active on the γ-aminobutyric aid (GABA) neurotransmission system. In humans the main toxic effects are tremor, coordination problems (especially with DDT), and convulsions (especially from the 'drins'), these being due to perturbation of GABA-mediated inhibitory neurotransmission. There have also been suggestions that exposure to organochlorines may be associated with an increase in the incidence of breast cancer in humans, but detailed consideration of the data indicated that there was no convincing evidence that organochlorine insecticides were associated with the development of breast cancer (COC 2004). The property that has brought this group of insecticides into disrepute is persistence: organochlorines are not easily degradable either in mammals or in the environment, and therefore they do not break down to non-toxic compounds easily. They tend to persist in human fat and are excreted in breast milk. As they are persistent in the environment, they pose a potential long-term threat to human health. There have been diverse concerns about ill-health in humans attributed to or associated with the use of organochlorine compounds. These concerns, although contentious to date, together with concerns of their persistence in, and effects on, the environment, have resulted in the banning of all these compounds in the EU. The last agricultural use of organochlorines in the EU was that of lindane but this has been revoked. DDT was very effective in destroying mosquitoes, the insects that transmit malaria, and the banning of DDT was associated with a very large increase in the incidence of malaria in several developing countries, therefore DDT is still used in some countries to protect public health.

15.7.1.2 Anticholinesterase agents: organophosphorus and carbamate insecticides

Acetylcholine is a neurotransmitter (chemical messenger) both in the central nervous system and the peripheral nervous system (see appendix for more details). It is a transmitter in the brain and the only known transmitter at autonomic ganglia, at the post-ganglionic nerve endings of the parasympathetic nervous system and some post-ganglionic fibres of the sympathetic nervous system, and at the skeletal neuromuscular junctions. The action of acetylcholine is limited in time and space by the enzyme acetylcholinesterase (AChE), which hydrolyses acetylcholine, thus inactivating it so that resting nerve activity is restored quickly after the passage of a nerve impulse and is ready to respond to another nerve impulse. This state is markedly disturbed when AChE is inhibited—it is made inactive by a process called phosphorylation, and can no longer hydrolyse and thereby inactivate acetylcholine. As a result, acetylcholine accumulates at all the sites where it is the neurotransmitter and this accumulation causes several well-defined and some less well-defined clinical syndromes and features. Anticholinesterases also inhibit esterases other than AChE. The main syndromes that follow inactivation of AChE by organophosphorus insecticides and, for that matter, by all organophosphorus compounds that inhibit this enzyme, which includes the chemical warfare agents or nerve agents tabun, sarin, and soman, include the following:

1. The acute cholinergic syndrome, which follows almost immediately after exposure, where there are increased secretions from all salivary and tear glands (lacrimation), urination, defecation, and gastric emesis (Salivation, Lachrymation, Urination, Defecation, Gastric Emesis (SLUDGE)) and usually slowing of the heart rate (bradycardia), muscle fasciculations, and constriction of the pupils (pinpoint pupils).

2. The intermediate syndrome, which sets in after the acute cholinergic syndrome. Recent published data from Sri Lanka has shown the intermediate syndrome to be a spectral disorder, with patients manifesting varying degrees of muscle weakness–from those of neck muscles to cranial nerves and only a few progressing to develop respiratory failure due to paralysis of the muscles of respiration (i.e. diaphragm, inter-costal muscles). Both these conditions are life-threatening and subjects who have been exposed to a large amount of organophosphorus compound(s) often require treatment in an intensive care unit. They also require the procedures discussed in Chapter 6 on the medical management of chemical incidents such as decontamination, prevention of further exposure, resuscitation, and administration of antidotes such as atropine. If the patient survives the initial management, recovery is almost always complete with the acute cholinergic syndrome and the intermediate syndrome. These organophosphorus insecticides also produce a third syndrome which is not related in any way to inhibition of AChE (organophosphate-induced delayed polyneuropathy [OPIDP]). This condition, which is not life-threatening, causes inter alia weakness of peripheral muscles in the limbs, i.e. the hands and particularly the feet. It is a polyneuropathy, which affects both motor and sensory nerves, and there is an upper motor neurone component so that spasticity is seen. It is called a delayed polyneuropathy because there is a latent period after poisoning before the syndrome develops. The syndrome is attributed to inactivation of the neuronal enzyme, neuropathy target esterase. Unfortunately, recovery from OPIDP is often incomplete and it causes long-term morbidity. Not all organophosphorus insecticides cause OPIDP. Those causing OPIDP are classed as neuropathic organophosphates and they cause a similar weakness or paralysis in hens. It is possible to test for such effects in a toxicity study in the hen and the policy in the EU is that, based on the hen test, compounds likely to causes OPIDP in humans will not be allowed on the market.

Carbamates produce an identical clinical picture as they too inhibit AChE but the binding of the carbamate to the enzyme is more readily reversible and thus the duration of poisoning shorter. Carbamates do not appear to cause the intermediate syndrome and OPIDP-like muscle weakness has not been observed. Some examples of organophosphorus insecticides are chlorpyrifos, dichlorvos, malathion (used widely in control of malaria at present), parathion, diazinon, and disulfoton. Some organophosphorus insecticides, e.g. trichlorfon/metrifonate, are used in tropical medicine. The related organophosphorus compounds which are grouped as nerve agents used in chemical warfare are discussed in Chapter 17 on chemical warfare agents. Important carbamates include aldicarb and carbaryl.

15.7.1.3 Pyrethrins and synthetic pyrethroids

Pyrethrins are natural products of pyrethrum plants (particularly from the flowers of *Tanacetum cinerariaefolium*, a plant of the chrysanthemum family). Synthetic pyrethroids are synthetic analogues that are more stable in sunlight (photostable). These substances are all of low toxicity to humans when taken orally or following dermal exposure. However, they are very toxic to fish. These agents are broadly grouped into two types on the basis of their parenteral toxicity to rodents.

Type I are those that produce tremors, for example permethrin and the (natural) pyrethrins. These lack an α-cyano group.

Type II synthetic pyrethroids have an α-cyano group and produce salivation and choreoathetosis (involuntary movements of limbs and fingers), for example deltamethrin, flumethrin, and cypermethrin. While of interest to mechanistic toxicologists, these syndromes are of no relevance to the toxic effects in humans, which are largely confined to paraesthesia after skin contact.

15.7.1.4 Nicotine and neonicotinoid compounds

Nicotine and the neonicotinoids target cholinergic transmission (transmission where acetylcholine is the key chemical messenger or neurotransmitter) as do the anticholinesterases. However, the mechanism is different and their effect is direct on cholinergic receptors, particularly nicotinic ones. Nicotine, from tobacco, was much used by Victorians as an insecticide but is quite toxic to mammals. The neonicotinoids are structurally related to nicotine, but are safer for humans, this reduced toxicity possibly being associated with different receptor binding characteristics. The most important of the neonicotinoids is imidacloprid. It is claimed that this compound specifically targets insect nicotinic receptors but data from both human poisonings and experimental animals suggest that imidacloprid is capable of producing cholinergic signs, so that specificity towards insects is clearly not complete. Nevertheless, imidacloprid has a good safety record but there have been suggestions that toxicity to bees may be a problem.

15.7.1.5 Insecticides that target structures/systems unique to insects

These include the insect growth regulators (juvenile hormone [JH] analogues) methoprene and hydroprene. JHs are a group of acyclic sesquiterpenoids that regulate development and reproduction. Insect growth regulators prevent reproduction by stopping metamorphosis of insect larvae into viable adults. Chitin synthesis inhibitors prevent growth in insects by stopping the synthesis of chitin, a modified polysaccharide containing nitrogen. Chitin is the main component of the exoskeletons of arthropods, including insects and crustaceans, and as they grow by repeatedly moulting and creating a new exoskeleton, chitin synthesis inhibition prevents growth. Neither JH nor chitin is found in mammals, hence these compounds are not intrinsically toxic to mammals: curiously what toxicity is observed is mainly to the mammalian haematological system. A third group of insecticides that interfere with structures specific to insects are those that mimic the action of ecdysone and bind to the ecdysone receptor. This causes an incomplete and premature unsuccessful moult, leading eventually to death. The main insecticides in this group are tebufenozide and methoxyfenozide. Unlike the other insect systems/structures discussed above, which are structurally unrelated to known mammalian hormones, ecdysone resembles hormones important in mammalian physiology. Both ecdysone and its metabolite 20-hydroxy ecdysone are steroids and unsurprisingly are pharmacologically active in mammals.

15.7.1.6 Other insecticides

Other insecticides do not fit into any of the above groups. Many are of natural origin, including avermectin and similar compounds which interfere with chemical messengers (GABA) while derris contains rotenone and interferes with the electron transport chain. An important synthetic insecticide that does not fall into any of the groups above is fipronil: this is a GABA antagonist. As GABA neurotransmission in adult mammals is inhibitory, the effect of fipronil in mammals is excitatory. At high doses in experimental animals, neurotoxicity was observed, while Mohamed et al. (2004) reported that poisoning was characterized by vomiting and agitation. Firponil is widely used in the UK as a cat flea treatment.

15.7.2 Fungicides

Fungicides are substances that kill fungi on plants or in wood. They comprise a chemically heterogeneous group of compounds. The main groups are as follows:

- Metallic fungicides, e.g. neutralized copper sulphate (Bordeaux mixture), which is the oldest commercially available fungicide and was originally used in viticulture. Other metallic fungicides include mercurous chloride and organometals such as methyl mercury, organotins (e.g. fentin), organocopper and organozinc compounds. Organification of metals makes them fat-soluble and able to cross biological membranes, notably the blood–brain barrier) and most metallic fungicides cause toxicity to the nervous system. Some of these compounds can also interfere with the immune system. Bordeaux mixture and mercury-containing fungicides are no longer used in the EU.

- Phenolic fungicides such as pentachlorophenol are acutely toxic and interfere with metabolic processes by uncoupling oxidative phosphorylation. This may give rise to an increase in body temperature, liver and kidney failure, and dehydration. Another effect of pentachlorphenol is to cause cataract. Pentachlorophenol was widely used in the past as a wood preservative. A related compound, dichlorophen, however, has very low oral and repeated dose toxicity (opacities in the lens of the eye). Azole fungicides such as hexaconazole, penconazole, and tebuconazole are used in agriculture and horticulture, and in human and veterinary medicine. They inhibit sterol synthesis in fungi. In experimental animals they can affect the liver, thyroid gland, blood, and reproductive system but they are well tolerated as drugs for humans.

♦ Carbamates fungicides include the dithiocarbamates and benzimidazole derivatives, The dithiocarbamates include three main groups of fungicides: the methyl dithiocarbamate (metam) the dimethyl dithiocarbamates (ferbam, thiram, and ziram) and the ethylenebis(dithiocarbamate)s. All dithiocarbamates seem to have the potential to be thyrotoxic, decreasing plasma thyroxine levels and increasing thyroid stimulating hormone levels.

15.7.3 Herbicides

Herbicides are substances that kill plants with variable degrees of specificity towards particular plants. Many are completely unselective, but a major exception is the organic acid group (see below).

15.7.3.1 Non-selective herbicides

The best-known herbicides are probably the bipyridilium compounds paraquat and diquat. These are non-selective. These compounds are toxic, especially paraquat, which can cause death in humans by toxicity to the lungs. Initially there is an acute alveolitis followed by fibrosis in which both type I and type II alveolar cells, as well as the clara cells, are destroyed. Infiltration with fibroblasts, alveolar oedema, perivascular and peribronchial oedema, and accumulation of neutrophils and macrophage are observed. Progressive fibrosis of lung tissue leads to respiratory failure and there is no known effective treatment to date. Lethal cases have almost all been the result of ingestion of the agricultural concentrate, usually with suicidal intent. Depending on the dose, death occurs up to three weeks after exposure, but after large doses are ingested, death may occur within 24 hours of ingestion. The local effects of paraquat ingestion are sore throat, pharyngitis, loss of voice (aphonia), eye damage, and skin damage. Diquat does not cause lung injury and the organ most affected by diquat is the kidney, with overdoses resulting in kidney failure. Glyphosate and glufosinate are organophosphorus compounds that are used as herbicides without any significant anticholinesterase activity. Glyphosate kills plants by inhibiting the pathway by which plants produce branched-chain amino acids. Glyphosate is not very toxic to humans or mammals because the pathway it affects for the synthesis of amino acids in plants is not present in humans. Large doses may cause stomach or gastric irritation, low blood pressure (hypotension), and poor lung function (pulmonary insufficiency). These toxic effects are thought to be due to the other constituents in the formulations and not due to glyphosate itself. Glufosinate also affects the synthesis of amino acids in plants. However, the pathway affected by glufosinate is also present in humans and overdoses cause toxicity of the nervous system (neurotoxicity), leading to convulsions or fits and tremors. There are many other herbicides (aniline compounds such as alachlor, propachlor, and propanil, triazines such as atrazine and simazine, and triazoles such as amitriole, diuron, and linuron).

15.7.3.2 Selective herbicides

The phenoxy herbicides such as 2,4-dichlorophenoxyacetic acid (2,4-D) are selective for broad leaved plants, so they can be used on grain crops such as wheat and maize: they are also used as selective lawn weed killers to kill daisies, dandelions etc. Their toxic effects include alterations in consciousness, decreased tone of the muscles, metabolic acidosis (increased acidity of the blood), muscle fasciculation, and coma. If the urine is made alkaline, there may be increased loss of these herbicides from the body, especially 2,4-D.

15.7.4 Rodenticides

The rodenticides are substances used to destroy or inhibit the action of rats, mice, or other rodents. Many such substances have been identified. Of particular note are the warfarins and coumarins, which act by preventing the clotting of blood. When taken by humans the toxic effects of these are similar and prolonged bleeding disorders usually result.

15.7.5 Molluscicides

Molluscicides, such as metaldehyde and methiocarb, are used to kill slugs and snails. The toxic effects of metaldehyde are related to those of acetaldehyde, of which it is atetramer. Salivation, facial flushing, fever, abdominal cramps, nausea, vomiting, drowsiness, tachycardia, spasms, irritability, and ataxia have been observed in humans at lower doses and convulsions, tremor, and coma and death at higher doses. Methiocarb is an anticholinesterase carbamate and causes the typical adverse effects of that group of compounds in mammals.

15.8 Conclusion

Pesticides are a trade-off between plant health and human health. Human health risk is kept low by an elaborate system of pre-marketing approval. There are rigid guidelines set by health authorities which permit only amounts considered safe for humans to be found as residues on food products. There are also guidelines for users of pesticides in the occupational setting. However, with the production of safer pesticides and public health education programmes for safe storage and use of pesticides along with legislative procedures to ban import/use of the more toxic pesticides, the incidence of ill-health associated with these agents has been decreased considerably.

15.9 References

COC. (2004) Breast cancer risk and exposure to organochlorine insecticides: consideration of the epidemiology data on dieldrin, DDT and certain hexachlorocyclohexane isomers. Committee on Carcinogenicity of Chemicals in Food, Consumer Products and the Environment. Department of Health, London. At http://cot.food.gov.uk/pdfs/cocsection.pdf Accessed 10/01/12.

Gunnell D, Eddleston M. (2003) Suicide by intentional ingestion of pesticides: a continuing tragedy in developing countries. *J Epidemiol* **23**:902–909.

Litchfield MH. (2005) Estimates of acute pesticide poisoning in agricultural workers in less developed countries. *Toxicol Rev* **24**:271–278.

UN Millennium Project. (2005) Coming to grips with malaria in the new millennium. Task Force on HIV/AIDS, Malaria, TB, and Access to Essential Medicines, Working Group on Malaria, New York.

UNICEF. (2007) Diarrhoeal diseases. Progress for Children: A World Fit for Children Statistical Review. Edition 6. New York, NY.

Whitehead R. (ed.) (2003) The UK Pesticide Guide. British Crop Protection Council, Farnham and CABI Publishing, Wallingford.

WHO. (2006) Pesticides are a leading suicide method. World Health Organization (UN Millennium Project, 2005). World Health Organization, Geneva.

15.10 Further reading

Ballantyne B, Marrs TC. (1992) Clinical and experimental toxicology of organophosphates and carbamates. Butterworth-Heinemann, Oxford.

Bismuth C, Hall AH. (eds) (2005) Paraquat poisoning: Mechanisms, Prevention, Treatment. Drug and Chemical Toxicology 10. M Dekker Inc, New York.

Gunnell D, Fernando R, Hewagama M, et al. (2007) The impact of pesticide regulations on suicide in Sri Lanka. *Int J Epidemiol* **36**(6):1235–1242.

Hayes WJ, Laws ER. (1991) Handbook of Pesticide Toxicology. Volume 1, General Principles. Academic Press, St Louis, MO.

Jayawardane P, Dawson AH, Weerasinghe V, Karalliedde L, Buckley NA, Senanayake N. (2008) The spectrum of intermediate syndrome following acute organophosphate poisoning: a prospective cohort study from Sri Lanka. *PLoS Medicine* **5**(7):e147:1–11.

Karalliedde L, Feldman S, Henry JA, Marrs TC. (eds) (2003) Organophosphates and Health. Imperial College Press, London.

Manuweera G, Eddleston M, Egodage S, Buckley NA. (2008) Do Targeted Bans of Insecticides to Prevent Deaths from Self-Poisoning Result in Reduced Agricultural Output? *Environ Health Persp* **116**(4):492–495.

Mohamed F, Senarathna L, Percy A, Abeyewardene M, Eaglesham G, Cheng R, Azher S, Hittarage A, Dissanayake W, Sheriff MH, Davies W, Buckley NA, Eddleston M (2004). Acute human self-poisoning with the N-phenylpyrazole insecticide fipronil—a GABAA-gated chloride channel blocker. *J Toxicol Clin Toxicol* **42**:955–963.

Chapter 16

Toxicology associated with traditional medicines

Lakshman Karalliedde

Learning outcomes

At the end of this chapter and any recommended reading the student should be able to:

1. discuss the use of traditional medicines, including the growing market in western cultures, and explain the concerns and issues associated with traditional medicines;

2. explain the potentially harmful constituents of herbal medicines, including heavy metals, allopathic medicines, toxic plants and plant constituents, animal and human body parts, and pesticides;

3. discuss the herbal traditional medicines that should be avoided by vulnerable population groups, e.g. pregnant women, breastfeeding mothers, the elderly, the immuno-suppressed;

4. evaluate policies and regulatory systems for traditional medicines, and some issues associated with integration with allopathic medicine;

5. apply acquired knowledge in the analysis and management of hazardous situations;

6. discuss the approaches and difficulties associated with the integration of allopathic and traditional medicines in healthcare systems.

16.1 Introduction

The World Health Organization (WHO) defines traditional medicine as 'health practices, approaches, knowledge and beliefs incorporating plant, animal and mineral based medicines, spiritual therapies, manual techniques and exercises applied solely or in combination to treat, diagnose and prevent illnesses or maintain well-being' (WHO 2003a). In industrialized countries, adaptations of traditional medicines are termed 'complementary' or 'alternative' (CAM). Traditional medicines developed over several thousands of years before the birth of Christ in Egypt, Mesopotamia, and Persia (Iran), and were documented by Greek and Roman scientists and physicians. In addition, communities in all parts of the world ranging from South America (the Incas) to Africa and the Pacific islands have been using forms of medical practice developed by their communities to manage ill-health, poisonings, and envenomings (e.g. snake bite, scorpion bite).

Complementary medicine use is growing in Western European countries (Zhang 1999). In the UK, a large-scale study of Scottish prescription data in 2003–2004 revealed that 49% of GPs prescribed homeopathic remedies and 32% prescribed herbal remedies (Ross et al. 2006). Waxman (2006) estimated 'that up to 80% of all patients with cancer take a complementary treatment or follow a dietary programme to help treat their cancer'.

The global market for herbal medicines currently stands at over US $60 billion annually and is growing. Estimates suggest that over 50% of the population in developed countries use some form of traditional medical practice at least once during their life times, either in addition to or instead of conventional medicine. Gardiner et al. (2006) reported that in the USA 21% of adult prescription medication users reported using non-vitamin dietary supplements (which includes herbal medicines) and that 69% of those did not discuss this use with a conventional medical practitioner.

Worldwide, WHO estimates that 70% and 40% of the populations of Canada and France, respectively, have tried complementary or alternative medicine, which often included herbal remedies (WHO 2003b). In Japan, 85% of doctors prescribe not only allopathic medicine but also traditional herbal medicine (called Kampo), which is covered by health insurance (Dharmananda 2003). WHO also report that 75% of patients suffering from a single, specific disease state, such as HIV/AIDS, are likely to use some form of traditional medicine, predominantly of plant origin, an estimate that is similar for patients in San Francisco, London, and South Africa (WHO 2003b).

Over one-third of the population in developing countries lack access to essential conventional (allopathic) medicines. In Africa, up to 80% of the population uses traditional medicine for primary health care and it is estimated that 65% of the population in rural India use Ayurveda and medicinal plants to help meet primary healthcare needs (WHO 2011). Of the traditional medicines in use today, Chinese, Ayurveda, siddha, and Unani (South Asian) medicines are probably the best known. Ayurveda, yoga, naturopathy, Unani, siddha, and homeopathy are systems which originated respectively in India, Asia, and Europe.

Medical pluralism—the use of multiple forms of health care—is widespread. Consumers practice integrated health care irrespective of whether integration is officially present. The challenge of integrated health care is to generate evidence on which illnesses are best treated through which approach. Simultaneous use of both types of treatment was so common that their individual contributions were difficult to assess. Asia has seen the most progress in incorporating its traditional health systems into national policy. Most of this began 30–40 years ago and has accelerated in the past 10 years. In some Asian countries, such as China, the development has been a response to mobilizing all healthcare resources in meeting national objectives for primary health care. In other countries, such as India and South Korea, change has come through politicization of the traditional health sector and a resultant change in national policy. Two basic policy models have been followed: an integrated approach, where modern and traditional medicine are integrated through medical education and practice (for example China and Vietnam), and a parallel approach, where modern and traditional medicine are separate within the national health system (for example India and South Korea).

One of the key reasons for the increased use of complementary medicine in developed countries is the generally accepted perception that 'natural' products are safe, have 'stood the test of time', and do not carry the risks inherent in newly developed conventional 'allopathic' medicines. However, there is insufficient awareness that the ingredients that make traditional medicines effective may also be capable of causing serious illness, such as allergy, liver or kidney malfunction, blindness, cancer, or even death. Herbal medicines should be used with the same degree of caution as conventional medicines but this is difficult given the lack of information available about effectiveness, optimum dose, or adverse effects.

The rapidly increasing use and growing popularity of traditional medicines in developed countries is intriguing and is to some extent being stimulated by increasing scientific interest in herbal medicine. Scientific evidence of efficacy is beginning to emerge from randomized controlled trials in which herbs compare favourably with placebo. Evidence is emerging for herbs such as St John's Wort (used for mild depression), ginkgo biloba (used for some forms of dementia), saw palmetto (used for benign prostatic hyperplasia), and horse chestnut (used for chronic venous insufficiency).

Complementary medicine is becoming more widespread with the surge in immigration, where communities are bringing with them their traditional medical practices. This has the potential to cause difficulties in diagnosis and management by allopathic practitioners in the developed countries to which these patients have migrated. For example, reports from many poisons centres in the USA illustrate the difficulties and the numbers of certain migrant populations that have been affected by the adverse effects of traditional medicines brought from their countries of origin (Haller et al. 2002). Even in Taiwan, where traditional medicines have been in use for centuries, a poison control centre reported experiencing difficulties in managing patients with poisonings associated with Chinese traditional medicines (Deng et al. 1997).

Thus information, at least on the potential dangers of traditional medicines and herbal medicines in particular, has become a necessity for the provision of appropriate and adequate health care to communities in both developed and developing countries.

16.2 Concerns and issues associated with traditional medicines

It is important to be aware of the factors that influence the safety of traditional medicines, particularly herbal medicines. These include the following:

1. The presence of intrinsically toxic constituents to which a patient may be exposed whilst using herbal medicines, and the potential for adulteration and contamination of herbal products. Practitioners or manufacturers may deliberately incorporate allopathic medications that may be banned in some countries or are only available on prescription from an allopathic practitioner in developed countries.

2. There may be disadvantages or danger of delays in seeking allopathic medical care that may be caused by the initial use of herbal medicines of doubtful efficacy for a particular disease state.

3. Some specific population groups may be vulnerable to adverse effects of herbal medicines. These include pregnant women, breast-feeding mothers, infants, and older people.

Such population groups should avoid using herbal preparations or take them only under close supervision.

4. There may be a risk of patients not revealing their use of herbal medicines to allopathic practitioners who may prescribe allopathic medicine prior to surgical interventions and investigations or to treat disease. The interaction of allopathic medicine with herbal medicine could render the allopathic medicine ineffective or could cause life-threatening adverse effects.

5. There may be significant variations in the concentrations of ingredients used in medicines prepared by different manufacturers or at different times and in the potency of those ingredients due to geographical variations, stage of maturity of the plant, or plant component and/or improper storage.

6. The labelling of some herbal medicines may be inaccurate, both in indicating the constituents and the amounts of the constituents used. In addition the labelling may be in a language not familiar to users or local medical practitioners.

7. Socio-cultural, religious, and other factors may result in different therapeutic regimens or dosages of very similar herbal medicines being used for a particular disease state.

8. There is seldom any biochemical or physiological evidence of the efficacy of a herbal medicine on disease state.

9. There is less stringent regulation of herbal medicine practitioners compared to allopathic practitioners. Although schemes for training and assessment of competence and knowledge for the practice of herbal or traditional medicine are being introduced or are already in use in many countries, there are no internationally accepted standards.

Although many countries have systems for monitoring adverse reactions to herbal medicines, for example the yellow card system in the UK, the adverse effects of many herbs are poorly documented, despite medical practitioners and patients being encouraged to report adverse effects. Another factor leading to poor understanding of toxic effects is manufacturers of unlicensed products not complying with normal safety monitoring requirements. In addition, adverse effects may not be attributed to the herbal medicine if the patient does not reveal such use to their doctor. Even when an adverse effect is attributed to the use of a herbal product, the identity and the quantities of the constituents may be uncertain.

16.3 Potentially harmful constituents of herbal medicines

A range of potentially toxic or harmful constituents have been identified in samples of herbal medicines (Ernst 2002; Ko 1998; Steenkamp et al. 2000). These include: heavy metals, allopathic medications (both prescription and over the counter), toxic plant constituents, animal and human body parts, and pesticides.

16.3.1 Heavy metals

One of the earliest published cases of heavy metal poisoning due to the use of a traditional medicine was in 1975 (Tay and Seah 1975). Since then there have been a large number of published reports of such poisonings. A survey of 5536 exposures to traditional medicines and food supplements reported to the National Poisons Unit in London from January 1983 to March 1989 and in 1991 included 657 (12%) reports of symptomatic cases and five confirmed cases of heavy metal poisoning resulting from the use of contaminated traditional remedies (Perharic et al. 1994). The same unit reported 12 cases of poisoning with lead, arsenic, or mercury between 1991 and 1995, nine of which were associated with herbal remedies from India and three with use of Indian cosmetics (Shaw et al. 1995). Lynch and Braithwaite (2005) published 31 cases of poisoning by lead, arsenic, mercury, and magnesium resulting from the use of Indian traditional medicines. The reports came from the UK, USA, Canada, Australia, India, Israel, Germany, The Netherlands, and Qatar. Seventy-one per cent of these patients were of an Indian ethnic origin and 10% were of white ethnic origin. The patients' ages ranged from 9 months to 70 years.

16.3.2 Allopathic adulterants

The prevalence of allopathic medicines in herbal preparations has been of particular concern in Asian countries with large Chinese populations. The Taiwanese Food and Drugs Administration reported that 30% of the antirheumatic and analgesic herbal products that they sampled contained a wide range of allopathic drugs, including analgesics and steroids (NLFD 1991). Another large-scale study in Taiwan analysed 2609 samples and found that 26% contained at least one adulterant, such as acetaminophen and prednisolone (Huang et al. 1997). In Hong Kong, the government laboratory carried out 65,748 tests on Chinese medicines in 2004 (GovHK 2004). Many of the proprietary Chinese medicines on sale for the treatment of obesity and impotence caused the most concern. They were found to contain sidenafil, tadalafil, sibutramine, and N-nitrosofenfluramine. In Malaysia in 1991, 83% of anti-arthritis preparations seized from Chinese medicine shops contained phenylbutazone. 'Black pills' for arthritis, known as 'Zhui Feng Tou Gu Wan' or 'Black Pearls', have also been reported to contain phenylbutazone (Ries and Sahud 1975).

Adulteration is a widespread practice and has been reported in Australia, Belgium, Canada, The Netherlands, New Zealand, the UK and the USA. In 1999, 8 out of 11 Chinese herbal creams available in London for the treatment of eczema were found to contain dexamethasone at concentrations inappropriate for use on the face or in children (Keane et al. 1999). The 1998 Californian survey of imported Asian patent medicines revealed that of the 257 products that were analysed for pharmaceuticals, 17 products contained pharmaceuticals that were not declared on the label (most commonly ephedrine, chlorpheniramine, methyltestosterone, and phenacetin) (Chan 2003). In India, 38% of 120 samples of alternative medicines that had been dispensed to patients suffering mainly from asthma and arthritis were found to be adulterated with steroids (Gupta et al. 2000).

16.3.3 Toxic plants and herbal medicines

Whilst most of the information on the toxicity of plants remains anecdotal, studies on the toxic components of plants have resulted as a result of serious 'unexplained' adverse effects, such as the occurrence of kidney disease (Box 16.1) or liver disease in groups of patients who received a particular form of herbal treatment. The concentrations of the toxic constituents in herbal preparations are an important consideration. The presence of

Box 16.1 Toxic effects on the kidney as a target organ

- **Herbs with direct renal toxicity:** Many traditional medicines and foods, especially in the tropical regions of Africa and Asia, contain plants that can cause renal toxicity. One of the better known plants is the djenkol bean. A traditional remedy in South Africa is 'impila', which is made from the roots of *Callilepis laureola*. It has marked liver and kidney toxicity.

- **Herbs that cause kidney toxicity due to oxalic acid content:** Some herbs high in oxalic acid content, such as rhubarb and star fruit, may increase the formation of kidney stones.

- **Herbs that cause changes in electrolyte (e.g. sodium and potassium) exchange in the kidney:** Licorice root in high doses for prolonged periods causes retention of sodium, which has the potential to increase blood pressure, and a loss of potassium, which leads to hypokalaemia and possibly symptoms such as muscle weakness. It also increases the toxicity of allopathic drugs such as digoxin.

- **Herbs with high potassium content:** The juice from the noni fruit (*Morinda citrifolia*) can cause an increase in blood and body potassium due to its high potassium content. Dandelion, stinging nettle, horsetail, and alfalfa are also high in potassium.

- **Herbs that cause an increase in volume of urine (diuresis):** Juniper berry, parsley, dandelion, horse tail, asparagus root, lovage root, golden rod, uva ursi, stinging nettle leaf, and alfalfa have been used traditionally as diuretics. These drugs should be used cautiously by patients who have compromised kidney function, particularly by those patients who require frequent renal dialysis.

- **Herbs in patients with renal transplants:** The success of renal transplants could be compromised by drugs such as St John's Wort, which decrease the effectiveness of immunosuppressants such as cyclosporin. Echinacea is an immune system modulator and caution is required in patients using immunosuppressants.

Source: Karalliedde and Gawarammana (2007).

a toxic component does not always imply that an adverse effect will follow intake. Thus the concentration of the toxic component, the amount of the herb taken (dosage), and the duration of intake are all important factors in defining the toxicity of plant medicines. For example, with herbal teas and honey, the amount or frequency of consumption is important. Large quantities may be consumed over a long periods, which can lead to toxic effects. Few toxicological studies have been done on herbal tea. It is possible that the method of preparation or formulation may lead to concentration of toxic constituents, especially water-soluble toxins in some herbal teas.

16.3.4 Presence of animal tissue

The inclusion of animal and human products in traditional herbal medicines can have two possible adverse consequences. Firstly, they may transmit infections to the user.

For example, the ingredients of Nu Bao have been found to include human placenta, deer antler, and donkey skin, which are all potential sources of bacteria and viruses. Secondly, some constituents that are used medicinally are toxins themselves, for example the venom extracted from the skin glands of certain species of toads (*Bufo marinus, Bufo alvarius*) used in some Chinese aphrodisiacs. The venom contains bufotoxins, which have similar molecular structure and pharmacological effects to digoxin. These preparations can cause symptoms and clinical findings very similar to digitalis overdose and toxicity, and have led to dangerous alterations in heart rhythm and even death.

16.3.5 Pesticide contaminants

Samples of green tea have been found to be contaminated with DDT pesticides, indicating that herbal preparations can contain pesticides and raising concerns about tea's possible role in the development of breast cancer (Barbee 2008).

Tagami et al. (2008) detected 56 pesticides in natural medicines. The 2004 Annual Report of the Government Laboratories in Hong Kong reported that about 1% of Chinese herbal medicine samples were found to contain levels of pesticides that were of concern (GovHK 2004). In early 2004, some ginseng powder products imported from Taiwan were found to be contaminated with organochlorine pesticide. Since then, all ginseng powder products imported from Taiwan have been screened for the presence of pesticide residues. Contamination of ginseng was also reported in 2002 on the ConsumerLab.com website. Of the 21 ginseng products tested, two had levels of pesticides 20 times more than allowed levels (Aschwanden 2001).

Cumin is commonly used in Egypt for childhood coughs, aches, or itching. A sample of seeds purchased from a local Egyptian market was found to contain the organophosphate insecticide profenfos at a concentration of 0.37 g/kg, which is nearly twice the residue the WHO and Codex Alimentarius Commission permit in vegetables (Karalliedde and Gawarammana 2007). This finding was of concern as children's low body weights may make them vulnerable to the toxicity from the pesticide.

16.4 Population subgroups that are at risk from herbal medicines

Traditional herbal remedies can have particularly serious effects on vulnerable patient subgroups.

16.4.1 During pregnancy

The following groups or classes of herbal medicines should be avoided during pregnancy:

1. those with a tendency to promote or regulate menstruation or cause abortions;
2. those that either directly or indirectly produce contractions of the smooth muscle of the uterus, e.g. laxatives, essential oils, and bitters. These may also cause adverse effects on the developing foetus, such as nervous system abnormalities.
3. those that produce hormonal effects that would either cause feminizing of a male foetus or masculinisation of a female foetus (oestrogenic and androgenic) herbs;

4. those that could cause malformation in the foetus (teratogenic herbs);

5. those that could cause changes in the genetic make-up of the foetus (mutagenic herbs) mutagens.

16.4.2 During breast-feeding

As a general rule, breast-feeding mothers should avoid:

1. remedies containing high doses of herbs containing alkaloids, particularly those that may affect the nervous system, e.g. the Chinese herbs coptis, philodendron (berberine alkaloids), sophora root (oxymantrine), ma-huang (ephedrine), and evodia (rutecarpine);

2. remedies containing high doses of herbs known to have hormonal effects, e.g. fennel, anise, liquorice;

3. herbs containing plant alkaloids known to cause liver and/or kidney damage, e.g. some herbs that contain toxic pyrrolizidine alkaloids are known to cause liver failure;

4. strong purgatives, e.g. aloe or rhubarb root, which can cause diarrhoea or colic in the infant;

5. herbs with a powerful immunosuppressive effect, e.g. tripterygium.

16.4.3 The elderly

Any form of drug therapy in the elderly, whether with allopathic or herbal medicines, is associated with an increased risk of side effects and of those side effects having serious consequences because of decreased metabolism and pre-existing organ damage. In addition, the risk of drug interactions is greater as older people tend to suffer from several diseases and often take a number of medications.

In old age, most functions of the vital organs are decreased and if kidney function is decreased, drugs are likely to be eliminated from the body more slowly, giving a risk of accumulation of drugs and thus of adverse effects and toxicity.

Specific problems include the following:

1. The metabolism of some drugs may be reduced in the elderly.

2. Altered mental activity often occurs in old age due to nerve cells having been lost or damaged or due to some defect in the production and effects of the chemical messengers (neurotransmitters). This results in many elderly patients becoming more sensitive to drugs that act on the nervous system, particularly nervous system depressants such as sedatives and pain killers.

3. Drugs which affect the heart and blood vessels are more likely to lead to low blood pressure and dangerous changes in heart rhythm as a result in older users. This is due to loss of elasticity of the blood vessels and degenerative changes in blood vessel walls and heart muscle cells that occur with ageing.

4. Adverse drug reaction may present differently in the elderly. Vague symptoms should not be ignored. Confusion is often a presenting symptom in older people.

5. Since falls are likely to have serious consequences for the elderly, all precautions should be taken to minimize side effects that might result in falls, such as a decrease in blood pressure or confusion.

16.5 Regulation of traditional medicines in the UK

Globally the preparation, distribution, and marketing of traditional medicines are largely unregulated, although this is changing in some countries. However, new European rules require all herbal medicines to be registered from 1 May 2011. Thus all traditional herbal medicines available in the EU, including the UK, in health food shops, pharmacies, and other outlets must be formally registered and approved before they can be sold. The new requirements are set out in the EU's Traditional Herbal Products Directive (Directive 2004/24/EC 2004), which was agreed in 2004. The directive gives manufacturers of traditional herbal remedies a seven-year transitional period to register their products already on sale in the EU with the relevant national authorities, which for the UK is the Medicines and Healthcare products Regulatory Agency (MHRA 2011). In summary, the new rules mean that only products whose use is 'plausible on the basis of longstanding use and experience' and whose quality and safety are guaranteed will be licensed.

16.6 Conclusions

It is now recognized that about half the population of industrialized countries regularly use complementary medicines. This growth in consumer demand and availability of services for complementary medicine has outpaced the development of regulatory policy by governments and health professions. As Western governments grapple with regulatory and funding policies for complementary medicine, many developing countries have long since addressed these issues. Their experience constitutes a valuable, although largely unexplored, pool of policy data.

There is little controversy that several traditional herbal remedies in particular have stood the test of time. It is also clear that documentation of efficacy and adverse effects, particularly of carcinogenicity and mutagenicity, is sparse when compared to allopathic medications. The variations in preparations, doses, and routes of intake are all influenced by cultural, social, and religious factors. Although herbal medicines will continue to provide affordable and accessible health care to the vast majority of the world population, there is an urgent public health necessity to ensure their safety and to scientifically validate their manufacture or production and usefulness using the criteria used for allopathic medications. In addition, from a health protection and public health perspective, it is necessary to be aware that 'epidemics' of most unusual disease states may occur due to the undeclared use of traditional herbal medicines.

16.7 References

Aschwanden C. (2001) Contamination problems. *B World Health Organ* **79**(7):692.

Barbee M. (2008) Excerpt from *Politically incorrect nutrition*, (Vital Health Publishing), quoted in Worldwide Health.com 28.3.2008. Available at: www.worldwidehealth.com.

Chan K. (2003) Some aspects of toxic contaminants in herbal medicines. *Chemosphere* **52**:1361–1371.

DEFRA. (2005) Project SID 5. Department for Environment, Food and Rural Affairs. Available at: www.defra.gov.uk.

Deng JF, Lin TJ, Kao WF, Chen SS. (1997) The difficulty in handling poisonings associated with Chinese traditional medicines: a poison control centre experience for 1991–1993. *Vet Hum Toxicol* **39**(2):106–114.

Dharmananda S. (2003) Kampo Medicine – The Practice of Chinese Herbal Medicine in Japan. Institute for Traditional Medicine, Portland, Oregon. Available at: http://www.itmonline.org/arts/kampo.htm.

Directive 2004/24/EC. (2004) Directive of the European Parliament and of the Council amending, as regards traditional herbal medicinal products, Directive 2001/83/EC on the Community code relating to medicinal products for human use 20.04.2004. Available at: http://eur-lex.europa.eu/LexUriServ/LexUriServ.do?uri=OJ:L:2004:136:0085:0090:en:PDF.

Ernst E. (2002) Toxic heavy metals and undeclared drugs in Asia herbal medicines. *Trends Pharmacol Science* **23**:136–139.

Gardiner P, Graham RE, Legedza TR, Eisenberg DM, Phillips RS. (2006) Factors associated with dietary supplement use among prescription medication users. *Arch Intern Med.* **166**(18):1968–1974.

GovHK (2004) Government Laboratory Annual Report 2004, Government of Hong Kong, Hong Kong.

Gupta SK, Kaleekal T, Joshi S. (2000) Misuse of corticosteroids in some of the drugs dispensed as preparations from alternative systems of medicine in India. *Pharmacoepidemiol Drug Saf* **9**(7):599–602.

Haller CA, Dyer JE, Ko R, Olson KR. (2002) Making a diagnosis of herbal-related hepatitis. *West J Med* **176**(1):39–44.

Huang WF, Wen KC, Hsiao ML. (1997) Adulteration by synthetic therapeutic substances of traditional Chinese medicines in Taiwan. *J Clin Pharmacol* **37**:344–350.

Karalliedde L, Gawarammana I. (eds) (2007) Traditional herbal medicines – a guide to their safer use. Hammersmith Press, London.

Keane FM, Munn SE, du Vivier AW, Taylor NF, Higgins EM. (1999) Analysis of Chinese herbal creams prescribed for dermatological conditions. *BMJ* **318**:563–564.

Ko RJ. (1998) Adulterants in Asian patent medicines. *N Engl J Med* **339**(12):847.

Lynch E, Braithwaite R. (2005) A review of the clinical and toxicological aspects of traditional (herbal) medicines adulterated with heavy metals. *Expert Opinion Drug Safety* **4**:769–778.

MHRA. (2011) Traditional Herbal Medicines Registration Scheme. Available at: http://www.mhra.gov.uk/Howweregulate/Medicines/Herbalmedicines/PlacingaherbalmedicineontheUKmarket/TraditionalHerbalMedicinesRegistrationScheme/index.htm.

NLFD. (1991) Annual report of National Laboratories of Food and Drugs. Department of Health. Taiwan, ROC.

Perharic I, Shaw D, Coldbridge M, House I, Leon C, Murray V. (1994) Toxicological problems resulting from exposure to traditional remedies and food supplements. *Drug Safety* **11**:284–294.

Ries CA, Sahud MA. (1975) Agranulocytosis caused by Chinese herbal medicines. Dangers of medications containing aminopyrine and phenylbutazone. *JAMA* **231**(4):352–355.

Ross S, Simpson CR, McLay JS. (2006) Homeopathic and herbal prescribing in general practice in Scotland. *Br J Clin Pharmacol* **62**(6):647–652; discussion 645–646. Epub June 23 2006.

Shaw D, House I, Kolev S, Murray V. (1995) Should herbal medicines be licensed? *BMJ* **311**(7002):451–452.

Steenkamp V, Stewart MJ, Zuckerman M. (2000) Clinical and analytical aspects of pyrrolizidine poisoning caused by South African traditional medicines. *Ther Drug Monit* **22**:302–306.

Tagami T, Kajimura K, Satsuki Y et al. (2008). Rapid analysis of 56 pesticide residues in natural medicines by GC/MS with negative chemical ionization. *J Natural Med* **62**(1):126–129.

Tay CH, Seah CS. (1975) Arsenic poisoning from antiasthmatic herbal preparations. *Med J Aust* **2**(11):424–428.

Waxman J. (2006) Shark cartilage in the water. *BMJ* **333**:1129.

WHO. (2003a) Traditional medicine. *Factsheet* 134. World Health Organization, Geneva.

WHO. (2003b) Traditional medicine – Report by the Secretariat. *56th World Health Assembly* A56/18. World Health Organization, Geneva.

WHO. (2006–2011) The WHO Country Cooperation Strategy. India – Supplement on Traditional Medicines WHO secretariat report on Traditional Medicine, 56th World Health Assembly.

Zhang, X. (1999) Traditional medicine worldwide: the role of the WHO. *Drug Info J* **33**:321–328.

16.8 Further reading

Bodeker G. (2001) Lessons on integration from the developing world's experience. Commonwealth Working Group on Traditional and Complementary Health Systems. *BMJ* **322**:164.

Chan TY, Critchley JA. (1996) Usage and adverse effects of Chinese herbal medicines. *Hum Exp Toxicol* **15**(1):5–12.

Corns C, Metcalfe K. (2002) Risks associated with herbal slimming remedies. *J R Soc Promotion Health* **122**(4):213–219.

Karalliedde L, Gawarammana I. (eds) (2007) Traditional herbal medicines – a guide to their safer use. Hammersmith Press, London.

Venter CP, Joubert PH. (1988) Aspects of poisoning with traditional medicines in Southern Africa. *Biomed Environ Sci* **1**:388–391.

Chapter 17

Chemical weapons: deliberate release of chemical agents

David Baker

Learning outcomes

At the end of this chapter the student should be able to:

1. discuss the history, nature, and classification of chemical warfare agents;

2. explain the essential properties of chemical agents and how these determine the management of an incident and the management of the patient;

3. describe and discuss the pathophysiological effects, signs, and symptoms of exposure to chemical agents;

4. explain the military and civil approaches to incident management;

5. evaluate and discuss policies for the management of the incident and the management of the patient, and

6. apply acquired knowledge in the analysis and management of hazardous situations.

17.1 Introduction

Most health professionals in developed nations today have little or no experience of managing victims of chemical warfare. In the early 20th century in Europe the situation was quite different. Chemical warfare was widely used in the static battlefield conditions of World War I and caused many hundreds of thousands of casualties on all sides. During this time, military doctors, nurses, and ambulance teams, most of who had come from civil life, would have been very familiar with the effects of chemical agents. This experience persisted into the period between the two wars. Although chemical weapons were not used in World War II in Europe there was considerable concern that they would be, particularly against civilians by aerial bombardment. During the brief years of peace the experience gained in World War I was put to use and there was detailed planning for managing gas attacks with the mass provision of respirators to civilians.

Following World War II public awareness of chemical weapons gradually diminished. Although they remained a major threat during the Cold War, this was only seen to be a military problem. Elsewhere, civil defence was abandoned and a new generation of health practitioners worked without any training to manage chemical warfare victims other that that they might have gained during military service, which was itself becoming a rarity, particularly in the UK.

Against this, chemical weapons were used in a number of campaigns around the world, notably in the Iran–Iraq War, often with considerable effect, particularly against unprotected civilians. Because of a growing fear of an unknown quantity and the atmosphere of widespread civilian involvement and fear that characterized the Cold War, chemical agents were increasingly seen as 'weapons of mass destruction' in the same light as nuclear and biological agents. It was believed that there was little that could be done for the mass casualties that would be the result of an attack using chemical agents on crowded cities. This view has persisted and has been fuelled by the use of chemical warfare agents by terrorists, highlighting again the vulnerability civil populations.

This situation is, however, at odds with reality. Release of chemicals in the urban environment is almost an everyday occurrence and casualties are managed routinely by the emergency services. However, when dangerous chemicals are released deliberately as a result of terrorist action, the incident takes on an aura that is disproportionate to the real hazards present. There is an element of fear and turbulence that surrounds any report of a possible urban chemical attack, which is often fuelled by the media. Targeted civil populations are vulnerable as a result of lack of organization, protection, and understanding of the real risks, and thus chemical releases lead to a multiplication of panic, which amplifies the effects of the incident. For the terrorist this is a desirable outcome and so the attractions of the release of chemical agents which are relatively easy to produce are magnified.

The objective of this chapter is to present the realities of chemical warfare agents in a simple way from the point of view of the immediate and longer term hazards to health that they present in a civilian setting. The classical and newer agents will be discussed in terms of their characteristics and their effects on the body. Management of any chemical release involves both management of the incident and management of the patient, and a clear understanding of both is essential if health professionals are not to become casualties themselves and the lives of victims are not to be lost as a result of inadequate or inappropriate medical care. Thus the importance of protection and decontamination, and the management of casualty flow will be considered, together with the essentials of life support and specific therapy.

17.2 Chemical warfare agents and weapons

17.2.1 Definitions

A chemical warfare agent may be defined as a chemical substance that is released deliberately to kill, seriously injure, or otherwise incapacitate humans through pathophysiological effects. For a chemical to cause harm either accidental or deliberate release is necessary. Chemical warfare agents, like many dangerous toxic industrial chemicals used in civil life, are not harmful if properly confined. In the military context, release of a chemical to cause harm is achieved by the use of a weapon to distribute it. Shells, bombs, and aerial spraying are the classic methods employed to disperse chemical. Experience in Japan in the 1990s has shown that chemical agents can be released directly in a civil setting by terrorists.

17.2.2 Chemical, biological, radiological, and nuclear agents

Chemical warfare agents have conventionally been considered along with biological and nuclear weapons as 'weapons of mass destruction'. A biological agent may be defined as a self-replicating organism (e.g. bacteria or viruses) deliberately released to cause harm to humans by infection. This results in a deliberate, calculated epidemic. Nuclear weapons cause harm by a massively powerful explosion, which is accompanied by the release of large quantities of radiation and radioisotope contamination.

After World War II, chemical weapons were classified along with biological and nuclear devices as nuclear, biological, and chemical (NBC) agents. This classification has now been expanded to chemical, biological, radiological, and nuclear weapons (CBRN) to include radioisotopes that may be released deliberately using a small conventional explosive charge.

It is important to realise that all CBRN weapons do not cause casualties in the same way. Chemical and biological agents are quite different in their properties, particularly in the time they take to act. Radiological agents are really chemicals that cause harm as a result of the effects of the radiation they release. Nuclear weapons cause harm in a substantially different way. They produce serious physical damage to humans and their environment from the effects of the powerful explosion in a similar way to high explosives but with secondary effects from the released radiation.

17.3 Poisoning in peace and war

Most health professionals are familiar with individual poisoning, either deliberate or suicidal. The use of chemical substances for this end has been known through the ages and is still a feature of modern life. Poisoning is often different from chemical agent release in that medical responders are not usually at risk from the poison. This is a different situation from chemical agent release, where medical teams may be in danger of themselves becoming casualties by being exposed to the released agent that persists on the casualty or his location. Chapter 6 discusses management of chemical incidents in healthcare settings in detail.

The use of chemicals in warfare had been considered for many centuries but it was not until World War I that mass release of chemical was used as part of military activity. Over 113,000 tons of chemicals were used in that war. Mass casualties were often caused when there was an element of surprise. The first major chemical attack was on 22 April 1915, when chlorine released as a cloud caused 15,000 Allied wounded, with 5000 fatalities. However, with the introduction of protective masks such mass fatalities were not usually repeated. The Russians, however, who had little or no protection, suffered over 500,000 casualties from chemical warfare, a fact that had great bearing on the subsequent organization of their army. Box 17.1 outlines the development of chemical agents.

Box 17.1 Development and use of chemical weapons

- 1915   Chlorine, phosgene used
- 1916   Hydrogen cyanide used
- 1917   Mustard gas used
              (many other compounds were tested during the period of WW1)
- 1919   Lewisite weaponized, but not used
- 1925   International treaty banning the use of chemical weapons
- 1936   Mustard gas used in Abyssinia
- 1936–1945   Nerve agents such as sarin developed and weaponized
- 1945–1991   Soviet development of nerve agents and new toxin agents
- 1980s   Mustard gas and nerve agent use in Iran–Iraq War
- 1988   Use of chemical agents against a civilian population in Hallubjah, Iraq
- 1995   First use of a chemical warfare agent by terrorists (Tokyo)
- 2000–   Further development of urban chemical agents and toxins by terrorists

Early chemical attacks in World War I probably fuelled the idea of chemical agents being weapons of mass destruction. In fact the ratio of dead to wounded was less than 8% and was lower than for any other weapon systems used during that war. Explosive shells, on the other hand, had a dead-to-wounded ratio of over 15% and were the cause of 59% of all fatalities on both sides. In later wars where chemical weapons were used, the dead-to-wounded ratio fell further. In the Iran–Iraq War in the 1980s the ratio among 27,000 casualties was less than 1%. By the time of the terrorist chemical attack on the Tokyo subway in 1995 the dead-to-wounded ratio was 0.25% among 5000 casualties. These figures highlight the fact that if modern respiratory and antidote care is available, casualties from chemical warfare agents can be successfully treated.

17.3.1 Medical and civil chemical releases

Most use of chemical agents has been in battle. Where used against unprotected civilians in countries with little or no medical resources, such as Abyssinia in 1936 and Kurdistan in 1988, there has been considerable loss of life. This highlights the major differences between chemical agent use in military and civil situations. These differences are outlined in Table 17.1.

17.3.2 Hazards and threats

The terms 'hazard' and 'threat' are often used interchangeably in the media but have distinct meanings in relation to the dangers from chemical weapons. As noted previously, hazardous chemicals are not dangerous while confined. For a chemical agent to cause

Table 17.1 Comparison of military and civilian exposures to chemical agents

Characteristics	Military	Civil
Chemical agent	Limited range of identified chemical warfare agents	Large range of toxic industrial chemicals—urban release of chemical warfare agents also possible
Nature of release	Expected and detected—deliberate attack	Unexpected and variable detection—accidental release or deliberate urban attack
Detection and identification	Tuned battlefield alarm system and identification systems	No fixed detection systems—mobile identification possible
	Evidence of attack from weapon characteristics	Detection of release usually based on presenting toxidromes
Response	Trained and protected physically fit population	Untrained, unprotected population
	Organized and protected medical response	Fear of attack a strong panic multiplier fuelled by media
		Limited protected medical responses in some areas

harm (1) it must be available to the user, (2) it must be deliverable through a weapon system, and (3) the assailant must have the intention and the ability to use it. Thus threat is a function of a number of factors, which may be expressed as follows:

$$threat = f \,(available\ hazard + delivery\ means + intention)$$

17.3.3 Chemical and biological hazards

Chemical and biological weapons (CBW) are usually considered to be separate. However, they can be regarded as a spectrum of hazards, ranging from low to high molecular weight substances through to self-replicating organisms (Box 17.2). The advantage of this concept medically is that agents with different physical properties can be grouped according to their pathophysiological effects and the medical responses that are available for treatment.

Examples of the pathophysiological effects of CBW agents are:

- cellular disruption—DNA cross linking;
- toxic pulmonary oedema;
- receptor binding (neuromuscular junction, nerve ion channels, GABA); and
- bacterial toxin release.

17.4 Toxicology of chemical warfare agents

Chemical warfare agents have been extensively tested over the years in laboratory animals but there are very few direct toxicological data available for humans. Thus expressions of toxicity in terms of LD_{50} are derived from experimental data (see Chapter 3 for details of determining toxicity experimentally). An expression commonly used for toxicity of inhaled agents is LCt_{50}. This is the chemical concentration in milligrams per cubic metre multiplied by the time of exposure in minutes to cause death in 50% of an exposed population.

Box 17.2 The chemical and biological weapon spectrum

Chemical agents————**Toxins** ————————— **Biological agents**

Small molecular	higher molecular	self-replicating
weight, simple	weight, complex	organism
e.g. sarin	e.g. botulinum toxin	e.g. smallpox

1. Uses of the CBW spectrum

Chemical and biological warfare agents are usually viewed as being separate weapons but in terms of their effects in humans they may be viewed as a continuous spectrum of hazards. The spectrum ranges from low molecular weight chemical agents through to self-replicating organisms such as viruses and bacteria. Toxins, which are chemicals with molecular weights ranging from 1000 to about 1,000,000, are chemical substances usually of biological origin (e.g. from bacteria, animals, or plants). The value of the CBW spectrum is that agents from different parts of the spectrum have common mechanisms or act at the same site. A good example of this is the nerve agents such as the chemical sarin, which blocks the neuromuscular junction, and botulinum toxin (produced by the organism *Clostridium botulinum*), which does the same but at a different receptor site. In terms of medical management, both lead to a failure of transmission of nerve impulses to muscle fibres and paralysis, and require common emergency life support measures.

2. Properties of agents of the CBW spectrum

Agents in the CBW spectrum each possess four distinct properties: toxicity, latency of action, persistency, and transmissibility.

◆ **Toxicity and latency of action:** determined by toxicodynamics and toxicokinetics.

◆ **Persistency and transmissibility:** determined by physico-chemical properties.

Expressions of toxicity for CW agents are discussed in the main text. Latency may be expressed as L_{50}, the time taken for signs to develop in 50% of an exposed population. This covers a time span ranging from seconds to hours for chemical agents and days in the case of biological agents (a period most familiar as 'incubation time'). Persistency and transmissibility are related to the physical properties of the agents and characterize the ability of agents to remain where they have been released and the risk of contamination or infection being passed to others. Toxicity and latency determine the management of the patient whereas persistency and transmissibility determine the management of the chemical agent released.

Data from Baker, The chemical–biological spectrum of toxic hazards, *Jane's Intelligence Review*, **5**(1), 1993.

The problem with the expression is that the amount of agent inhaled depends on the rate and depth of breathing: persons breathing quickly and deeply will inspire a greater quantity of agent than those breathing normally. However, LCt_{50} is a useful comparison of the effective toxicity to humans of different chemical warfare agents. Toxicity values of a range of chemical agents are shown in Box 17.3.

Box 17.3 Chemical warfare agents: expressions of toxicity

Expressions commonly used to measure toxicity:

- LD_{50} Lethal dose required to kill 50% of test animals, extrapolated to humans. Expressed as weight of chemical per kilogram bodyweight (mg/kg).

- LCt_{50} Lethal dose required to kill 50% of test animals over time. Usual expression for inhalational pathway. Expressed as concentration × time for 50% lethality $(mg.min/m^3)$ The product of concentration × time is known as the 'lethal index'.

Toxicity of CBW agents in LCt_{50} values $(mg.min/m^3)$

- GA (tabun): 150
- GB (sarin): 70–100
- GD (soman): 40–60
- Phosgene: 3200
- Sulphur mustard: 1500
- Lewisite: 1200
- Hydrogen cyanide: 3000

Botulinum toxin

- Based on experimental toxicology botulinum toxin (BoTx) is 15,000 times more toxic than VX and 100,000 times more toxic than GB.

Data from Marrs et al. (eds), Chemical warfare agents: toxicology and treatment, 2nd edition, John Wiley and Sons, 2007.

17.4.1 Pathophysiological effects of chemical warfare agents

Chemical warfare agents have effects on all the functional systems of the body, including the central and peripheral nervous systems, the skin and mucus membranes, the gastro-intestinal and urinary systems, the blood and bone marrow, and the cardiac and respiratory systems. The effects on the respiratory system are the most important since these lead to respiratory failure and subsequent cardiac arrest. Effects on the respiratory system may be on the airway, alveolar gas exchange, or on the control and muscular activity of dia-phragm and chest wall movement. Such effects are mediated via the autonomic and vol-untary nervous system. Respiratory failure is the final pathway leading to death from chemical warfare agents.

17.5 Classification of chemical warfare agents

It is convenient to consider chemical warfare agents in terms of the conventional military classification but it should be remembered that this classification serves just as well as models for many industrial chemicals that cause similar pathophysiology. Box 17.4 lists the conventional military classification.

Box 17.4 Classification of chemical warfare agents

- **Nerve agents**
  - Tabun, sarin, soman, VX
- **Lung-damaging agents (choking agents)**
  - Chlorine, phosgene
- **Agents affecting tissue respiration ('blood' agents)**
  - Hydrogen cyanide, cyanogens
- **Vesicants**
  - Mustard gas, Lewisite
- **Disabling and knock-down agents**
  - Tear gases, ?opioids

Data from MOD, Medical Manual of Defence Against Chemical Agents, 1987.

17.5.1 Nerve agents

These are highly toxic organophosphate compounds developed as chemical warfare agents from pesticide research by Schrader in 1936. Following secret development during World War II, nerve agents became a major threat during the Cold War. A nerve agent was almost certainly used in the attack against Kurds in Hallabjah, Iraq, in 1988. The nerve agent sarin was used in the terrorist attack in Tokyo in 1995.

17.5.1.1 Actions

Acetyl cholinesterase (AChE) is a key enzyme at all sites in the nervous system where acetyl choline (ACh) is the chemical transmitter. Chemical nerve agents can cause non-reversible inhibition of AChE throughout the cholinergic system, leading to a build up of ACh and a continuous overstimulation of the synapses. The increased concentrations of ACh at muscarinic and nicotinic sites give rise to signs and symptoms related to the basic pharmacology of the cholinergic nervous system (see Chapter 2 and the appendix for further information). As a result there are acute, intermediate, and long-term effects of organophosphate poisoning. Acutely excessive stimulation of the autonomic nerve system produces excess secretions with airway blockage, bronchospasm, bradycardia, gastric, and urinary effects. Excessive stimulation of the neuromuscular junction produces initial fasciculation (twitching of groups of muscle fibres) and flaccid (depolarizing) muscle paralysis requiring ventilation, which may resolve following oxime therapy.

Following an initial recovery there may be renewed paralysis after 24 hours in 20% of cases. This may last several days and is of a different type to the initial paralysis (non-depolarization paralysis).

17.5.1.2 Toxins

Neurotoxins can block the transmission of impulses along the nerves. Many natural neurotoxins are produced by insects, reptiles, and marine organisms but few are feasible as CBW agents. An example is saxitoxin, which is produced by a small marine organism and blocks the sodium channels in the nerve on which normal transmission of impulses depends.

Botulinum toxin, from the bacterium *Clostridium botulinum*, acts by inhibition of release of ACh at the nerve terminal, causing failure of cholinergic nerve transmission. The classic pattern of botulism is a gradual paralysis setting in several hours after eating contaminated food. Botulinum toxin is the most toxic substance known to humans but its toxicity is greatly reduced by life support and antitoxin intervention.

17.5.2 Lung damaging agents (pulmonary oedemagens)

Lung-damaging agents were used as chemical weapons during World War I. Chlorine was first used in 1915 and was followed by phosgene, the properties of which are described in Box 17.5. These agents caused both upper and lower damage to the airways and lungs, and were fatal due to the onset of pulmonary oedema, where the lung alveoli fill with fluid and normal oxygenation of the blood fails. Lung-damaging agents were eclipsed during the Cold War by more toxic agents such as nerve agents but a new threat arose from per-fluoro isobutylene (PFIB), which is known in the civil context as a by-product of heating Teflon.

Box 17.5 Properties of phosgene

Uses of phosgene

- Chemical warfare gas and major industrial use.
- Liquid/vapour can be formed accidentally by decomposition of chlorinated hydrocarbons.

Symptoms of phosgene exposure

- Acute and chronic exposure causes toxic pulmonary oedema (PE).
- Exposure causes initial upper respiratory symptoms of pronounced cough, dyspnoea, and 'choking'.
- The latent period between exposure and symptoms is dose dependent:
  - high dose: 1–4 hours;
  - low dose: 8–24 hours.

Toxic effects and dose

- 1 ppm chronically: chronic lung disease (NB: below odour threshold).
- >25 ppm.min: acute lung effects.
- 50–150 ppm.min: initial inflammatory response, which may be followed by PE.
- >150 ppm.min: clinically significant and life-threatening PE.
- 800 ppm for 2 minutes: lethal.

Data from Marrs et al. (eds), Chemical warfare agents: toxicology and treatment, 2nd edition, John Wiley and Sons, 2007.

There are many toxic industrial chemicals which cause pulmonary oedema. Both phosgene and chlorine are widely used in the chemical industry. In addition, isocyanates are also used in many synthetic processes. A release of methyl-isocyanate in Bhopal, India (1984) caused over 5000 deaths from pulmonary oedema.

17.5.3 Vesicant agents

Chemical warfare agents which attacked the skin and mucous membranes were also developed and used during World War I. The best known, mustard gas (which is actually an oily liquid at normal temperatures), caused many hundreds of thousands of casualties, mostly with disabling rather than fatal injuries. Mustard gas was used again in the Iran–Iraq War during the 1980s.

The signs and symptoms of mustard gas poisoning are shown in Box 17.6. Characteristic effects include severe conjunctivitis, vesication, and ulceration of the skin, an example of which can be seen in Figure 17.1.

17.5.4 Agents affecting tissue respiration (cyanides)

Cyanide agents include the gas hydrogen cyanide (HCN) and the cyanogens. Following inhalation they act very quickly (short latency) and in high concentrations cause death by interfering with the normal function of oxygen at the mitochondria in the body cells. Early antidote therapy is essential for management. This involves either producing a variant of haemoglobin in the red cells of the blood (methaemoglobin), which binds to cyanide and renders it ineffective, or accelerating the breakdown of HCN by the enzyme rhodonase, which can be achieved by providing sodium thiosulphate. Another approach is to use dicobalt edetate. HCN combines with heavy metals and the cobalt ions in this compound act to remove HCN. The properties of cyanide are described in Box 17.7.

17.6 Practical realities for the emergency medical management of chemical casualties

Exposure to chemical warfare agents is a rare event that is unfamiliar to most emergency responders in the UK. However, there are many lessons which apply to the management of

Box 17.6 Signs and symptoms of mustard gas poisoning

- Early smell of garlic, then latent sign-free period.
- After 2–6 hours: nausea, fatigue, headache, eye inflammation and pain, lachrymation, blepharospasm, photophobia, and rhinorrhoea.
- Hoarse voice and development of erythema to skin.
- Exacerbation of above symptoms with blister formation to inner thighs, perineum, and other sweat areas.
- Development of chemical bronchiolitis in high-temperature exposure.

Data from MOD, Medical Manual of Defence Against Chemical Agents, 1987.

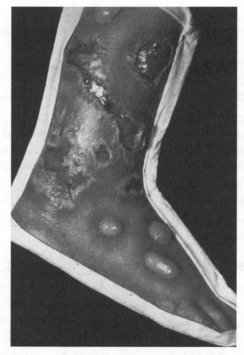

Fig. 17.1 Mustard gas vesication with ulceration. Courtesy of the Ministry of Defence, London (MOD 1987).

accidental chemical release in the civil arena that are direct parallels of the measures required for the safe management of chemical warfare agent casualties. The key issues are (1) to ensure the safety of the responders and to prevent secondary casualties, and (2) to provide essential life support and antidotes to casualties to prevent loss of life from respiratory failure.

Chemical agent release management can therefore be divided into (1) management of the incident and (2) management of the patient.

The key steps in management are:

- planning
- incident management

Box 17.7 Actions of hydrogen cyanide

- Short latency.
- Binds to Fe^{3+} atom on cytochrome oxidase in mitochondria, uncouples electron receptor action of oxygen, and disrupts production of ATP.
- Cellular tissue oxygen concentrations are initially normal.
- Advanced life-support measures may not be effective.
- Early antidote therapy essential.

Data from Marrs et al. (eds), Chemical warfare agents: toxicology and treatment, 2nd edition, John Wiley and Sons, 2007.

- protection
- triage
- resuscitation and immediate therapy
- decontamination, and
- continuing care.

17.6.1 Chemical incidents: the civil Hazmat response

To respond safely to contaminated casualties following chemical agent release, protection of the medical responders is essential. Medical and paramedical staff are now trained and equipped in many countries to be able to wear level C protection (Figure 17.2). This consists of a filtration respirator, which filters the contaminated atmosphere through activated charcoal, and a protective suit and gloves. The length of time such a suit can be worn in a contaminated zone depends on the level of contamination. The level C suit is the civilian equivalent of the military NBC suit, which is worn to protect troops against the most toxic chemical warfare agents.

In the civil context, chemical releases are managed by describing zones around the release. These are (1) the hot zone around the site of release, where direct contamination risk is highest, (2) the warm zone outside the hot zone, where contamination is usually secondary and transmitted by contaminated persons leaving the hot zone, and (3) the cold zone outside the warm zone, where contamination is minimal. Between the warm and cold zones is the decontamination unit, where patients are decontaminated before

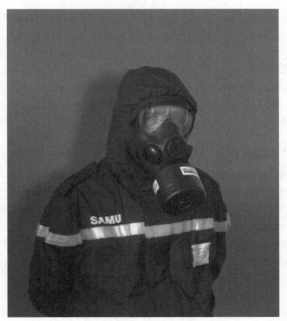

Fig. 17.2 Level C protective equipment worn by a medical officer of the Paris Emergency Medical Service. Courtesy of SAMU de Paris.

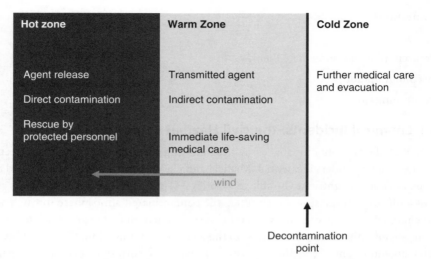

Hot zone	Warm Zone	Cold Zone
Agent release	Transmitted agent	Further medical care and evacuation
Direct contamination	Indirect contamination	
Rescue by protected personnel	Immediate life-saving medical care	

wind →

Decontamination point

Fig. 17.3 Arrangement of contamination and zones following a chemical release.

being evacuated further. Figure 17.3 shows the standard arrangement of these zones following chemical agent release in the civil setting.

The hot zone contains the highest level of contamination. Victims are rescued by protected fire personnel and taken to the warm zone to await decontamination. Here protected medical responders may have to provide essential life support before patients are decontaminated: this is the basis of the UK hazardous area response teams (HART), who provide early treatment dynamically integrated with decontamination. The HART teams, which were set up in 2006, provide specially trained and equipped paramedic teams who can operate safely in a contaminated zone (Figure 17.4). They are trained to administer specific antidotes for chemical agents and to provide airway and ventilatory support. Equipment includes a full range of protective equipment, antidotes, airway management devices, and an automatic ventilator designed to operate in a contaminated zone (Figure 17.5).

17.6.2 Practical aspects of the treatment for chemical casualties

Early advanced life support and antidote therapy must be provided by specially trained medical and paramedical personnel working in the contaminated zone wearing level C protection. This care includes essential provision of airway and ventilatory support for victims with impending respiratory arrest, which is the main cause of death following chemical agent exposure. Triage of patients is also required in the contaminated zone to give priority of decontamination and evacuation to those who are most seriously injured.

Care given prior to decontamination is termed TOXALS (the provision of advanced life support in a contaminated area). This is an extension of the familiar ABC (airway, breathing, and circulatory support) of basic and advanced life support. The elements of TOXALS are shown in Box 17.8.

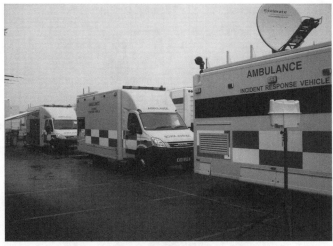

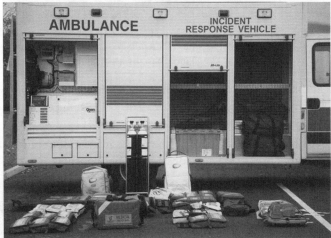

Fig. 17.4 HART team response vehicles, 2006. Courtesy of HART team response vehicles, 2011.

Once a patient has been decontaminated and stabilized, continuing airway, ventilatory, and antidote treatment through to the hospital emergency room and, for severely affected cases, the intensive care unit is essential.

17.7 Chemical agent release in a civil setting: some lessons from recent history

In recent years, chemical agents have been used by urban terrorists. Chemical agent exposure should therefore now be regarded as a civil as well as a military hazard. Examples are:

♦ Tokyo, 1995: the nerve gas sarin was released into the underground railway system (Box 17.9).

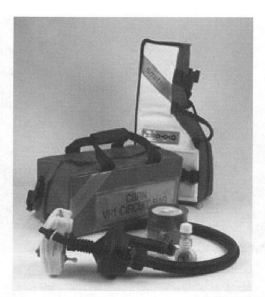

Fig. 17.5 Life support in a contaminated area, 2012: the Pneupac VR1 ventilator with patient circuit filtration. Courtesy of Pneupac Ventilation, Smiths Medical International, Luton, UK.

◆ USA, 2001: anthrax spores were sent through the post. Anthrax is a biological warfare agent that kills by producing anthrax toxin. This can also be considered a chemical agent in its own right.

◆ Moscow, 2003: in order to end a siege by terrorists in a theatre, security forces used a chemical compound producing rapid onset of unconsciousness (a knock-down agent)

Box 17.8 Life support for chemical warfare agent casualties (TOXALS)

Assessment (patient and site)

Airway

Breathing (requirement for artifical ventilation)

Circulation—control of haemorrhage and cardiac abnormalities

Disability (level of unconsciousness)

Drugs and antidotes

Decontamination

Evacuation to hospital care

Reproduced from Baker, Advanced life support for acute toxic injury (TOXALS), *Eur J Emerg Med* 3(4):256–62, 1996 with permission from Lippincott, Williams and Wilkins.

Box 17.9 Case study: the Tokyo sarin incident, 1995

Primary casualties

- 688 victims were transported to hospitals by ambulance.
- >4000 casualties reached hospitals either on foot or by private transport.
- 5510 sought medical attention in 278 hospitals and clinics.
- 12 patients died from respiratory failure.

Occupational health consequences

- Of 1364 fire emergency personnel who were at the incident, 135 (9.9%) showed acute symptoms and received medical treatment.
- 23% of staff at St Luke's Hospital had secondary exposure and developed signs and symptoms:
  - 39.3% of nurse assistants
  - 26.5% of nurses
  - 21.8% of doctors
  - 18.2% of clerks.

Medical lessons learnt from the Tokyo sarin incident

1. Many contaminated patients left the release site and came to hospital, where they contaminated the medical and nursing staff.
2. Careful cordon control of contaminated persons is required and decontamination should be carried out before sending patients on to hospital.
3. Strain on medical and ventilation resources may occur. The most severely injured patients require life support with artificial ventilation to survive.
4. Patients with severe and moderate poisoning required follow-up with evaluation to determine long-term adverse health effects, including neurotoxic and behavioural effects.
5. Disaster planning should include mass casualties from chemical exposure: both acute and chronic effects.

Data from Okumura et al., The Dark Morning in Marrs et al. (eds) Chemical warfare agents: toxicology and treatment, 2nd edition, John Wiley and Sons, 2007, pp. 277–286, 2007.

which was claimed to be an opioid of the fentanyl class, a compound used widely during general anaesthesia. The agent was non-persistent but responders wore protective equipment and respirators. Due to poor management of casualties, there were deaths among both terrorists and hostages from acute respiratory failure.

These incidents, and the continuing concern that terrorists will strike again using chemical agents, underline the importance of understanding the risks and management of chemical agent releases by all healthcare workers.

17.8 Conclusions

Chemical agents are part of a chemical–biological toxic agent spectrum. Release of CBW agents by terrorists in civilian settings has been shown to be possible and medical services should be prepared to respond accordingly. The essential characteristics of toxic agents determine both the incident and casualty management, and careful site management is essential to avoid secondary casualties. CBW casualties can be managed using standard medical skills but protection and training of emergency and healthcare personnel is essential. Good incident management and early life support affects the prognosis and can break the link between mass injury and mass loss of life.

17.9 References

Baker DJ. (1993) The chemical—biological spectrum of toxic hazards, Jane's Intelligence Review **5**(1).

Baker DJ. (1996) Advanced life support for acute toxic injury (TOXALS). Eur J Emerg Med **3**(4):256–262.

Marrs TC, Maynard RL, Sidell FR (eds) (2007) *Chemical warfare agents: toxicology and treatment*, 2nd edn. John Wiley and Sons, Chichester, UK, Chapter 13, pp 277–286.

Ministry of Defence. (1987) *Medical Manual of Defence Against Chemical Agents*. D/Med (F and S) (2)/10/1/1 p1–1. HMSO, London.

Okumura T, Nomura T, Suzuki T et al. (2007) The Dark Morning: The Experiences and Lessons Learned from the Tokyo Subway Sarin attack. In: Chemical Warfare Agents: Toxicology and Treatment, Marrs T, Maynard R and Sidell F (eds). Wiley and Sons Ltd, Chichester, UK, Chapter 13, pp 277–286.

17.10 Further reading

Harris R, Paxman J. (2003) *A higher form of killing. (Dark Shadows)*, 2nd edn. Arrow Books, London.

Kaplan D, Marshall A. (1996) The Cult at the End of the World. Random House, New York.

Zaitchuk R, Bellamy RF (eds) (1997) *Medical Aspects of Chemical and Biological Warfare*. United States Army Textbook of Military Medicine, Department of the Army, Office of the Surgeon General, Borden Institute, Washington, DC.

Chapter 18

Combustion toxicology

James C. Wakefield and Robert L. Maynard

Learning outcomes

At the end of this chapter and any recommended reading the student should be able to:

1. understand types of fires and smoke composition;
2. describe the properties of common toxic combustion products;
3. understand the formation of hazardous combustion products as a function of the fuel producing them;
4. apply acquired knowledge to the analysis of hazardous situations arising from products of combustion.

18.1 Introduction

The pyrolysis and combustion of materials can result in the generation of smoke containing many toxic products. These products of combustion can cause irritation, incapacitation, systemic toxicity, and asphyxiation, and may be lethal following acute exposures. Some of the common toxic chemicals which may be present in fire effluent include asphyxiant gases, such as carbon monoxide (CO) and hydrogen cyanide (HCN), irritant gases such as hydrogen chloride (HCl), oxides of nitrogen (NO_x), acrolein, and phosgene, as well as complex molecules such as polycyclic aromatic hydrocarbons (PAHs). The amounts of toxic products evolved during combustion vary with the type of combustion, the availability of oxygen, the temperature, and the materials involved. Therefore, the conditions of combustion will affect the severity of the adverse health effects in those exposed to the products of combustion.

18.2 Types of fires and smoke composition

The thermal breakdown of materials can occur under a number of different conditions (availability of oxygen, availability of combustible materials, and temperature), which can affect how complete the degradation of the material may be.

Thermal degradation can be classified into four main types:

- flaming combustion, well ventilated;
- flaming combustion, ventilation-controlled;

- oxidative pyrolysis (smouldering);
- anaerobic pyrolysis.

Thermal breakdown of materials in a 'normal oxygen' environment in the presence of flaming can be described as well ventilated, flaming combustion. Flaming combustion is the highly efficient burning of materials above the auto-ignition temperature in the presence of sufficient oxygen (Norris and Ballantyne 1999). Flaming combustion of a material in a normal oxygen environment produces complete oxidation of that material, producing only water and carbon dioxide. However, in most cases carbon dioxide and water will not be the only products of combustion under these conditions because of the presence of other elements in the atmosphere and in the fuel for the fire. For example, in a normal oxygen environment, nitrogen in the combustion atmosphere will also undergo oxidation to form nitrogen dioxide. Initially, under the conditions of well-ventilated combustion, the production of smoke and toxic compounds tends to be low, with more toxic products formed as the fire develops (Department of Health 1996).

Thermal degradation of materials in a low oxygen environment in the presence of flaming can be described as ventilation-controlled flaming combustion. Ventilation-controlled fires occur when the air supply is restricted compared with the amount of fuel available for combustion. Most fires in confined spaces (such as in buildings) become ventilation controlled fairly early on in the stages of combustion. Ventilation-controlled fires may be either small enclosed fires or large post-flashover fires. The reduction in oxygen present in these types of fires leads to the production of high yields of carbon monoxide, carbon dioxide, hydrogen cyanide, other organic and inorganic gases, and smoke (Department of Health 1996; Norris and Ballantyne 1999).

Oxidative pyrolysis or smouldering is the thermal breakdown and chemical conversion of materials in a normal oxygen environment, but in the absence of flaming. Smouldering combustion progresses at a much slower rate than flaming combustion, most commonly involves a porous fuel material, and is sustained by the heat given off during oxidation at the fuel surface (Ohlemiller 2002). Pyrolysis occurs at much lower temperatures than flaming combustion and is defined as the thermal degradation of a material below the auto-ignition temperature (Norris and Ballantyne 1999). During pyrolysis, oxidation occurs at the surface of the solid material, in contrast to flaming combustion in which it occurs within the gas phase around the material. Smouldering combustion may occur in the initial stage of a fire and can provide a pathway to flaming combustion from a heat source that is insufficient, per se, to produce a flame (Ohlemiller 2002). Smouldering is a form of incomplete combustion due to the lower temperatures involved, and therefore may yield a much greater quantity of toxic products than flaming combustion (Department of Health 1996; Ohlemiller 2002).

Anaerobic pyrolysis can be described as thermal degradation of materials in a low oxygen environment and the absence of flaming (Norris and Ballantyne 1999). This type of combustion may be initiated as oxidative pyrolysis, but can continue in a low oxygen environment, such as may occur following depletion of oxygen during pyrolysis in a closed compartment. In this situation, the higher the temperature of the combustion environment, the lower the amount of oxygen required. Anaerobic pyrolysis is similar to smouldering combustion in that the chemical conversion is incomplete and will therefore produce much greater quantities of toxic products than flaming combustion. However, because of the further limitation of oxygen in the case of anaerobic pyrolysis, this situation may yield more toxic compounds than oxidative smouldering. There is no infallible sign to distinguish the progression from oxidative pyrolysis to anaerobic pyrolysis, and therefore both cases of pyrolysis are commonly described as smouldering or non-flaming fires (Department of Health 1996; Ohlemiller 2002).

These four types of fire may occur simultaneously at different locations within the fire environment or one may be prevalent (Norris and Ballantyne 1999). The composition of smoke in a combustion environment depends on a number of variables and can be complex due to the dynamic nature of a fire. Some of the principal factors affecting smoke composition include the nature of the fuels (chemical composition, structure, and formulation), the stage of combustion (smouldering, flaming, or post-flashover), the temperature of combustion, and the availability of oxygen and ventilation in the fire environment (Norris and Ballantyne 1999; Levin and Kuligowski 2006; Tewarson 1996).

18.3 Common toxic combustion products

The gaseous products formed during the combustion of most organic materials can be divided into two main categories on the basis of their toxicity. The first category relates to fire smoke components which have asphyxiant properties; depletion of the ambient air of oxygen also falls into this category. The second category includes components which cause irritation, either as sensory irritants affecting the eyes and upper respiratory tract (nose, mouth, and throat) or as pulmonary irritants (affecting the lungs), although in many cases sensory and pulmonary irritation may be present simultaneously. A third category is occasionally used to describe products which may give rise to effects unlike those produced by the two main categories. There are, however, few documented cases of specific toxic combustion products which fall into this third category (Hartzell 1996). Also included in this third category are toxic chemicals which may be present at the site of the fire and do not undergo decomposition in the combustion atmosphere. This may be an important consideration in scenarios such as a fire at a chemicals factory or warehouse.

18.3.1 Asphyxiant gases

Asphyxiant gases cause collapse, unconsciousness, and death by depriving the body of oxygen (Purser 1992; Hartzell 1996). The principal asphyxiants produced during the combustion of organic materials are carbon monoxide, hydrogen cyanide, and carbon dioxide; ambient air with a significantly reduced oxygen content is also regarded as an asphyxiant (Purser 1992; Department of Health. 1996; Hartzell 1996; Norris and Ballantyne 1999). These can interact, producing additive effects.

Chemical asphyxiants prevent the normal uptake of oxygen by tissues by interfering with specific elements in oxygen delivery and metabolic processes, such as carbon monoxide and hydrogen cyanide. Simple asphyxiants are physiologically inert gases that, if inhaled, displace oxygen from the alveoli and lead to hypoxia, such as carbon dioxide, nitrogen, and methane.

18.3.1.1 Carbon monoxide

Carbon monoxide (CO) is the most common asphyxiant product in most fire environments and is formed during both smouldering and flaming combustion of all organic materials (Purser and Berrill 1983; Hartzell 1996. The production of CO in a fire is dependent upon the availability of oxygen, with an increase in CO formation with decreasing availability of O_2 (Hartzell 1996). The production of CO is therefore greater in cases of ventilation-controlled combustion. At the point of flashover, the production of CO increases significantly due to the combustion becoming ventilation-controlled and the rapid increase in the mass burning rate (Hartzell 1996).

Carbon monoxide causes tissue hypoxia by reducing oxygen transport by, and release from, haemoglobin. The affinity of carbon monoxide for haemoglobin is 200–250 times that of oxygen. Each molecule of fully oxygenated haemoglobin carries four molecules of oxygen; as each molecule is released the likelihood of another molecule being released is increased, producing the well-known sigmoid dissociation curve. Binding of carbon monoxide in precisely the same way as oxygen not only reduces the number of oxygen molecules that can be transported but also interferes with the release of such oxygen molecules as are carried and causes a left-shift of the dissociation curve, thus reducing the availability of oxygen to the tissues (Hartzell 1996; Maynard and Waller 1999; Norris and Ballantyne 1999). The concentration of COHb in the blood will be elevated in most cases in individuals exposed to a combustion atmosphere, with the concentration of COHb being dependent on the duration of exposure and the concentration of CO in the fire environment. The presence of COHb in low concentrations in the blood of individuals exposed to a fire atmosphere may be difficult to interpret, since environmental factors (e.g. an urban environment or tobacco smoking) may be associated with raised levels of COHb (Norris and Ballantyne 1999). Most fatalities following inhalation of CO have a concentration of COHb in the blood greater than 50% (Kaplan and Hartzell 1984; Norris and Ballantyne 1999; Health Protection Agency 2007a). A post-mortem COHb concentration of greater than or equal to 70% following acute exposure to CO can be associated with fatality caused directly by CO poisoning alone. A COHb concentration in the range of 30–70% is likely to be associated with a cause of death due to a combination of CO poisoning and other factors, such as the presence of additional toxic combustion products. For a fatality in which there is a COHb concentration of less than 30%, the main cause of death is likely to be due to effects other than CO poisoning (Maeda et al. 1996).

Acute health effects resulting from CO-induced hypoxia at concentrations below that causing lethality can include neurological effects such as headache, dizziness, confusion, disorientation, loss of coordination, memory loss, fainting, cerebral oedema, and coma (International Programme on Chemical Safety 1999; Norris and Ballantyne 1999). These neurological effects of CO exposure in a fire environment may hinder the ability to perform tasks, recognize danger, and escape from a hazardous fire situation (Norris and Ballantyne 1999). Neurological symptoms following severe acute toxicity may appear

2–40 days post exposure and include lethargy, irritability, and lack of concentration, and possible severe effects including dementia and psychosis, which may not all be related to CO-induced hypoxia (Health Protection Agency 2007a). Inhalation of CO is also likely to give rise to metabolic acidosis (International Programme on Chemical Safety 1999; Norris and Ballantyne 1999). The heart is particularly sensitive to the effects of CO, and acute exposure may give rise to cardiovascular effects, including heart failure, myocardial function, hypotension, cardiac arrhythmias, shock, circulatory failure, and cardiac arrest (Stewart 1975; Institute for Environment and Health 1998). Pregnant women, the foetus *in utero*, and newborn infants are at an increased risk from CO exposure. CO readily crosses the placenta and binds to foetal haemoglobin with a higher affinity than for maternal haemoglobin. CO is also cleared from foetal blood much slower than from maternal blood, resulting in a 10–15% increase in COHb formation in the foetus relative to the mother (Health Protection Agency 2007a).

The reader is referred to Chapter 13 for further information on CO poisoning.

18.3.1.2 Hydrogen cyanide

Any organic material containing carbon and nitrogen will produce hydrogen cyanide (HCN) during combustion under most conditions. Polymers such as nylons, polyurethanes, and polyacrylonitrile are all known to be prominent sources of HCN on thermal decomposition or combustion (Bertol et al. 1983; Purser and Wooley 1983; Norris and Ballantyne 1999). The yield of HCN from the combustion of materials containing nitrogen is dependent on the temperature and availability of oxygen in the fire environment. In an oxygen-limited environment, the generation of HCN is initiated at high temperatures, with the yield increasing with further increases in temperature. In air, the evolution of HCN begins at much lower temperatures than in an anaerobic environment, with the yield increasing with temperature up to around 625°C. However, at temperatures in the range of approximately 625–925°C the yield of HCN decreases, followed by a secondary increase as the temperature rises above this range (Urhas and Kullik 1977; Norris and Ballantyne 1999). One study has shown that the generation of HCN is proportional to the nitrogen content of the polymer involved in the combustion (Morikawa 1978). However, there is also evidence to suggest that the yield of HCN may not be proportional to the nitrogen content of the burning material since the yield of HCN from polyacrylonitrile (1500 ppm) has been shown to be around 7.5 times greater than from wool (200 ppm), although the nitrogen content of the two materials is similar (19% and 14.3%, respectively) (Bertol et al. 1983).

Following exposure and systemic uptake, HCN undergoes dissociation in the blood to form the cyanide ion. The cyanide ion is readily distributed within the body and is responsible for the toxicity of HCN by reducing the cellular utilization of oxygen (cellular respiration). The cyanide ion binds to cytochrome oxidase, a principal enzyme involved in the utilization of oxygen, and inhibits it by forming a cytochrome oxidase–cyanide complex. The inhibition of cytochrome oxidase results in a rapid onset of cytotoxic hypoxia and loss of cellular function. The heart and brain are particularly susceptible to the effects of cyanide on cellular respiration. The most common cause of death from HCN intoxication is due to depression of respiration resulting from the effect of the cyanide ion on the central nervous system, but effects on the heart may also be a cause of death (Hartzell 1996). Some features of acute exposure to HCN at less than fatal concentrations include headache, nausea, dizziness, confusion, muscle weakness, loss of coordination, hyperventilation, cardiac arrhythmia, bradycardia, rapid loss of consciousness, and coma (Hartzell 1996; Norris and Ballantyne 1999; World Health Organization 2004). These acute effects of HCN inhalation may impede escape from a fire environment.

The concentration of HCN that is fatal to humans following inhalation is dependent on the duration of exposure. It has been widely reported that a concentration of 130 ppm for 30 minutes is likely to be fatal, a concentration of 180 ppm HCN is likely to be fatal after just 10 minutes, and a HCN concentration of 270 ppm is considered to be immediately fatal (Kimmerle 1974; World Health Organization 2004). A blood cyanide concentration of greater than 1 µg/ml in blood samples taken post mortem from fire fatalities is considered to suggest significant toxicity of HCN. Blood cyanide levels of 3 µg/ml or greater are considered to be lethal levels of cyanide (Hartzell 1996). However, measurements of blood cyanide levels can be problematic and analysis should be cautious with respect to factors including the time between sample removal and analysis, and the storage method (Ballantyne 1976).

The majority of fire fatalities cannot be attributed to inhalation of HCN alone because in a combustion atmosphere many additional toxic products are also likely to be evolved. CO is produced in all fires involving organic materials and there is likely to be a toxicological interaction between CO and HCN, causing hypoxia by two separate mechanisms. In a combustion environment where both CO and HCN are present at sublethal doses, the combination of the two toxicants has an additive effect that can prove fatal (Lundquist et al. 1989; Moore et al. 1991; Hartzell 1996). Hyperventilation resulting from acute inhalation of HCN could also give rise to increased toxicity of CO, reducing the time to death by increasing the amount of CO respired (Norris and Ballantyne 1999). Therefore, in many cases of fatalities resulting from smoke inhalation it is difficult to attribute death to either CO or HCN.

18.3.1.3 Carbon dioxide

Carbon dioxide (CO_2) is generated in all fires involving organic materials; its rate of production is largely dependent upon the availability of oxygen in the fire environment. As the level of oxygen present in a fire environment diminishes, there is a shift from production of CO_2 to CO. In this respect, the highest rate of generation of CO_2 occurs when combustion is complete due to sufficient ventilation (Tewarson1996).

An increase in the amount of CO_2 inhaled at concentrations such as those likely to be generated in a fire is not considered to cause significant toxicity on its own. However, the inhalation of CO_2 in a fire atmosphere will give rise to physiological effects which enhance the toxicity of other combustion products. An increase in CO_2 concentration will stimulate the rate and depth of respiration, increasing the respiratory minute volume (Hartzell 1996). This leads to an increase in the amount of any toxicants present that are inspired over a given period. A concentration of 2% CO_2 has been shown to increase the respiratory minute volume by 50%, whilst 10% CO_2 may increase the volume of air respired in one minute by as much as 10-fold (Hartzell 1996). Human volunteers exposed to 7.5% CO_2 for 15 minutes have also reported difficulty breathing, headache, sweating, increased heart rate, restlessness, disorientation, and visual distortion (Busby 1968). Prolonged exposure over a few hours to similar concentrations of CO_2 (7–10%) can cause the onset of severe distress and nausea, and may lead to a loss of consciousness (Department of Health 1996).

The presence of CO_2 has been shown to potentiate the toxicity of CO by increasing the formation of COHb due to an increase in the volume of CO inspired (Levin et al. 1987; Norris and Ballantyne 1999). Additionally, exposure to elevated levels of CO_2 will give rise to respiratory acidosis, which in conjunction with metabolic acidosis caused by CO will result in severe acidosis, with a prolonged recovery period following cessation of exposure (Levin et al. 1987).

18.3.1.4 Low oxygen concentration

In a combustion atmosphere, as oxygen is consumed by the fire, the level of oxygen is depleted, particularly if the fire is in a closed environment. The depletion of oxygen below normal levels (21%) in a fire environment can give rise to adverse health effects. Therefore, a reduction in oxygen levels might also be considered to be a dangerous effect of combustion (Hartzell 1996). A reduction in the concentration of oxygen of only 4% (17% O_2) can lead to an impairment of motor co-ordination. Further reduction of the level of oxygen in the combustion environment to around 14–10% can lead to fatigue and an increased likelihood of making faulty judgements. These effects of low oxygen concentration could seriously hinder the escape from a hazardous fire situation. If the level of oxygen falls below approximately 10%, it is likely that an exposed individual will become unconscious and to prevent fatality will require immediate removal to fresh air or treatment with oxygen (Einhorn 1975; Hartzell 1996).

The effects of a reduction of the oxygen concentration in a combustion environment are due to hypoxic hypoxia caused by a decrease in the partial pressure of oxygen (PO_2) in the arterial blood (Norris and Ballantyne 1999). Depletion of oxygen in a fire environment could potentially enhance the toxicity of the asphyxiant gases produced during combustion. As CO and HCN also give rise to hypoxia, a reduction in the level of atmospheric oxygen will be likely to reduce the concentrations of these substances at which significant toxicity may be observed, compared to a normal oxygen environment, due to a further reduction in the availability of oxygen for cellular respiration. Low oxygen concentration in addition to raised carbon dioxide levels has a marked effect on breathing. Physical exertion such as may be required to escape a hazardous fire environment will increase the individual's demand for oxygen, which may also accelerate the onset of hypoxia (Hartzell 1996).

18.3.2 Irritant gases

The combustion of most commonly used materials, ranging from wood to synthetic plastics and polymers, will result in the generation of irritant gases, therefore irritant gases are present in most fire atmospheres, irrespective of whether the combustion is smouldering, flaming, or ventilation-controlled (Prien and Traber 1988; Hartzell 1996). The irritant gases evolved and the rate of generation may, however, depend on the mode of combustion, relative to temperature and ventilation. Irritant gases produced during combustion can be divided into two main groups by their chemical composition: inorganic irritant gases and organic irritants. The injury following exposure to an irritant gas depends on the chemical involved, its concentration, the exposure duration, and its solubility. The initial effect of exposure to irritant gases is likely to be sensory irritation (Prien and Traber 1988; Hartzell 1996). Irritation of the eyes will cause pain and stinging of the eyes, initiation of the blinking reflex, and lachrymation (Hartzell 1996). The severity of sensory irritation is dependent on the concentration of the irritant present and independent of the duration of exposure. An individual exposed to irritant gases in a combustion atmosphere with the effect of stinging or burning of the eyes and throat may shut their eyes and hold their breath to alleviate the irritation, hindering their ability to escape from the hazard (Hartzell 1996). An additional characteristic sign of exposure to irritant gases is a burning sensation of the mucous membranes of the upper respiratory tract, including the nose, mouth, and throat (Prien and Traber 1988; Department of Health 1996; Hartzell 1996). Pulmonary irritation will commonly occur following sensory irritation because of inhalation of the irritant into the lungs. Irritation of the airways gives rise to bronchoconstriction, coughing, and breathing difficulties. Unlike sensory irritation, the severity of pulmonary irritation is dependent on both the concentration and the duration of exposure to the irritant. Exposure to high concentrations of irritant gases can cause inflammation of the lung tissues and pulmonary oedema, and could potentially be fatal in a period of between 6 and 48 hours after removal from the exposure (Hartzell 1996).

18.3.2.1 Inorganic acid gases

The most common inorganic acid gases evolved during combustion include the halogen acids (HCl, HF, HBr) and oxides of sulphur, nitrogen, and phosphorus (Department of Health 1996). Production of these gases will be dependent on the chemical composition of the materials involved.

Hydrogen chloride Hydrogen chloride (HCl) is the most important halogen acid gas likely to be evolved during combustion (Hartzell 1996). Because of the chlorine content of many commonly used materials, including plastics and polymers such as polyvinylchloride (PVC), combustion of these materials will be likely to result in the generation of HCl. In experimental combustion PVC has been shown to release as much as 50% of its weight as HCl (Marongiu et al. 2003).

HCl is a strong sensory and respiratory irritant, with the main targets being the eyes, skin, nose, mouth, throat, and trachea. Exposure to HCl at 35 ppm has been reported to induce sneezing, chest pain, hoarseness, laryngitis, and a feeling of suffocation (Einhorn 1975; International Programme on Chemical Safety 1982). Inhalation of HCl at around 50 ppm is strongly irritating to the eyes, nose, and throat, causing pain, coughing, inflammation, and oedema of the upper respiratory tract; concentrations of about 100 ppm have been described as being extremely irritating and excruciatingly painful to the upper respiratory tract (Department of Health 1996; Hartzell 1996). Exposure to HCl in the range of around 50–100 ppm is considered to be barely tolerable (Einhorn 1975). Because of the high water solubility of HCl, irritation of the upper respiratory tract occurs predominantly. However, pulmonary irritation can occur following exposure to higher concentrations of HCl, resulting in damage to the alveolae and, consequently, pulmonary oedema (Prien and Traber 1988). Inhalation of high concentrations of HCl has also been associated with corrosive burns to the eyes, nose, mouth, and throat, ulceration of the nasal septum, tachypnoea, bronchoconstriction, and laryngeal spasm (International Programme on Chemical Safety 1982; Department of Health 1996; Hartzell 1996). Exposure to high levels that are sufficient to produce pulmonary toxicity may lead to the development of reactive airways dysfunction syndrome (RADS). Brief exposure of humans to concentrations of HCl of may potentially br fatal (Department of Health 1996).

Hydrogen bromide Hydrogen bromide (HBr) is another gas that may be generated during combustion, particularly of synthetic polymeric materials. Flame-retardant compounds containing halogens are commonly added to many plastics and polymers to reduce their flammability, an example being brominated flame retardants such as decabromodiphenyl ether (deca-BDPE), which is used in high-impact polystyrene (eg, television casings) (International Programme on Chemical Safety 1997a; Agency for Toxic Substances and Disease Registry 2004a). On combustion of such flame-retarded polymeric materials, the bromine present is liberated as HBr (Clarke 1999; Levin and Kuligowski 2006).

Only very limited data are available on the irritant effects of HBr. The effects are expected to be similar to those caused by HCl at comparable concentrations (Hartzell 1996). Exposure of six volunteers to HBr at 5 ppm resulted in nasal irritation in all of the subjects and throat irritation in one (American Conference of Governmental and Industrial Hygienists 1991). Exposure to concentrations between 1300 and 2000 ppm has resulted in death (National Library of Medicine 1992). It has been suggested that the sensory irritation produced by exposure to HBr at 200 ppm may be sufficient to impede escape from a hazardous combustion environment (Purser 1988).

Hydrogen fluoride The combustion of synthetic fluorine-containing polymers, such as polytetrafluoroethylene (PTFE), perfluoroalkoxy (PFA), fluorinated ethylene-propylene (FEP), and polyvinylidene fluoride (PVDF), leading to the liberation of fluorine on decomposition, is likely to result in the production of hydrogen fluoride (HF) (Young 1976; Oberdorster 2000).

HF is a strong sensory irritant and corrosive gas: inhalation for 1 hour at concentrations of just 0.5 ppm has been shown to cause irritation and corrosion of the mucous membranes of the nose, mouth, and throat. Inhalation of higher concentrations is likely to result in injury to the lungs, with the onset of pulmonary oedema, which may be delayed for 24–48 hours after exposure (International Programme on Chemical Safety 1990; Lund et al. 1997). Studies in volunteers showed some relatively low sensory and lower airways irritancy at 0.2–2.9 ppm, including chest tightness, soreness, coughing, expectoration, and wheezing. At 3.0–6.3 ppm more severe effects were reported (Expert Panel on Air Quality Standards 2006). HF is the most potent irritant of the halogen acid gases based on animal lethality data, but has equivalent potency to HCl and HBr based on sensory irritancy. However, less HF than HCl is likely to be produced by combustion.

Sulphur dioxide Sulphur dioxide (SO_2) is an inorganic irritant gas that is commonly produced by the combustion of fossil fuels, but may also be formed during the thermal decomposition of any sulphur-containing compounds, such as vulcanized rubber, which is used in the manufacture of tyres.

SO_2 is a respiratory irritant and may cause tightening of the airways. Individuals with asthma are significantly more sensitive to SO_2 than people who do not suffer from this condition. WHO suggest that exposure to 0.4 ppm of SO_2 may lead to significant narrowing of the airways in those suffering from asthma. In most, the effect would not be expected to be large, but some individuals may be clinically affected (Committee on the Medical Effects of Air Pollutants 1998). Inhalation of SO_2 at 1 ppm for 1–6 hours has been shown to increase airway resistance and decrease forced expiratory volume and forced expiratory flow in healthy patients (Agency for Toxic Substances and Disease Registry 1998a). SO_2 is readily absorbed by the mucosa of the upper respiratory tract, with irritation of the nose and mouth being the most common effect following inhalation (International Programme on Chemical Safety 1979; Agency for Toxic Substances and Disease Registry 1998a). At concentrations of about 10 ppm SO_2 causes moderate to severe eye irritation with lachrimation (Agency for Toxic Substances and Disease Registry 1998a). The irritation effect of SO_2 is due to its conversion to sulphuric acid in the presence of water on the mucous membranes of the upper respiratory tract end eyes. Sulphur dioxide also stimulates pain/irritant receptors, which are present as fibres in the epithelium (Widdicombe 1982). Exposure to high concentrations of SO_2 can be fatal because of asphyxiation caused by blockage of the upper respiratory tract as a result of severe irritation and local oedema (Einhorn 1975).

Oxides of nitrogen Nitrogen oxides such as nitric oxide (NO) and nitrogen dioxide (NO_2) are commonly present as mixtures in combustion atmospheres and can be denoted collectively as NO_x (International Programme on Chemical Safety 1997b). Oxides of nitrogen are likely to be generated during the combustion of any nitrogen-containing materials, with the formation of each being dependent on the availability of oxygen in the fire environment. Atmospheric nitrogen is oxidized to NO_x at high temperatures (International Programme on Chemical Safety 1997b; Thomas 1997; Glarborg et al. 2003; Levin and Kuligowski 2006). Burning coal, wood, tobacco, oil, and gas generates nitrogen oxides. Nitrogen oxide is formed first and then oxidized to nitrogen dioxide.

Nitrogen oxides are less soluble than most irritant gases and are therefore more likely to reach the bronchioles and alveoli following inhalation, giving rise to pulmonary damage (International Programme on Chemical Safety 1992a).

Nitric oxide Of the nitrogen oxides present in combustion effluents, NO is expected to be present only in close proximity to the fire or in oxygen-limited atmospheres.

The possible health effects arising from exposure to NO have been relatively little studied, but it is recognized to be significantly less active as an airways irritant than NO_2 (Committee on the Medical Effects of Air Pollutants 2004). NO is irritating to the eyes and upper respiratory tract. Deep inhalation can result in the delayed onset of pulmonary oedema occurring a few hours post exposure and may be aggravated by physical exertion (International Programme on Chemical Safety 1998a). Controlled exposure of healthy human volunteers to NO at concentrations above approximately 20 ppm (24.6 mg/m³) have demonstrated a significant increase (~10%) in total airway resistance (International Programme on Chemical Safety 1997b).

Nitrogen dioxide Nitrogen dioxide is most likely to be present in smoke as it moves away from the fire and when sufficient oxygen is present as NO will be converted to NO_2 in air. Nitrogen dioxide is an irritant and an oxidant, which produces inflammation and oedema of the lungs if inhaled in high concentrations.

The potency of NO_2 as an irritant is approximately five times greater than that of NO (Hartzell 1996). The irritant effect of NO_2 is due to the conversion of NO_2 in the presence of water into nitric acid (HNO_3) and nitrous acid (HNO_2) in the mucous membranes of the respiratory tract (International Programme on Chemical Safety 1992a; Levin and Kuligowski 2006). Low concentrations of NO_2 may cause cough, headache, difficulty breathing, nausea, vertigo, and fatigue (Leikauf and Prows 2001). NO_2 has been shown to cause significant increases in airway resistance in healthy individuals at exposure concentrations as low as 2.5 ppm (International Programme on Chemical Safety 1997b). Exposure to high concentrations of NO_2 have resulted in sudden death due to severe constriction of the airways and larynx (Horvath et al. 1978). Severe pulmonary oedema may occur within a few hours following removal from exposure to NO_2 (Horvath et al. 1978; Leikauf and Prows 2001). During pulmonary oedema the oxygen tension of arterial blood (PaO_2) may fall due to impairment of diffusion capacity (Horvath et al. 1978). Breathing CO_2 increases the effects of NO_2 by increasing the minute volume. Studies in healthy individuals have shown a threshold of effect of around 2 ppm. Individuals with asthma are more sensitive, with a threshold of around 0.2 ppm (Expert Panel on Air Quality Standards 1996).

Phosphorus pentoxide The combustion of any compounds containing phosphorus may lead to the formation of phosphorus pentoxide (P_2O_5) and phosphoric acid. Many traditional flame retardants contain halogen groups and there has been a drive to replace these with halogen-free products (Jeng et al. 2002; Zhang and Horrocks 2003). Phosphorus is a common constituent of many halogen-free flame retardants, such as the isopropylated triphenyl phosphates often incorporated in polyurethane foam. Some halogen-containing flame retardants, such as tris(2-chloropropyl) phosphate, may also incorporate phosphorus to enhance the flame-retardant effect (Zhang and Horrocks 2003). Such phosphorus-containing flame retardants are incorporated into the casings and housing of electronic components (e.g. televisions) in place of halogenated compounds.

Phosphorus pentoxide is corrosive to the eyes and upper respiratory tract: it reacts with moisture to form orthophosphoric acid. Inhalation of P_2O_5 may also lead to pulmonary oedema, the onset of which may be delayed for a few hours following cessation of exposure (International Programme on Chemical Safety 1997c; Bingham 2001).

18.3.2.2 Organic irritants

The combustion of organic compounds also results in the formation of organic irritant products in the fire effluent. The incomplete combustion or pyrolysis of materials including wood, fossil fuels, synthetic and natural polymers, and foodstuffs gives rise to a range of aldehydes (International Programme on Chemical Safety 1991). Of this group, acrolein and formaldehyde are the best known, although it is highly unlikely that these will be the sole organic irritants present in fire smoke, which may also include compounds such as acetaldehyde and butyraldehyde (Einhorn 1975).

Acrolein The combustion of cellulose-based materials such as wood, cotton, and paper has been demonstrated to produce significant quantities of acrolein (Zikria et al. 1972). Acrolein generated during the combustion of wood may represent up to 13% of the total aldehydes in the fire effluent (International Programme on Chemical Safety 1991). Studies to investigate the amount of acrolein generated during combustion have measured acrolein at up to 50 ppm in wood smoke and 60 ppm in smoke generated during the combustion of cotton (Einhorn 1975). Acrolein has also been shown to be generated from polyurethane foams, especially during incomplete combustion. The complete combustion of polyethylene foam was shown to evolve acrolein in the range of 2–23 ppm, whilst incomplete combustion (smouldering fires) generated between 76 and 180 ppm acrolein (Potts et al. 1978).

Acrolein is the most potent of the irritants. It is severely irritating to the respiratory tract and eyes, and is a potent lachrymatory agent. Concentrations of acrolein of 0.5–5 ppm have been shown to cause the onset of lachrymation and eye irritation in humans within a 10-minute exposure period (Kane and Alarie 1977). Acrolein at 1.2 ppm has also been reported to cause lachrimation in humans within just 5 seconds of commencing exposure (Sim and Pattle 1957). Volunteers exposed to a steadily increasing concentration of acrolein reported nose irritation at 0.26 ppm, throat irritation at 0.43 ppm, and a reduction in respiratory rate at 0.6 ppm (Agency for Toxic Substances and Disease Registry 2007). Exposure to acrolein may result in the onset of pulmonary oedema, which may not manifest until a few hours post exposure (Hales et al. 1992; International Programme on Chemical Safety 2001). Pulmonary oedema is due to inflammation in the respiratory mucosa resulting from protein denaturation caused by acrolein (Prien and Traber 1988). Eye irritation resulting from exposure to acrolein has been observed at concentrations as low as 0.06 ppm, and nasal irritation has resulted from exposure to 0.15 ppm. A reduction in respiratory rate has been observed in male volunteers exposed to acrolein at 0.3 ppm for 40 minutes. Respiratory effects including coughing, chest pain, and difficulty breathing have been reported following exposure to 0.26 ppm acrolein. Most individuals are unable to tolerate acrolein in air at above 2 ppm for more than 2 minutes (International Programme on Chemical Safety 2002a). Exposure to acrolein at concentrations above 10 ppm has been shown to fatal within just a few minutes (Einhorn 1975).

Formaldehyde Formaldehyde is likely to be generated under similar conditions of combustion to acrolein. The combustion of wood has been shown to produce formaldehyde in the fire effluent at up to 80 ppm and the combustion of cotton has been shown to generate up to 70 ppm formaldehyde (Einhorn 1975). Formaldehyde is also commonly present as a smoke product from the combustion of many polymers and plastics, particularly during incomplete combustion (International Programme on Chemical Safety 1989a).

Formaldehyde is a potent sensory irritant, causing mild to moderate irritation of the upper respiratory tract and eyes at concentrations in the range of 0.2–3 ppm (Agency for Toxic Substances and Disease Registry 1999). In both normal subjects and asthmatics, no significant clinically detrimental effects were seen in lung function at up to 3 ppm for 3 hours (International Programme on Chemical Safety 2002b). Formaldehyde inhalation at high concentrations will give rise to respiratory effects, including bronchospasm, dyspnoea, respiratory depression, and laryngeal spasm. Inhalation of formaldehyde at high concentrations may also cause laryngeal and pulmonary oedema, which may be potentially fatal and may be delayed for a few hours post exposure (International Programme on Chemical Safety 1989a, 2004). Upper respiratory tract irritation has been reported following exposure to formaldehyde in the rather wide concentration range of 0.1–25.0 ppm, and lower respiratory tract and pulmonary irritation resulting from exposure to 5.0–30.0 ppm. Pulmonary oedema, inflammation, and pneumonia have been reported following exposure to formaldehyde at 50–100 ppm, and concentrations greater than 100 ppm may be fatal (Committee on the Medical Effects of Air Pollutants 2004).

18.3.2.3 Other inorganic irritants

The combustion of many polymeric materials is also likely to generate irritants additional to those previously described. These irritants do not fall within the previous category of inorganic acid gases. Inorganic irritants commonly produced by the combustion of natural and synthetic materials include ammonia, chlorine, and phosgene.

Ammonia Ammonia (NH_3) is likely to be present in the fire effluent of the combustion of any nitrogen-containing materials, including wood, coal, paper, and household waste. Ammonia may be generated in significant amounts during the incomplete combustion (pyrolysis) of low rank coals (containing water and impurities due to inadequate pressure, heat, or time during formation) and biomass (Glarborg et al. 2003).

Ammonia is severely irritating and corrosive to the respiratory tract and eyes, and causes lachrimation and respiratory distress (International Programme on Chemical Safety 1986). Ammonia reacts with the water present in the eyes and mucous membranes of the respiratory tract to form ammonium hydroxide, resulting in necrosis of the cells with which it comes into contact due to its alkaline properties (Agency for Toxic Substances and Disease Registry 2004b). Exposure to ammonia at 50 ppm results in the immediate onset of moderate irritation to the eyes, nose, and throat (Agency for Toxic Substances and Disease Registry 2004b). Exposure to higher concentrations of ammonia in the region of 400 ppm have been demonstrated to cause severe irritation of the nose and throat, 500 ppm ammonia has been shown to increase the rate of breathing, and concentrations of 1700 ppm are reported to induce coughing (Silverman et al. 1949; International Programme on Chemical Safety 1986). Exposure to ammonia at high concentrations above 1500 ppm may be associated with the onset of pulmonary oedema, which may be delayed for up to 24 hours post exposure (Flury et al. 1983; Agency for Toxic Substances and Disease Registry 2004b). Inhalation of very high concentrations of ammonia (~5000 ppm and above) may be rapidly fatal due to obstruction of the airways (Agency for Toxic Substances and Disease Registry 2004b).

Chlorine The generation of chlorine during combustion is likely to occur in similar situations to those in which HCl is formed, with both substances likely to be present. The combustion of any chlorine-containing compounds, including plastics, polymers, and synthetic rubbers such as polyvinylchloride, and bleaches such as sodium hypochlorite, may result in the presence of chlorine in the fire effluent.

Exposure to chlorine causes severe irritation to the eyes, nose, throat, and upper respiratory tract. Concentrations of chlorine in the range of 1–3 ppm are associated with mild irritation of the eyes and the mucous membranes of the nose and throat, coughing, difficulty breathing, and headache (International Programme on Chemical Safety 1982, 1996; Health Protection Agency 2007b). Moderate irritation of the upper respiratory tract and eyes is caused by exposure to concentrations of 5–15 ppm. Exposure to higher concentrations of about 30 ppm results in immediate chest pain, vomiting, and coughing, with the onset of toxic pneumonitis and pulmonary oedema resulting from exposure to 40–60 ppm chlorine (International Programme on Chemical Safety 1996; Health Protection Agency 2007b). The onset of pulmonary oedema may be delayed for several hours post exposure (Teitelbaum 2001). Exposure to chlorine at concentrations greater than 430 ppm for 30 minutes can be fatal, whilst concentrations above 1000 ppm may be fatal in just a few minutes due to respiratory failure (International Programme on Chemical Safety 1996; Teitelbaum 2001; Health Protection Agency 2007b).

Phosgene Phosgene ($COCl_2$) is likely to be evolved from the combustion of any chlorinated organic compounds, for example chlorinated solvents such as chloroform and plastics and polymers such as polyvinylchloride. The requirement for oxygen for the formation of phosgene during the combustion of materials containing chlorine and carbon suggests that it is likely to be formed in the greatest quantities during fire situations where ventilation is not a limiting factor.

Phosgene is a potent irritant, particularly of the lower respiratory tract. Acute exposure to a concentration of 3 ppm results in irritation of the eyes and upper respiratory tract (International Programme on Chemical Safety 1997d). Phosgene will also penetrate into and irritate the deep lung following inhalation because of its relative insolubility in water and thus limited absorption in the upper airway, with onset of lung damage occurring at exposures of greater than 300 ppm/minute (Teitelbaum 2001). Exposure to phosgene can cause fatal pulmonary oedema at concentrations above 150 ppm/minute (International Programme on Chemical Safety 1997d). The clinical effects of phosgene following an acute exposure in the range of 30–300 ppm/minute typically display three phases. The first is reflex characterized by irritation to the eyes and respiratory tract, pain, difficulty breathing, and coughing which occurs during exposure and usually subsides once withdrawn from exposure. The second is a latent phase in which the exposed individual experiences no symptoms and generally feels he/she has recovered. The duration of the latent phase may be between 30 minutes and 24 hours, and depends on the severity of phosgene exposure, with a shorter latent period as the concentration or duration increases. The final phase of phosgene toxicity is the clinical oedema stage, which involves the manifestation of pulmonary oedema and is associated with shortness of breath, coughing, cyanosis, shock, and respiratory arrest (Teitelbaum 2001; International Programme on Chemical Safety 1997d). In cases of phosgene exposure in the lethal range (above 300 ppm/minute), the latent period may be abbreviated or non-existent, with immediate onset of pulmonary oedema (International Programme on Chemical Safety 1997d). Exercise is particularly dangerous in people exposed to phosgene as it exacerbates the adverse effects.

18.3.3 Complex molecules

The combustion of many organic materials may, particularly if it is incomplete, give rise to the formation of complex molecules characterized by long chains or connected ring formations of carbon atoms. The acute toxicity of these compounds is generally low and may not pose a direct health hazard during exposure. However, some of these compounds, in particular those from the polycyclic aromatic hydrocarbon groups, are recognized mutagens and carcinogens. The risks from single (acute) exposure are very small (and unquantifiable). Others give rise to concern because of a possible effect on the reproductive system (e.g. dioxins) (International Agency for Research on Cancer 1983; International Programme on Chemical Safety 1998b; Lewtas 2007).

18.3.3.1 Polycyclic aromatic hydrocarbons

Polycyclic aromatic hydrocarbons (PAHs) are a large group (over 100) of organic compounds containing a minimum of two fused benzene rings. Some of the best known PAHs include benzo[a]pyrene, naphthalene, and anthracene (International Programme on Chemical Safety 1998b). PAHs may be evolved in the fire effluent from all combustion processes, with the largest quantities likely to be generated during the slow, incomplete combustion of organic materials (International Programme on Chemical Safety 1998b; Lewtas 2007). PAHs are present as complex mixtures rather than as individual compounds.

Little information is available on the adverse health effects of an acute exposure to PAHs. Much of the data regarding the acute toxicity of PAHs relates to reports of accidental exposure of naphthalene (International Programme on Chemical Safety 1998b), which may cause headaches, nausea, vomiting, confusion, profuse sweating, nose, throat and eye irritation, and corneal damage. Acute haemolytic anaemia, particularly in individuals with glucose 6-phosphate dehydrogenase deficiency, is a characteristic feature of acute exposure to naphthalene, which may be delayed post exposure (International Programme on Chemical Safety 1998b; Agency for Toxic Substances and Disease Registry 2005).

Concern regarding the health effects following exposure to mixtures of PAHs focuses on the fact that many of these compounds are known to have the potential to be carcinogenic, based on animal experiments or data from occupational exposures to mixtures of PAHs (e.g. coke oven workers) (International Programme on Chemical Safety 1998b). In most cases the carcinogenic compounds also have mutagenic potential and they are considered 'genotoxic carcinogens'. An exception is naphthalene, which is an animal carcinogen, but has no significant mutagenic potential. Some commonly known PAHs which are classified by IARC as being probably carcinogenic to humans (group 2a), include benzo[a]pyrene, dibenz[a,h]anthracene, and benz[a]anthracene (International Agency for Research on Cancer 1987). PAHs which are classified as possibly carcinogenic to humans (group 2b) include naphthalene, indeno[1,2,3-cd]pyrene, and benzo[b]fluoranthene, whilst compounds including chrysene, fluorine, and anthracene are not classifiable as to their carcinogenicity in humans (group 3) (International Agency for Research on Cancer 1987). The experimental data relating to carcinogenicity of PAHs is mainly from chronic (long-term) exposure studies in animals. Any risks from a single acute exposure are likely to be very small.

18.3.3.2 Dioxins/dibenzofurans

Polychlorinated dibenzo-p-dioxins (PCDDs) and polychlorinated dibenzofurans (PCDFs) are large groups (75 dioxin isomers, 135 furan isomers) of polychlorinated tricyclic aromatic compounds that have very similar structures. PCDDs and PCDFs are formed mainly during the incomplete combustion of any materials containing carbon, oxygen, and chlorine, and are therefore commonly found as emissions in fire effluents (International Programme on Chemical Safety 1989b; Stanmore 2004; Pelclova et al. 2006). The pyrolysis of organochlorine polymers such as polyvinylchloride has been shown to give rise to the formation of both PCDDs and PCDFs at temperatures ranging from 500 to 700°C (National Institute for Occupational Safety and Health 1986; Carroll 1996; Levchik and Weil 2005). Once formed, PCDDs and PCDFs are relatively resistant to thermal decomposition and are only destroyed after heating to 800°C for a prolonged period (International Programme on Chemical Safety 1989b). PCDDs and PCDFs present in combustion effluents are most likely to be present as complex mixtures. The amounts of dioxins and dibenzofurans produced during combustion will depend largely on the material involved. Data on the total emissions of PCDDs and PCDFs from municipal solid waste incinerators suggest that the amounts are very small, in the range of a few to several thousand ng/m^3 (International Programme on Chemical Safety 1989b). However, it has been demonstrated that the formation of PCDDs and PCDFs from the combustion of chlorine-containing plastics increased dramatically in the presence of copper (Cu) in the form of electrical wire (Nakao et al. 2006). The combustion of plastics containing polychlorinated biphenyls (PCBs) was known to be a source of PCDFs and PCDDs, although the use of PCBs has been restricted since the late 1970s (International Programme on Chemical Safety 1992b). However, fires involving PCB-containing materials, such as electrical transformers and capacitors manufactured prior to the beginning of the 1980s, could potentially form PCDFs and PCDDs in the combustion effluent. The most commonly known of the PCDDs is 2,3,7,8-tetrachlorodibenzo-*p*-dioxin (2,3,7,8-TCDD) as it is one of the most toxic and most extensively studied of the dioxins (Agency for Toxic Substances and Disease Registry 1998b). Many of the other isomers are very much less potent than TCDD and have low toxicity, e.g. the fully chlorinated derivative. The toxicity of mixtures of PCDDs is often expressed in terms of TCDD equivalents, with TCDD being the standard. The most toxic PCDFs are those which have chlorine atoms substituted at the 2, 3, 7, and 8 carbon positions, particularly 2,3,4,7,8-pentachlorodibenzofuran (2,3,4,7,8-pentaCDF) and 2,3,7,8-tetrachlorodibenzofuran (2,3,7,8-TCDF) (Agency for Toxic Substances and Disease Registry 1994).

The most commonly documented adverse health effect following exposure to dioxins is the gradual onset of chloracne, which may appear within days or even months post exposure (International Programme on Chemical Safety 1989b; Agency for Toxic Substances and Disease Registry 1998b; Pelclova et al. 2006). Chloracne is typically characterized by comedones, epidermal cysts, and inflamed papules with hyperpigmentation (Pelclova et al. 2006). The distribution of chloracne differs from that typically observed in cases of adolescent acne, and is more commonly associated with areas of contact. Some additional adverse health effects which may occur following acute exposure to dioxins include transient hepatotoxicity, hypertension, hyperlipidaemia, and possible peripheral and central neurotoxicity (Pelclova et al. 2006). Studies in firefighters involved in PCB transformer fires (considered to be the worst-case scenario, with respect to dioxin formation) did not detect any observable health effects after 1 year post exposure, although PCDD levels were slightly elevated (International Programme on Chemical Safety 1989b). Data from animal studies indicate that dioxins have adverse effects on the reproductive system, including teratogenicity, and that the most sensitive and consistent effect is on the developing reproductive system in the male offspring. Exposure to chlorinated dibenzofurans appears to give rise to similar adverse effects as those observed following exposure to 2,3,7,8-TCDD, but the potency of these dibenzofurans and other chlorinated dioxins is much lower. There have been no reports of human fatalities due solely to acute exposure to dioxins (Agency for Toxic Substances and Disease Registry 1998b). However, 2,3,7,8-TCDD has been evaluated as carcinogenic to humans (group 1) by the IARC (International Agency for Research on Cancer 1997). Polychlorinated dibenzo-*p*-dioxins other than 2,3,7,8-TCDD and polychlorinated dibenzofurans are not classifiable as to their carcinogenicity to humans (group 3) (International Agency for Research on Cancer 1997). However, TCDD and other dioxins do not have significant mutagenic properties and prolonged exposure is likely to be necessary for the promoter effects to induce carcinogenicity. Risks from single exposure, if any, would be expected to be very low.

18.3.3.3 Isocyanates

Thermal decomposition of polyurethane foams and plastics is known to produce isocyanates due to dissociation of the urethane monomer (Paabo and Levin 1987; Tinnerberg 1997). Polyurethane foams are widely used and may therefore be present as materials in many combustion situations. Flexible polyurethane foams are used in many common domestic materials, including furniture, bedding, and carpet underlay, semi-flexible foams are employed widely in motor vehicle interiors, whilst rigid foams are commonly used as insulation for central heating tanks and pipes, and in appliances such as refrigerators (Esperanza et al. 1999). The amount of isocyanates formed in combustion effluents is expected to be greater from polyurethane foams which contain unreacted isocyanate. The combustion of polyurethane will not only yield isocyanates, but is also likely to result in the formation of greater yields of aromatic compounds such as benzene and toluene (Paabo and Levin 1987; Esperanza et al. 1999). The isocyanates present as products of combustion will vary depending upon the composition of the material involved and the combustion conditions, but may include relatively simple compounds such as methyl isocyanate, and more complex compounds such as toluene diisocyanate.

Methyl isocyanate is a severe irritant of eyes and mucous membranes. Studies in volunteers indicated eye irritation and lachrymation in all individuals exposed to 1 ppm for 5 minutes. Nose and throat irritation was reported in some at this exposure level. A large amount of data is available on the effects of methyl isocyanates resulting from the Bhopal accident, which resulted in over 2000 deaths with more than 100,000 people being affected. The most frequently reported symptoms were burning/watering of the eyes, coughing, respiratory distress from pulmonary congestion, nausea, muscle weakness, and CNS effects secondary to hypoxia. However, insufficient details are available regarding the levels of exposure producing these effects, although those living near the discharge point are likely to have been exposed to high concentrations. There is also evidence that methyl isocyanate produces allergic sensitization reactions. Animal studies indicate that exposure to pregnant animals at 2 ppm produces fetotoxic effects (reduced body weight) whilst having no effects on the maternal animals, indicating that an acute exposure may harm the unborn child (Cohrssen 2001).

Toluene diisocyanate is severely irritating to the eyes and throat with exposure to 0.5 ppm for 30 minutes producing lachrymation. Exposure to 1.3 ppm was intolerable for 10 minutes; several hours later cold-like symptoms with cough persisted. Studies in pregnant animals indicated no adverse effects on development at exposure levels that were not toxic to maternal animals (International Programme on Chemical Safety 1997e; Cohrssen 2001). Data from experimental exposure have clearly established that toluene diisocyanate is a potent allergic sensitizer following inhalation exposure, producing an asthma-like reaction. Persons previously sensitized would be expected to have such reactions following exposure to very low levels of toluene diisocyanate (International Programme on Chemical Safety 1997e).

Inhalation of isocyanates can lead to the delayed onset of potentially fatal pulmonary oedema, which may develop 12–48 hours post exposure (International Programme on Chemical Safety 1997e; Cohrssen 2001).

18.3.3.4 Perfluoroisobutylene

Perfluoroisobutylene (PFIB) is formed during the thermal decomposition of fluorine-containing polymers, such as PTFE (Waritz 1975; Smith et al. 1982; Wang et al. 2001).

A study of the combustion products from PTFE has identified that PFIB is produced at temperatures greater than 475°C (Waritz 1975). PFIB may therefore be present as a product in the effluent following thermal degradation of polymers such as PTFE at relatively low combustion temperatures.

Inhalation of PFIB is extremely irritating to the respiratory tract. The adverse health effects of exposure to PFIB are similar to those of phosgene, but the toxic potency of PFIB is approximately ten times greater than phosgene (Patocka and Bajgar 1998; Jugg et al. 1999). In addition to the sensory and respiratory irritant effects, exposure to vapours of PFIB may give rise to headache, cough, chest pain, and dyspnoea. Inhalation of sufficient amounts of PFIB can also lead to the onset of potentially fatal pulmonary oedema, which may be delayed up to 8 hours post exposure (Maidment and Upshall 1992; Patocka and Bajgar 1998).

18.3.3.5 Particulate matter

Particles of organic and inorganic matter are likely to be released during all types of fires involving organic materials, particularly under conditions of incomplete combustion. The ambient aerosol comprises a complex mixture of different particle types and particles sizes. Particles of less than 10 µm aerodynamic diameter can pass through the larynx and a proportion will be deposited in the airways and alveolar spaces of the lung. These particles make up the 'thoracic fraction' of the ambient aerosol and are monitored as PM10: the mass per cubic metre of particles of, generally, less than 10 µm aerodynamic diameter. A smaller size fraction, PM4, represents the 'respirable fraction' and PM2.5 represents the 'high-risk respirable fraction'. Particles measured both as PM10 and PM2.5 have been found to be associated with a wide range of effects on health (Donaldson et al. 2005; Duffin et al. 2007; US Environmental Protection Agency 2004) Ultrafine or nanoparticles with diameter in at least one dimension of less than 100 nm have been suggested to be the most active component of the ambient aerosol (US Environmental Protection Agency 2004). It has been suggested that such particles may cross from the lung to the blood. Knowledge of the health effects of PM10 comes mainly from epidemiology studies relating to the effect of air pollution. A large number of such studies have shown that PM10 levels are associated with effects on health with no apparent threshold of effect. These effects include increased daily deaths, increased admissions to hospital in patients suffering from heart and lung disorders, and a worsening of conditions in those with asthma. It is believed by some authorities that these effects on the respiratory and cardiovascular system are caused predominately by the very small particles usually referred to as ultrafine (or nanoparticles), i.e. those smaller than 100 nm in diameter.

On deposition in the lungs, some PM and especially the ultrafine particles, produce free radicals, which may provoke local and systemic oxidative stress. This oxidative stress can contribute to inflammation in the lung tissue and may exacerbate any pre-existing lung condition such as asthma (Stenfors et al. 2004; Duffin et al. 2007). Ultrafine particles that are able to migrate from the lungs into the blood have also been implicated in causing adverse effects on the cardiovascular system (Committee on the Medical Effects of Air Pollutants 2006). There are two main theories as to how effects on the cardiovascular system may be induced. The first argues that ultrafine particles destabilize atheromatous plaques and thus cause myocardial infarction; the second argues that potentially danger-ous changes in the regulation of the heart beat may be induced reflexly from the lung (Committee on the Medical Effects of Air Pollutants 2006; Duffin et al. 2007). In contrast to many of the other combustion products highlighted in this review, the degree of adverse effects observed following exposure to particulate matter may not be directly related to the external exposure concentration, but may be more closely related to the size and surface area of the particles deposited at the target organ (US Environmental Protection Agency 2004). PAHs are some of the most common toxic compounds present in combustion derived particulate matter, which may also include nitrogen-substituted polycyclic aromatic hydrocarbons (nitro-PAHs) and nitro-PAH lactones, many of which are highly mutagenic and carcinogenic (Lewtas 2007). Particulate matter may also include metals such as lead, arsenic, cadmium, and nickel (European Commission 1997, 2001).

18.3.4 Health Issues for vulnerable groups

The individuals who are most at risk from exposure to combustion products are those who have pre-existing respiratory diseases, such as asthma or chronic obstructive pulmonary disease. The presence of an existing respiratory condition increases the susceptibility of the individual to the adverse effects of exposure to asphyxiant gases such as CO (International Programme on Chemical Safety 1999). Acute exposure to smoke containing mixtures of asphyxiant and irritant gases is therefore likely to exacerbate these conditions.

Pregnant women are particularly at risk following exposure to smoke, as unborn infants are particularly susceptible to carboxyhaemoglobin due to CO. Other combustion prod-ucts such as methyl isocyanates give rise to concern because of adverse effects following *in utero* exposure.

Elderly individuals exposed to hazardous combustion products would also be expected to be at greater risk of potentially life-threatening health effects due to conditions associ-ated with age, including reduced in lung function and cardiovascular reserve. Any reduc-tion in the utilization of oxygen increases the individual's risk to hypoxia resulting from exposure to asphyxiant gases such as CO, HCN, and low oxygen concentration.

Infants, children, elderly individuals, and those with physical or mental illnesses may be less able to escape from an environment containing hazardous combustion products, thereby increasing their duration of exposure and thus increasing the potential for adverse effects.

Individuals who smoke are also likely to be at greater risk to toxicity following inhala-tion of combustion products as their baseline level of COHb is likely to be greater than would be observed in non-smokers.

18.4 Hazardous combustion products formed by fuel type

The products formed during combustion processes can vary greatly depending on the material involved. The compounds generated during each individual fire scenario should be viewed on a case-by-case basis because of the large number of variables affecting the products formed. However, general predictions of the products most likely to present a hazard to health can be made if the materials involved are known.

18.4.1 Fires involving polymeric materials

Polymeric materials such as plastics, resins, fibres, and foams are likely to produce significant quantities of CO on combustion. The presence of a high level of CO is, however, likely to be of most concern within the immediate vicinity of the fire, particularly if the fire is enclosed within a building and is ventilation controlled.

The combustion of polymers which contain large quantities of nitrogen, such as nylons, polyurethanes, and polyacrylonitriles, is likely to yield significant amounts of HCN, NO_x and NH_3. However, HCN, NO_x and NH_3 are not exclusively formed from the combustion of nitrogen-containing plastics, but may also be present to a lesser extent during the combustion of non-nitrogen-containing plastics due to the incorporation of atmospheric nitrogen. In this case, the incorporation of atmospheric nitrogen to form HCN and NO_x will be largely dependent upon its availability in the combustion environment and the temperature.

Many plastics contain a considerable proportion of halogens, which can be released as irritant gases or as more complex molecules. HCl is released in large quantities during the combustion of plastic such as polyvinylchloride, with the majority of the chlorine present in the plastic being released as HCl. In addition to HCl, some chlorinated plastics may also release phosgene and small amounts of PCDDs and PCDFs. HBr is likely to be generated during the combustion of many plastics used for electrical applications due to the addition of bromine as a flame retardant. Fluorine-containing polymers, such as PTFE, are known to liberate HF on combustion, and if the combustion is incomplete can also generate PFIB, which is an extremely potent irritant. Many more recent flame-retardant plastics have been produced which do not contain halogens, but instead contain phosphorous. The combustion of these phosphorous-containing plastics may therefore yield oxides of phosphorous such as P_2O_5 and phosphoric acid. The combustion of polyurethane foams commonly used in furnishings have been shown to generate isocyanates and their derivatives.

As the composition of polymers such as plastics, resins, fibres, and foams can vary greatly, this will influence the products formed and it may not be possible to identify all of the types of plastic that may be involved during an individual combustion situation.

In general for fires involving plastics the greatest hazard to public health outside the immediate vicinity of the fire will be from inorganic and organic irritant gases, particulate matter, and other more complex organic compounds. The asphyxiant gases generated during plastic combustion are most likely to be of greatest concern to health within the same compartment/building as the fire.

18.4.2 Fires involving wood

The combustion of cellulose-containing materials such as wood, either as vegetation, such as in forest fires, or that used in construction and furnishings, will be likely to lead to the formation of organic irritants such as acrolein and formaldehyde. However, depending on the conditions, relatively small amounts of PAHs, particulate matter, and more complex exotic molecules may be formed, particularly during incomplete combustion, all of which may present a concern to public health.

Asphyxiant gases such as CO will be generated during the combustion of wood, although its presence is only likely to be of concern in the immediate vicinity of the source of the fire. The formation of CO from the combustion of wood in the open environment, such as that seen in the case of forest fires, is less likely to be a concern than in building fires due to the greater availability of oxygen and the greater potential for dispersion of the fire effluent.

In addition to the hazardous products from the combustion of wood, burning of wood incorporating preservatives, such as the heavy-metal-containing preservative chromate copper arsenate, may lead to the liberation of heavy metals as oxides such as chromium trioxide and arsenic trioxide (Lundholm et al. 2007).

The main hazard to public health following exposure to products from wood fires is due to the generation of organic irritant gases. These irritant compounds are more likely to be present in the effluent plume away from the source than gases such as CO, which are only expected to be present in significant quantities in the immediate vicinity/compartment of the fire.

18.4.3 Fires involving rubber/tyres

Fires which involve large quantities of rubber, such as tyre fires, may give rise to the generation of significant yields of SO_2 due to the high sulphur content resulting from the vulcanization process.

The combustion of rubber is also likely to give rise to the formation of CO, organic irritants, inorganic irritants, PAHs, some complex organic molecules and particulate matter. Some rubber compounds contain organophoshate-based flame retardants, which on combustion may additionally yield phosphorous pentoxide (P_2O_5).

The compounds most likely to pose a hazard to the health of individuals outside the immediate vicinity of the fire might be expected to be irritants such as SO_2 and organic irritants such as acrolein.

18.4.4 Fires involving oil/petrol

Fires involving oil or petrol in an external environment might be expected to undergo extensive combustion due to the high temperature and availability of oxygen, with carbonaceous particles being a prominent product. In this fire situation the generation of particulate matter may therefore be significant. Such a fire would also be expected to result in the generation of some PAHs, other complex compounds, and organic irritants, which would be present in the greatest quantities at the combustion source. If the temperatures are high enough, these more complex organic chemicals may be completely broken down. The health hazard that these compounds pose will be reduced as the distance from the source increases, but could be of concern for individuals directly exposed to the plume.

The combustion of petrol or oil will most likely lead to the generation of irritants and particulate matter in the effluent plume, which may be expected to be the greatest hazard to the health of individuals outside the immediate vicinity of the source.

18.4.5 Fires involving hazardous chemicals (chemical/pesticide manufacturer/storage)

This scenario involves a fire at a facility concerned with the manufacture or storage of hazardous chemicals, such as an industrial chemical or pesticide manufacturer. In such a situation the hazardous materials present may be evolved unchanged during the fire. Specific examples of hazardous chemicals which may be present either unchanged or as hazardous decomposition products in a smoke plume include organophosphorous and organochlorine pesticides. The compounds and products occurring in the smoke will depend on those present and will vary from location to location. Pesticides containing chlorine, for example, are unlikely to undergo complete decomposition under most combustion conditions, giving rise to the presence of hazardous organochlorine compounds in the smoke plume.

In general, if the quantity of these specialized chemicals in a fire situation is small and any emissions are well dispersed, there is unlikely to be any significant additional risk to that arising from the smoke from any large building fire.

18.4.6 Fires involving asbestos

Large-scale fires in which the fabric of the building may contain asbestos, e.g. from asbestos cement roofing, give rise to significant concern for the public regarding exposure to asbestos. However, there is considerable data to show that providing appropriate clean-up procedures are followed, there is no significant public health risk resulting from asbestos (Health Protection Agency 2007c).

18.5 Summary

The prediction of toxic combustion products is a complex area and there is the potential for the generation of a huge range of pyrolysis products depending on the nature of the fire and the conditions of burning. Although each fire will have individual characteristics and will ultimately need to be considered on a case-by-case basis, there are commonalities, particularly with regard to the most important components relating to toxicity.

♦ Asphyxiant gases (CO, HCN, and CO_2) and low oxygen concentration are most likely to be of concern to individuals within the fire compartment/building, but are less likely to pose a major hazard to public health to individuals outside the immediate compartment of the fire, because of dispersion and dilution.

♦ The most common potential hazards to individuals outside the immediate compartment of the fire from all considered sources are:
  • organic irritants, including acrolein and formaldehyde
  • complex molecules, including dioxins, dibenzofurans, isocyanates
  • particulate matter.

♦ Scenarios in which the combustion is considered to be incomplete, due to low temperature, lack of ventilation, and absence of flaming, would be expected to form the greatest quantities of hazardous combustion products.

These generalizations may assist in rapidly identifying which hazardous combustion products are likely to be of most concern to public health during a fire depending on the materials involved.

18.6 References

Agency for Toxic Substances and Disease Registry. (1994) *Toxicological profile for chlorodibenzofurans.* US Department of Health and Human Services, Atlanta, GA.

Agency for Toxic Substances and Disease Registry. (1998a) *Toxicological profile for sulfur dioxide.* US Department of Health and Human Services, Atlanta.

Agency for Toxic Substances and Disease Registry. (1998b) *Toxicological profile for chlorinated dibenzo-p-dioxins.* US Department of Health and Human Services, Atlanta, GA.

Agency for Toxic Substances and Disease Registry. (1999) *Toxicological profile for formaldehyde.* US Department of Health and Human Services, Atlanta, GA.

Agency for Toxic Substances and Disease Registry. (2004a) *Toxicological profile for polybrominated biphenyls and polybrominated diphenyl ethers.* US Department of Health and Human Services, Atlanta, GA.

Agency for Toxic Substances and Disease Registry. (2004b) *Toxicological profile for ammonia.* US Department of Health and Human Services, Atlanta, GA.

Agency for Toxic Substances and Disease Registry. (2005) *Toxicological profile for naphthalene, 1-methylnaphthalene and 2-methylnaphthalene.* US Department of Health and Human Services, Atlanta, GA.

Agency for Toxic Substances and Disease Registry. (2007) *Toxicological profile for acrolein.* US Department of Health and Human Services, Atlanta, GA.

American Conference of Governmental and Industrial Hygienists. (1991) *Documentation of the threshold limit values and biological exposure indices*, 6th edn. ACGIH, Cincinnati, OH.

Ballantyne B. (1976) Changes in blood cyanide as a function of storage time and temperature. *J Forensic Sci Soc* **16**(4):305–310.

Bertol E, Mari F, Orzalesi G and Volpato I. (1983) Combustion products from various kinds of fibres: Toxicological hazards from smoke exposure. *Forensic Sci Int* **22**:111–116.

Bingham E. (2001) Phosphorous, selenium, tellurium, and sulfur. In: *Patty's Toxicology, 5th* edn, Volume **3**, Bingham E, Cohrssen B, Powell CH (eds). John Wiley and Sons, New York.

Busby DE. (1968) Carbon dioxide toxicity. *Space Clin Med* **1**:381–419.

Carroll Jr WF. (1996) Is PVC in house fires the great unknown source of dioxin? *Fire and Materials* **20**(4):161.

Clarke FB. (1999) Effects of brominated flame retardants on the elements of fire hazard: A re-examination of earlier results. *Fire Mater* **23**(3):109.

Cohrssen B. (2001) Cyanides and nitriles. In: *Patty's Toxicology, 5th* edn, Volume **3**, Bingham E, Cohrssen B, Powell CH (eds). John Wiley & Sons, New York.

Committee on the Medical Effects of Air Pollutants. (1998) *COMEAP statement on the banding of air quality.* Department of Health, London.

Committee on the Medical Effects of Air Pollutants. (2004) *Guidance on the health effects of indoor air pollutants.* Department of Health, London.

Committee on the Medical Effects of Air Pollutants. (2006) *Cardiovascualr Disease and Air Pollution; A report by the Committee on the Medical Effects of Air Pollutants.* Department of Health, London.

Department of Health. (1996) *Health advisory group on chemical contamination incidents: Smoke toxins.* Department of Health, London.

Donaldson K, Tran L, Jimenez LA, Duffin R, Newby DE, Mills N, MacNee W, and Stone V. (2005) Combustion-derived nanoparticles: A review of their toxicology following inhalation exposure. *Part Fibre Toxicol* **2**(10).

Duffin R, Mills NL, Donaldson K. (2007) Nanoparticles—A thoracic toxicology perspective. *Yonsei Med J* **48**(4):561.

Einhorn IN. (1975) Physiological and toxicological aspects of smoke produced during the combustion of polymeric materials. *Environ Health Persp* **11**:163–189.

Esperanza MM, Garcia AN, Font R, and Conesa JA. (1999) Pyrolysis of varnish wastes based on a polyurethane. *J Anal Appl Pyrolysis* **52**(2):151.

European Commission. (1997) *DG XI, Working Group on Lead, Air Quality Daughter Directives— Position Paper on Lead.* Office for Official Publications of the European Communities, Luxembourg.

European Commission. (2001) *DG Environment, Working Group on Arsenic, Cadmium and Nickel Compounds, Ambient Air Pollution by As, Cd and Ni compounds-Position Paper.* Office for Official Publications of the European Communities, Luxembourg.

Expert Panel on Air Quality Standards. (1996) *Nitrogen Dioxide.* Department for Environment, Food and Rural Affairs, London.

Expert Panel on Air Quality Standards. (2006) *Guidelines for Halogens and Hydrogen Halides in Ambient Air for Protecting Human Health against Acute Irritancy Effects.* Department for Environment, Food and Rural Affairs, London.

Flury KE, Dines DE, Rodarte JR, and Rodgers R. (1983) Airway obstruction due to inhalation of ammonia. *Mayo Clin Proc.* **58**(6):389.

Glarborg P, Jensen AD, Johnsson JE. (2003) Fuel nitrogen conversion in solid fuel fired systems. *Prog Energ Combust Sci.* **29**(2):89.

Hales CA, Musto SW, Janssens S, Jung W, Quinn DA, and Witten M. (1992) Smoke aldehyde component influences pulmonary edema. *J Appl Physiol* **72**(2):555.

Hartzell GE. (1996) Overview of combustion toxicology. *Toxicology* **115**(1–3):7.

Health Protection Agency. (2007a) Carbon Monoxide, Toxicological Overview. In: *HPA Compendium of Chemical Hazards.* Health Protection Agency, London.

Health Protection Agency. (2007b) Chlorine, Toxicological Overview. In: *HPA Compendium of Chemical Hazards.* Health Protection Agency, London.

Health Protection Agency. (2007c) *The Public Health Significance of Asbestos Exposures from Large Scale Fires. HPA-CHaPD-003.* Health Protection Agency.

Horvath EP, doPico GA, Barbee RA, and Dickie HA. (1978) Nitrogen dioxide-induced pulmonary disease: five new cases and a review of the literature. *J Occup Med* **20**(2):103–110.

Institute for Environment and Health. (1998) *IEH assessment on Indoor Air Quality in the Home (2): Carbon Monoxide.* Medical Research Council, London.

International Agency for Research on Cancer. (1983) Polynuclear Aromatic Compounds, Part 1, Chemical, Environmental and Experimental Data. *IARC Monographs on the Evaluation of Carcinogenic Risk to Humans* **32**.

International Agency for Research on Cancer. (1987) Overall Evaluations of Carcinogenicity: An Updating of IARC Monographs Volumes 1 to 42. *IARC Monographs on the Evaluation of Carcinogenic Risk to Humans* Supplement 7.

International Agency for Research on Cancer. (1997) Polychlorinated dibenzo-para-dioxins and polychlorinated dibenzofurans. *IARC Monographs on the Evaluation of Carcinogenic Risk to Humans* **69**.

International Programme on Chemical Safety. (1979) *Sulfur Oxides and Suspended Particulate Matter. Environmental Health Criteria 8.* WHO, Geneva.

International Programme on Chemical Safety. (1982) *Chlorine and Hydrogen Chloride. Environmental Health Criteria 21.* WHO, Geneva.

International Programme on Chemical Safety. (1986) *Ammonia. Environmental Health Criteria 54.* WHO, Geneva.

International Programme on Chemical Safety. (1989a) *Formaldehyde. Environmental Health Criteria 89.* WHO, Geneva.

International Programme on Chemical Safety. (1989b) *Polychlorinated dibenzo-p-dioxins and dibenzofurans. Environmental Health Criteria 88.* WHO, Geneva.

International Programme on Chemical Safety. (1990) *Hydrogen Fluoride. Poisons Information Monograph. PIM 268.* WHO, Geneva.

International Programme on Chemical Safety. (1991) *Acrolein. Environmental Health Criteria 127.* WHO, Geneva.

International Programme on Chemical Safety. (1992a) *Nitrogen Oxides. Poisons Infomation Monograph: PIM G017.*, WHO: Geneva.

International Programme on Chemical Safety. (1992b) *Polychlorinated biphenyls and terphenyls. Environmental Health Criteria 140, 2nd edn.* WHO, Geneva.

International Programme on Chemical Safety. (1996) *Chlorine. Poisons Infomation Monograph: PIM 947.* WHO, Geneva.

International Programme on Chemical Safety. (1997a) *Flame Retardants. Environmental Health Criteria 192.* WHO, Geneva.

International Programme on Chemical Safety. (1997b) *Nitrogen, Oxides of Environmental Health Criteria 188, 2nd edn.* WHO: Geneva.

International Programme on Chemical Safety. (1997c) *Phosphorus Pentoxide. International Chemical Safety Card: 0545.* WHO, Geneva.

International Programme on Chemical Safety. (1997d) *Phosgene. Environmental Health Criteria 193.* WHO, Geneva.

International Programme on Chemical Safety. (1997e) *Toluene 2,4-diisocyanate (TDI). Poisons Infomation Monograph: PIM 534.* WHO, Geneva.

International Programme on Chemical Safety. (1998a) *Nitric Oxide. International Chemical Safety Card: 1311.* WHO, Geneva.

International Programme on Chemical Safety. (1998b) *Selected Non-heterocyclic Polycyclic Aromatic Hydrocarbons. Environmental Health Criteria 202.* WHO, Geneva.

International Programme on Chemical Safety. (1999) *Carbon monoxide. Environmental Health Criteria 213.* WHO, Geneva.

International Programme on Chemical Safety. (2001) *Acrolein. International Chemical Safety Card: 0090.* WHO, Geneva.

International Programme on Chemical Safety. (2002a) *Acrolein. Concise International Chemical Assessment Document 43.* WHO, Geneva.

International Programme on Chemical Safety. (2002b) *Formaldehyde. Concise International Chemical Assessment Document 40.* WHO, Geneva.

International Programme on Chemical Safety. (2004) *Formaldehyde. International Chemical Safety Card: 0275.* WHO, Geneva.

Jeng R-J, Shau S-M, Lin J-J, Su W-C, and Chiu Y-S. (2002) Flame retardant epoxy polymers based on all phosphorus-containing components. *Eur Polymer J* **38**(4):683.

Jugg B, Jenner J, Rice P. (1999) The effect of perfluoroisobutene and phosgene on rat lavage fluid surfactant phospholipids. *Hum Exp Toxicol* **18**(11):659.

Kane LE, Alarie Y. (1977) Sensory irritation to formaldehyde and acrolein during single and repeated exposures in mice. *Am Ind Hygiene Assoc J* **38**(10):509–522.

Kaplan HL, Hartzell G.E. (1984) Modeling of toxicological effects of fire gases: I. incapacitating effects of narcotic fire gases. *J Fire Sci* **2**:286–305.

Kimmerle G. (1974) Aspects and methodology for the evaluation of toxicological parameters during fire exposure. *J Fire Flammability Combustion Toxicology Supplement* **1**:42.

Leikauf GD, Prows DR, (2001) Inorganic compounds of carbon, nitrogen, and oxygen. In: *Patty's Toxicology*, 5th edn, Volume **3**, Bingham E, Cohrssen B, Powell CH, (eds). John Wiley & Sons, New York.

Levchik SV, Weil ED. (2005) Overview of the recent literature on flame retardancy and smoke suppression in PVC. *Polymers Adv Technol* **16**(10):707.

Levin BC, Kuligowski ED. (2006) Toxicology of fire and smoke. In: *Inhalation Toxicology*, 2nd edn, Salem H, Katz SA (eds). Taylor & Francis, Boca Raton, pp 205–228.

Levin BC, Paabo M, Gurman JL, Harris SE and Braun E. (1987) Toxicological interactions between carbon monoxide and carbon dioxide. *Toxicology* **47**(1–2):135–164.

Lewtas J. (2007) Air pollution combustion emissions: Characterization of causative agents and mechanisms associated with cancer, reproductive, and cardiovascular effects. *Mutat Res* **636**(1–3):95–133.

Lund K, Ekstrand J, Boe J, Sostrand P, and Kongerud J. (1997) Exposure to hydrogen fluoride: an experimental study in humans of concentrations of fluoride in plasma, symptoms, and lung function. *Occup Environ Med* **54**(1):32–37.

Lundholm K, Bostrom D, Nordin A, and Shchukarev A. (2007) Fate of Cu, Cr, and As During Combustion of Impregnated Wood with and without Peat Additive. *Environ Sci Technol* **41**(18):6534–6540.

Lundquist P, Rammer L, Sorbo B. (1989) The role of hydrogen cyanide and carbon monoxide in fire casualties: a prospective study. *Forensic Sci Int* **43**(1):9–14.

Maeda H, Fukita K, Oritani S, Nagai K, and Zhu BL. (1996) Evaluation of post-mortem oxymetry in fire victims. *Forensic Sci Int* **81**(2–3):201–209.

Maidment MP, Upshall DG. (1992) Retention of inhaled perfluoroisobutene in the rat. *J Appl Toxicol* **12**(6):393.

Marongiu A, Faravelli T, Bozzano G, Dente M and Ranzi E. (2003) Thermal degradation of poly(vinyl chloride). *J Anal Appl Pyrolysis* **70**(2):519.

Maynard RL, Waller R. (1999) Carbon monoxide. In: *Air Pollution and Health*, Holgate ST, Samet JM, Koren HS, and Maynard RL (eds). Academic Press, London. pp 749–796.

Moore SJ, Ho IK, Hume AS. (1991) Severe hypoxia produced by concomitant intoxication with sublethal doses of carbon monoxide and cyanide. *Toxicol Appl Pharm* **109**(3):412–420.

Morikawa T. (1978) Evaluation of hydrogen cyanide during combustion and pyrolysis. *J Combust Toxicol* **5**:315–338.

Nakao T, Aozasa O, Ohta S, and Miyata H. (2006) Formation of toxic chemicals including dioxin-related compounds by combustion from a small home waste incinerator. *Chemosphere* **62**(3):459–468.

National Institute for Occupational Safety and Health. (1986) *DHHS (NIOSH) Publication No. 86-111. Current Intelligence Bulletin 45. Polychlorinated Biphenyls (PCB's): Potential Health Hazards from Electrical Equipment Fires or Failures.* United States Department of Health and Human Services, Washington, DC.

National Library of Medicine. (1992) *Hazardous substance data bank: Hydrogen bromide.* National Library of Medicine, Bethesda, MD.

Norris JC, Ballantyne B. (1999) Toxicology and implications of the products of combustion. In: *General and Applied Toxicology*, 2nd edn, Ballantyne B., Marrs T., Syversen T. (eds). Macmillan Reference,: London, pp 1915–1933.

Oberdorster G. (2000) Toxicology of ultrafine particles: in vivo studies. *Phil Trans Roy Soc A* **358**(1775):2719–2740.

Ohlemiller TJ. (2002) Smoldering combustion. In: SFPE Handbook of Fire Protection Engineering, 3rd edn, DiNenno PJ, Drysdale D, Beyler CL, Walton WD, and Quincy MA (eds). National Fire Protection Association.

Paabo M, Levin BC.(1987) A review of the literature on the gaseous products and toxicity generated from the pyrolysis and combustion of rigid polyurethane foams. *Fire and Materials* **11**(1):1.

Patocka J, Bajgar J. (1998) Toxicology of perfluoroisobutylene. *ASA Newsletter* **22**.

Pelclova D, Urban P, Preiss J, Lukas E, Fenclova Z, Navratil T, Dubska Z, and Senholdova Z. (2006) Adverse health effects in humans exposed to 2,3,7,8-tetrachlorodibenzo-p-dioxin (TCDD). *Rev Environ Health* **21**(2):119–138.

Potts WJ, Lederer TS, Quast JF. (1978) A study of the inhalation toxicity of smoke produced upon pyrolysis and combustion of polyethylene foams. Part I. Laboratory studies. *J Combustion Toxicol* **5**:408–433.

Prien T, Traber D.L. (1988) Toxic smoke compounds and inhalation injury—a review. *Burns* **14**(6):451–460.

Purser DA. (1988) *Toxicity assessment of combustion products*. SFPE Handbook of Fire Protection Engineering, 2nd edn. National Fire Protection Association, Boston, p. 85–146.

Purser DA. (1992) The evolution of toxic effluents in fires and the assessment of toxic hazard. *Toxicology Lett* **64/65**:247–255.

Purser DA, Berrill KR. (1983) Effects of carbon monoxide on behavior in monkeys in relation to human fire hazard. *Arch Environ Health* **38**(5):308–315.

Purser DA, Wooley WD. (1983) Biological studies of combustion atmospheres. *J Fire Sci* **1**:118–144.

Silverman L, Whittenberger JL, Muller J. (1949) Physiological response of man to ammonia in low concentrations. *J Ind Hygiene Toxicol* **31**(2):74–78.

Sim VM, Pattle RE. (1957) Effect of possible smog irritants on human subjects. *J Am Med Assoc* **165**(15):1908–1913.

Smith LW, Gardner RJ, Kennedy Jr GL. (1982) Short-term inhalation toxicity of perfluoroisobutylene. *Drug Chem Toxicol* **5**(3):295.

Stanmore BR. (2004) The formation of dioxins in combustion systems. *Combust Flame* **136**:398–427.

Stenfors N, Nordenhall C, Salvi SS, Mudway I, Soderberg M, Blomberg A, Helleday R, Levin JO, Holgate ST, Kelly FJ, Frew AJ, and Sandstrom T. (2004) Different airway inflammatory responses in asthmatic and healthy humans exposed to diesel. *Eur Respir J* **23**(1):82.

Stewart RD. (1975) The effect of carbon monoxide on humans. *Ann Rev Pharmacol* **15**:409–423.

Teitelbaum DT. (2001) The halogens. In: *Patty's Toxicology*, 5th edn, Volume **3**, Bingham E, Cohrssen B, Powell CH (eds). John Wiley & Sons, New York.

Tewarson A.(1996) Ventilation effects on combustion products. *Toxicology* **115**(1–3):145–156.

Thomas KM. (1997) The release of nitrogen oxides during char combustion. *Fuel* **76**(6):457.

Tinnerberg H, Spanne M, Dalene M, and Skarping G. (1997) Determination of complex mixtures of airborne isocyanates and amines. Part 3. Methylenediphenyl diisocyanate, methylenediphenylamino isocyanate and methylenediphenyldiamine and structural analogues after thermal degradation of polyurethane. *Analyst* **122**(3):275–278.

Urhas E, Kullik E. (1977) Pyrolysis gas chromatographic analysis of some toxic compounds from nitrogen-containing fibres. *J Chromatogr* **137**:210–214.

US Environmental Protection Agency. (2004) *Air quality criteria for particulate matter*. National Center for Environmental Assessment-RTP Office, Research Triangle Park, NC.

Wang H, Ding R, Ruan J, Yuan B, Sun X, Zhang X, Yu S, and Qu W. (2001) Perfluoroisobutylene-induced acute lung injury and mortality are heralded by neutrophil sequestration and accumulation. *J Occup Health* **43**(6):331.

Waritz RS. (1975) An industrial approach to evaluation of pyrolysis and combustion hazards. *Environ Health Perspect* **11**:197–202.

Widdicombe JG. (1982) Pulmonary and respiratory tract receptors. *J Exp Biol* **100**:41.

World Health Organization. (2004) Hydrogen Cyanide and Cyanides: Human Health Aspects. Concise International Chemical Assessment Document: 61. WHO, Geneva.

Young W, Hilando CJ, Kourtides DA, and Parker DS. (1976) A study of the toxicity of pyrolysis gases from synthetic polymers. *J Combustion Toxicol* **3**:157–165.

Zhang S, Horrocks AR. (2003) A review of flame retardant polypropylene fibres. *Progr Polymer Sci* **28**(11):1517.

Zikria BA, Ferrer JM, Floch HF. (1972) The chemical factors contributing to pulmonary damage in "smoke poisoning". *Surgery* **71**(5):704–709.

Chapter 19

Nanotoxicology: current activities and considerations

Vicki Stone

Learning outcomes

At the end of this chapter and any recommended reading the student should be able to:

1. define nanotechnology and nanomaterials;

2. provide examples of synthetic nanomaterials;

3. explain why there is a need to investigate the risks posed by new technologies such as nanotechnology;

4. describe uses of nanomaterials that might lead to human or environmental exposure;

5. explain why concerns about nanomaterials were first suggested;

6. describe the different physical and chemical characteristics of nanomaterials that might influence their biological reactivity;

7. describe models that can be used to assess nanomaterial hazard.

19.1 Defining nanotechnology

Nanotechnology involves the production and handling of structures at the nanoscale, which means between 1 and 100 nm. A nanometer is one billionth (10^{-9}) of a metre, which is such a small dimension that it is difficult to imagine. A human hair is 30,000–50,000 nm in diameter, while a red blood cell is 6000–8000 nm in diameter, but you have to go down to the scale of proteins or DNA, which are just a few nanometers in size, before you reach the nanoscale.

The reason that objects are being made in the nanoscale is because materials change their physical and chemical properties at this size range. For example, gold is a yellow and relatively inert hard metal, but not when it is made as a nanoparticle. Instead, nanoparticle gold is red, pink, or purple depending on the particle size. In addition, gold changes from being inert to very reactive nanoparticles, allowing it to be used as a catalyst in chemical reactions. Gold nanoparticles are not a new invention; colloidal gold has been used to colour stained-glass windows for centuries. Now such gold particles are being used for many applications, including in medicine, where they are used to deliver drugs to specific targets in the body, as well as to image structures such as tumours (Powell et al. 2010). The main focus of nanotechnology is to exploit the unusual properties exhibited at the nanoscale to make useful, new, and exciting products.

19.2 Nanomaterials—definitions and applications

Nanomaterials come in many shapes, sizes, and compositions. Shapes can vary from spherical to rods or tubes, even to rather complex structures such as flowers. Material size may vary between 1 and 100 nm. However, to be defined as a nanomaterial only one dimension needs to be in this size range, therefore nanomaterials might include large plate-like structures. A nano-object is defined as having two dimensions in the nanoscale and so could include the rods and tubes mentioned above, while a nanoparticle such as a sphere or cube has all three dimensions within the nanoscale (British Standards 2007).

The uses of nanomaterials are extremely diverse, covering almost any product imaginable. Examples include medicines, medical diagnostics, sunscreens, cosmetics, food additives, food packaging, clothing, paints, electronics, and construction materials. Nanomaterials used as sunscreens include titanium dioxide and zinc oxide, because of their ability to reflect UV light (Osmond and McCall 2010). Both materials when generated as larger particles are white and opaque, whereas the nanoscale versions are clear and transparent, which is often considered to be more attractive by users. A number of nanomaterials have also been developed because of their antimicrobial properties (e.g. silver and titanium dioxide), which has led to the incorporation of nanomaterials in hospital equipment, wound dressings, food preparation surfaces, food packaging, and clothing (Chen and Schluesener 2008). Arguably, one of the most useful applications of nanotechnology is in the development of filters for the purification of water for drinking in remote locations. Such a cheap and portable device could save many lives.

There is a wide array of fibre-shaped nano-objects available, including tubes, wires, rods, and whiskers. They come in a variety of chemistries, including metals (e.g. silver, gold, and nickel), metal oxides (e.g. titanium dioxide), carbon, polymers, and organic materials. Within this group of nanomaterials, carbon nanotubes have received a lot of attention with respect to their development and use in a wide array of consumer products, but also due to their potential toxicity. Carbon nanotubes essentially consist of tubes made from graphene, which are single-walled carbon nanotubes that have just one layer of carbon; multi-walled carbon nanotubes have multiple layers stacked inside each other. Nanotube diameter is always within the nanoscale, whereas length can vary from the nanoscale up to centimetres in length. Like other fibres, these nanotubes are relatively strong, but light. In fact they are much stronger than larger fibre types, allowing them to be used in cars, planes, paints, sports equipment, and medical implants. In addition to being very strong, they are also semi-conductors, hence when incorporated into other materials these materials (e.g. plastic or fabrics) can conduct electricity.

19.3 **Risk assessment of nanomaterials**

Nanotechnology clearly has the potential to impact on our daily activities and to improve our quality of life. There are currently over 1300 products containing nanomaterials on the market (http://www.nanotechproject.org), suggesting that humans and the environment are likely to come into contact with nanomaterials in many forms. Some of these nano-materials will enter the body, perhaps via inhalation, ingestion, dermal penetration, or even direct injection. A proportion of these exposures will be intentional (e.g. medicines and food) but others may be incidental or unplanned. In addition to human exposure, we also need to consider release into the environment, both intentionally and incidentally through use of the product or its disposal. Intentional releases to the environment include iron nanoparticles used to break down contaminants in the environment, a process known as remediation (Zhang 2003). Incidental release includes the washing of products into waste water. In order to assess the risks of such new technologies we need to understand if there is any exposure to the individual or environment, and then whether or not there is any hazard (toxicity) associated with this exposure. This knowledge allows users and regulators to manage the potential risk in an appropriate manner.

19.4 **Nanoparticles in air pollution**

Although the term 'nanotoxicology' did not really exist prior to 2004, research into the hazards of particles within the nanoscale did exist. Much of this research was focused on the potential risks associated with inhalation of particulate air pollution known as PM_{10}. PM stands for particulate matter, while the 10 refers to 10 μm, the largest particle size that can be inhaled past the larynx and enter the small terminal airways of the lung. PM_{10} is the mass of particles generally less than 10 μm in diameter per cubic metre of air. Elevated PM_{10} is associated with a number of adverse health effects, including increased asthma symptoms and asthma medication usage, increased hospital admissions and an increase in the death rate (Pope 2000). The increases in hospital admissions and deaths include respiratory causes such as asthma, smoking-related lung disease (chronic obstructive pulmonary disease, COPD), and bronchitis. The respiratory system is an obvious target for an inhaled pollutant, but surprisingly a relatively large proportion of hospital admissions and deaths are due to cardiovascular causes such as heart attacks and strokes.

A large proportion of the particles within the PM_{10} spectrum are below 100 nm in size, and historically these have been called ultrafine particles. A significant number of research studies indicate that these ultrafine particles are relatively more reactive than larger par-ticles with respect to their ability to promote responses in lung epithelial and immune cells, which promote activation of the immune system and inflammation. Inflammation involves the influx of immune cells such as neutrophils and macrophages in order to ingest and clear the particles from the lung surface. Clearance takes place via either reloca-tion to the lymphatic system or migration along with mucus out of the respiratory tract. Such mechanisms protect the lungs from infection and pollutant exposure. However, on occasion these mechanisms may not work effectively, leading to reduced clearance of the pollutant or infective agent as well as prolonged inflammation. Prolonged inflammation is problematic, especially in individuals who already exhibit diseases driven via inflammation, for example asthma, COPD, bronchitis, and cardiovascular disease.

The ultrafine particles were proposed to be problematic due to their relatively large number per exposure mass and their small size (Donaldson et al. 2005). Ultrafine particles made from carbon and other low-toxicity materials were demonstrated to generate reactive oxygen species (ROS), which can either induce oxidative stress (depletion of antioxidants and oxidative damage of macromolecules) and/or activation of intracellular signalling pathways that promote the production of cytokine proteins that drive inflammation. It is hypothesized that this ultrafine particle derived inflammation is sufficient to worsen the symptoms of pre-existing disease, leading to increased medication use, hospitalization, or even death.

These observations and hypotheses led to concern that synthetic nanomaterials could induce similar health problems; for this reason the new field of nanotoxicology has now developed. Nanotoxicology not only includes consideration of inhalation as a route of exposure, but also ingestion, dermal absorption, and direct injection into the body. Furthermore, nanotoxicology includes a variety of target species in addition to humans in order to address the potential environmental impacts.

19.5 Relating the physical and chemical characteristics of nanomaterials to their toxicity

It is important to note that not all nanomaterials are equally toxic. There seems to be a wide variation in the biological reactivity of different nanomaterials, therefore there is much work underway to ascertain what makes a nanomaterial more or less likely to be toxic. This work is focusing on the identification of physical and chemical characteristics of the nanomaterials and trying to map these to biological responses. There are thousands of different nanomaterials already available, which is far too many to be tested on a case-by-case basis for both ethical and financial reasons. Instead scientists need to be able to predict nanomaterial toxicity. Current research aims to generate computer-based models that will predict toxicity from the known physical and chemical characteristics. This is also known as a 'structure–activity relationship', as is done for pharmaceutical agents.

Nanomaterials possess unusual properties because of their small size. Within any structure, the constituent atoms are held together by a series of bonds. These bonds occur at angles between the different atoms which are energetically favourable. Within a nanostructured object, the space available for these bonds to occur becomes restricted, forcing some bond angles to be less than favourable, resulting in a greater propensity to break and react with the surrounding environment. For this reason the behaviour of the material is modified, including the toxicity. It is therefore not possible to infer the toxicity of a nanomaterial directly from its chemistry alone. It is this surface reactivity that is responsible for some nanoparticles producing ROS and oxidative stress.

The introduction to this chapter has already detailed the variations between nanomaterials in relation to size, shape, and composition, but this is just the beginning of the potential complexities that exist. With respect to composition, nanomaterials can be made from almost any element within the periodic table. Sometimes the composition is simple, being limited to mainly one element (e.g. a metal or carbon) or perhaps an oxide of that element, but increasingly a single nanomaterial is made from several different combined materials. For example, a quantum dot, which is a light-emitting particle used for molecular imaging, can consist of a core of cadmium telluride, coated with zinc sulphate to encapsulate the toxic cadmium, and then decorated with protein or antibody to target it to a specific molecule within a biological specimen.

In addition, there are a number of other physical characteristics that can be varied between particles, such as surface area, charge, crystallinity, electrical conductance, solubility (also known as dissolution), and strength or durability.

Surface area is clearly related to particle size: smaller particles possess a greater relative surface area than larger particles of the same total weight. Since it is usually the surface of the particles that interacts with the biological system in which the particles are situated, the surface area clearly influences the dose experienced by that system. For low-solubility materials that are also of low toxicity, such as titanium dioxide and carbon, the surface area of particles has been linked to the ability of the particles to induce inflammation in the lungs of laboratory animals, oxidative stress in macrophages *in vitro*, and pro-inflammatory cytokine production by lung epithelial cells in culture. However, for more toxic particles, for example crystalline silica, which has a highly reactive surface, additional factors other than surface area clearly influence toxicity (Duffin et al. 2002).

Particle surface charge seems to influence particle uptake and toxicity into cells, although this is not yet completely understood. Many studies report positively charged particles to be more toxic than neutral or negatively charged particles (Arvizo et al. 2010). Within the body many molecules are charged. For example, many proteins have a net negative charge, therefore particle surface charge could influence molecular interactions. In addition, the lipid bilayer that makes up the cell surface is negatively charged, and there is a potential difference across the cell membrane of living cells, with the inside being negative compared to the outside. Again, each of these charge differentials can influence particle behaviour in the body that might lead to toxicity. Arvizo et al. (2010), using gold nanoparticles, were able to show that positively charged nanoparticles induced membrane depolarization of cells, leading to a calcium influx. Neural or negatively charged particles did not have this effect. Research using carbon black nanoparticles demonstrated that calcium influx is responsible for pro-inflammatory cytokine expression by macrophages (Brown et al. 2004). This study did not measure charge, but perhaps some nanoparticles induce some of their pro-inflammatory effects via alterations in membrane potential; this needs to be investigated further.

Crystallinity can vary between particles of the same chemical composition. Silica can be amorphous or crystalline. Titanium dioxide nanoparticles can include rutile or/and anatase forms of this metal oxide. For silica the crystalline form is clearly more toxic to the respiratory system for particles larger than the nanoscale. Crystalline silica particles are associated with fibrosis (silicosis) and lung cancer. For titanium dioxide the anatase form of this metal oxide has been found to be more toxic than the rutile form *in vitro* (Sayes et al. 2006), while *in vivo*, in the rat lung model, a higher anatase content has been associated with a greater inflammatory response than for pure rutile titanium dioxide (Warheit et al. 2007).

The relationship between electrical conductance and particle toxicity has not been investigated. However, because of the use of electrical potential difference and charge movement within biological systems for normal physiological function, conductivity is something that may need to be addressed.

Dissolution or solubility of particles is important for two reasons. Dissolution within a biologically relevant medium suggests that the particle is unlikely to be bio-persistent, hence dissolution could be a mechanism of clearance that would reduce the likelihood of particle-related toxicity. Alternatively, if the particle is made from a toxic substance, such as the cadmium in quantum dots, then dissolution results in mobilization of a component that results in adverse effects. When a particle enters the body there are a number of body fluids of different composition that it may interact with, such as the highly acidic gastric contents, the relatively neutral plasma of the blood, or the lipid-rich environment of the lung lining. Solubility may vary considerably between these different environments. Furthermore, if nanoparticles are internalized into cells by processes such as phagocytosis, they are likely to be compartmentalized into the relatively aggressive environment of the lysosomes, which have a pH of 4–5. A particle may therefore remain relatively stable within the extracellular environment, yet on entering the cell the intracellular environment may result in dissolution and release of toxic soluble components directly into the cell. Two particle types which appear to have some of their toxicity related to the dissolution of toxic ions include silver and zinc oxide. For silver there seems to be great variation between studies in terms of the relative solubility of the nanomaterial used, varying from less than 1% to 90%. This is likely to be due to different production, storage, and experimental set-ups, but such variation can clearly impact the toxicity data obtained for the particle tested.

Nanomaterial shape has already been mentioned briefly, with nanomaterials found to have many different morphologies. Fibre shape, also known as high aspect ratio, appears to play an important role in determining the toxic potential of respirable particles. Asbestos fibres (which are not nanomaterials) are related to lung fibrosis (scar tissue formation) and cancer, in particular a rather aggressive form of cancer known as mesothelioma. Mesothelioma occurs in the pleural space between the outer lung surface and the inner wall of the rib cage. The tumour is slow growing, sometimes taking 40 years to generate discernable symptoms, by which time it is so far progressed that treatment is not possible and life expectancy is often under one year. Asbestos-related diseases currently kill more than 2000 people per year due to the widespread historical use of this material. The death rate is anticipated to increase further over the next decade, and there is currently no known cure for such diseases.

For many years macrophages have been demonstrated to play a key role in the pathogenesis of these fibres. Macrophages are responsible for clearing inhaled particles from the respiratory system. These cells are approximately 15 µm in diameter, which means that as fibres increase in length above 10–15 µm they become increasingly difficult to ingest via phagocytosis. This situation results in frustrated phagocytosis with the cell failing to engulf the particle and clear it from the lung, leading to bio-persistence. Instead the cell stretches along the fibre length; in fact some studies have identified several macrophages along the length of a single asbestos fibre. As the cell ingests a particle, it generates ROS such as superoxide anion radicals, in an attempt to 'kill' the particle, as the particle may be a pathogen. Since the invagination in the cell surface remains open to the external environment, the ROS production continues, coming into contact with surrounding molecules and cells, leading to oxidative stress and potentially oxidative damage, often associated with further inflammation. The inflammatory and oxidative environment can also cause tissue damage, resulting in increased cell proliferation and mutagenesis, which when combined can result in an increased risk of carcinogenesis (Donaldson et al. 2011).

It is worth noting that fibres that are soluble, such as glass wool fibres, are easily dissolved within the lung environment, preventing bio-persistence and a continued inflammatory and oxidative environment. For this reason, fibres which are not durable are less problematic.

A number of nanomaterials could be considered as durable fibres, and are often of respirable dimensions. For this reason, concerns about the potential health effects of high aspect ratio nanomaterials have been raised. There are many different types of high aspect ratio nanomaterials, such as carbon nanotubes and a number of different metal and metal oxide nanorods, wires, and whiskers. With respect to toxicological assessment, so far the majority of work has been conducted using multi-walled carbon nanotubes. Studies include inhalation and instillation studies, but the results are diverse due to differences in the characteristics of the nanotubes (lengths, purity, defects, and shape), the mode of delivery (aerosol versus suspension), level of agglomeration (nanotubes are often highly agglomerated), and model employed (rat, mouse, and cell lines). Comparisons between different studies are difficult to make, but such contrasts seem to suggest that the more agglomerated forms are associated with greater pathological responses, such as granuloma formation.

Comparisons have been made between the ability of asbestos and nanotubes to invoke a mesothelial response in the peritoneal cavity of mice (Poland et al. 2008). The peritoneal cavity is lined with mesothelial cells which are comparable to those within the pleural space. The peritoneal cavity is much easier to inject into and study than the pleural space. These studies clearly show that long and relatively straight carbon nanotubes behave like long asbestos in that they induce an influx of inflammatory cells, thickening of the peritoneal mesothelium, and collagen deposition, all reactions associated with disease progression. In contrast, entangled nanotubes and short asbestos did not induce any significant response, clearly demonstrating the importance of dimensions and shape.

Recently, it has also been shown in animal models that asbestos fibres and long multiwalled carbon nanotubes injected directly into the pleural space become trapped due to their dimensions (Murphy et al. 2011). Lymph fluid naturally flows from the lung tissue into the pleural space and out into the lymphatic system via a number of holes known as stomata. These stomata are typically 10 µm in size, causing particles of greater than 10 µm to collect at the stomata without draining into the lymphatic system, leading to a local accumulation of the particles and interaction with the mesothelial cells lining the pleural cavity.

19.6 Toxicokinetics of nanomaterials

It is relatively difficult to study the toxicokinetics (absorption, distribution, metabolism, and excretion) of nanomaterials. In order to study the absorption and distribution of a chemical, toxicologists can simply measure the concentration of chemical in relevant tissues. However, the presence of the chemical constituents of a nanomaterial within a tissue sample does not allow identification of intact particle presence. A number of labelling techniques have been employed, including infrared light-emitting materials (e.g. some forms of gold nanorods) detectable via positron emission tomography (PET) scanners, contrast agents (e.g. iron oxide) detectable via magnetic resonance imaging (MRI) or radiolabels. With each technique it is necessary to ensure the stability of the label and that it remains attached to the particle. This is less of a problem for particles made directly from the labelling material, but is more of a problem for particles in which the label has been added subsequent to manufacture. For the infrared and MRI labels, the data provided is qualitative but not quantitative, which means you can see where the material goes but you cannot determine the actual amounts absorbed and distributed to specific locations. Radioactivity is quantitative, but is sometimes associated with potential release from the particulate material.

Very sensitive studies have been conducted using materials that can be neutron activated, such as gold (Semmler-Behnke et al. 2008). This work has demonstrated uptake into the body following instillation into the lung of particles suspended in liquid as well as by inhalation and ingestion. The proportion of uptake following ingestion is very low (less than 1%), but in all studies there is clear accumulation of nanoparticles in a number of organs, including the liver. Following direct injection into the blood, a small proportion of the nanoparticles were found within the faeces, suggesting that there is a route of excretion from the blood via the liver into bile.

19.7 Protein corona

When a foreign particle of any size enters the body, via any route, it immediately becomes coated with biological molecules such as proteins. This coating has been termed the 'protein corona' (Monopoli et al. 2011) and has been suggested to be important in determining the uptake, fate, and behaviour of the nanomaterial within the biological system. It is likely that this protein corona varies with particle type, and so it is the original particle characteristics which may ultimately determine the uptake, fate, and behaviour. However, knowledge about the corona and how it changes over time will help to elucidate the mechanisms by which different particles behave in the body.

19.8 Study design

Until 2004, much of the work conducted on nanoparticle toxicity focused on the respiratory route of exposure, therefore *in vivo* models included either inhalation or instillation experiments in rodents, while *in vitro* studies used bronchial and alveolar epithelial cell types as well as macrophages. As described earlier, there is now a need to address potential toxicity following exposure via ingestion, dermal application, and direct injection, and the models employed have therefore diversified accordingly to include these various exposure routes.

In addition, the demonstration that nanoparticles can translocate from organs such as the lung and gastrointestinal tract, as well as the medical injection of nanomaterials, has led to the need to study a wider array of target organs, such as the liver, brain, and cardiovascular system. Animal models remain important since this is predictive toxicology rather than reactive toxicology. Here scientists are not starting with a known disease for which they are trying to identify a cause; instead they are trying to predict whether there might be any adverse effects, therefore the target and disease scope for consideration is large, diverse, and complex. Using single-cell-type or tissue-type models does not allow for such complex questions to be addressed. There are European projects funded to generate models to mimic multiple tissue types and how they might interact. For example, the project InLiveTox (http://www.inlivetox.eu/) includes gastrointestinal epithelium, endothelial cells, and hepatocytes in a connected microfluidics system. From the air pollution literature, it is clear that healthy humans are relatively low risk in terms of pollution particle induced health effects, where as those with pre-existing disease are more susceptible. Models of susceptibility, both animal and *in vitro*, are also important to develop. There are some well-established models currently available, such as the ApoE mouse as a model for cardiovascular disease, but more are required. With respect to *in vitro* models, generating a pro-inflammatory environment may be more relevant, but this is seldom done. Again, InLiveTox is addressing this by using an inflamed gastrointestinal model for some of the studies.

Most studies require the preparation of nanomaterials in a liquid-based delivery agent prior to use. There is currently much debate about how to disperse nanomaterials in a relevant manner that will not lead to bias or irrelevant results. Such dispersions should be relevant in terms of the agglomeration status of the nanomaterial, i.e. what is the person likely to be exposed to? Many researchers recognize the need to include a dispersant to aid the de-agglomeration of nanoparticles, but the nature of the dispersant used varies, as does the point in the protocol at which it is added. Many *in vitro* studies use the standard serum concentration required for healthy cell growth to disperse the particles. The protein content of serum appears to be relatively efficient at providing good dispersion and stability to many particles. However, the dispersion protocol often involves sonication for anything up to 30 minutes. It is possible that sonication, or the heat generated by sonication, could impact on the serum, altering its stability and composition. Other studies disperse/sonicate the particles in water and then add this to the serum-containing medium. Some projects sonicate in a low serum content medium or water and then add to the experimental medium with the relevant higher concentration of serum present. Serum, however, is not the only dispersant used, for example it may not be considered to be relevant for some cell types such as those from the lung. Instead phospholipids, lung surfactant, detergents, and organic solvents have all been used. Organic solvents such as tetrahydrofuran, used with fullerenes, have been shown to influence toxicity results, hence are often avoided. In general, there are currently no clear answers, but most discussion is based on trying to make a protocol that is relevant and reproducible.

The dose of nanomaterials used in a study is also of great importance. It is difficult to publish an article in a peer-reviewed journal with irrelevant high doses, although researchers are not always clear what relevant doses may be because of the current lack of available exposure information. There is a need for dose–response relationships for nanomaterials to be provided, not just for cytotoxicity, but for sub-lethal effects too. Some studies have interestingly observed different effects at relatively low concentrations compared to high concentrations, presumably due to differences in the agglomeration of the particles. A lower dose therefore does not always mean less toxicity.

19.9 Ecotoxicology of nanomaterials

The ecotoxicology of nanomaterials has expanded rapidly to include studies on freshwater, marine and terrestrial invertebrates, vertebrates, plants, primary producers, and micro-organisms, therefore a review of this literature is beyond the scope of this chapter. Instead, it is worth considering that some of the same issues that concern human toxicology studies are also extremely relevant for these environmental models. For example, exposures to environmentally relevant particles, dispersed in an environmentally relevant manner, are extremely important. Most studies focus on healthy organisms, but a wider array of target models may need to be considered. What is interesting is that there seems to be some parity between human and environmentally relevant models in terms of the relative toxicity of nanomaterials. For example, a study investigating silver and cerium dioxide particles of nanoscale and larger recently demonstrated the same order of toxicity ranking across *Daphnia magna* (freshwater invertebrate), Carp (*Cyprius carpio*; freshwater fish), Carp hepatotocyes, a human hepatocytes cell line, and a human intestinal cell line (Caco-2) (Gaiser et al. 2011). In this study the silver was always more toxic than the cerium dioxide, and the nanoscale version was the most toxic.

19.10 Conclusion

A large body of toxicology data is now being generated for nanomaterials using a wide variety of models, protocols, and endpoints. It is clear that not all nanomaterials are equally toxic, and that there are variations based on their physical and chemical characteristics. Databases are being developed both in Europe (Napirahub) and the USA (NanoTAB) to act as central repositories for this data. These databases provide the opportunity for a variety of different analyses to be made, ranging from the relatively simple, such as all of the known toxic effects of a particular particle type, to relatively complex issues, such as the generation of models to allow structure–activity relationships to be generated, so that in the future we can hopefully predict the toxicity of new nanomaterials. However, such an ambition is probably still many years away, and so in the shorter term there is also a need to develop further relevant animal and non-animal models to try to predict the hazard of relevant doses of nanomaterials, dispersed using relevant methods, all of which requires more work.

19.11 References

Arvizo RR, Miranda OR, Thompson MA, Pabelick CM, Bhattacharya R, Robertson JD, Rotello VM, Prakash YS, Mukherjee P. (2010) Effect of nanoparticle surface charge at the plasma membrane and beyond. *Nano Lett* **10**(7):2543–2548.

British Standards. (2007) Terminology for nanomaterials. PAS 136. Ref Type: Report. British Standards Institution, London.

Brown DM, Donaldson K, Borm PJ, Schins RP, Denhart M, Gilmour P, Jimenez LA, Stone V. (2004) Calcium and reactive oxygen species-mediated activation of transcription factors and TNFa cytokine gene expression in macrophages exposed to ultrafine particles. *Am J Physiol Lung Cell Mol Physiol* **286**:L344–L353.

Chen X, Schluesener HJ. (2008) Nanosilver: A nanoproduct in medical application. *Toxicol Lett* **176**(1):1–12.

Donaldson K, Tran CL, Jimenez LA, Duffin R, Newby D, Mills N, MacNee W, Stone V. (2005) Combustion-derived nanoparticles: A critical review of their toxicology following inhalation exposure. *Particle Fibre Toxicol* **2**(10):1–14.

Donaldson K, Murphy F, Schinwald A, Duffin R, Poland CA. (2011) Identifying the pulmonary hazard of high aspect ratio nanoparticles to enable their safety-by-design. *Nanomedicine (Lond)* **6**(1):143–156.

Duffin R, Tran CL, Clouter A, Brown DM, MacNee W, Stone V, Donaldson K. (2002) The importance of surface area and specific reactivity in the acute pulmonary inflammatory response to particles. *Ann Occup Hyg* **46**(Suppl. 1):242–245.

Gaiser B, Fernandes TF, Jepson MA, Lead JR, Tyler CR, Baalousha M, Biswas A, Britton GJ, Cole PA, Johnston BD, Ju-Nam Y, Rosenkranz P, Scown TM, Stone V. (2011) Interspecies comparisons on the uptake and toxicity of silver and cerium dioxide nanoparticles. *Environ Toxicol Chem* **in press**.

Monopoli MP, Walczyk D, Campbell A, Elia G, Lynch I, Bombelli FB, Dawson KA. (2011) Physical-chemical aspects of protein corona: relevance to in vitro and in vivo biological impacts of nanoparticles. *J Am Chem Soc* **133**(8):2525–2534.

Murphy F et al. (2011) (manuscript submitted).

Osmond MJ, McCall MJ. (2010) Zinc oxide nanoparticles in modern sunscreens: an analysis of potential exposure and hazard. *Nanotoxicology* **4**(1):15–41.

Poland CA, Duffin R, Kinloch I, Maynard A, Wallace WA, Seaton A, Stone V, Brown S, MacNee W, Donaldson K. (2008) Carbon nanotubes introduced into the abdominal cavity of mice show asbestos-like pathogenicity in a pilot study. *Nat Nanotechnol* **3**(7):423–428.

Pope CA III. (2000) Epidemiology of fine particulate air pollution and human health: biologic mechanisms and who's at risk? *Environ Health Perspect* **108**(Suppl 4):713–723.

Powell AC, Paciotti GF, Libutti SK. (2010) Colloidal gold: a novel nanoparticle for targeted cancer therapeutics. *Methods Mol Biol* **624**:375–384.

Sayes CM, Wahi R, Kurian PA, Liu Y, West JL, Ausman KD, Warheit DB, Colvin VL. (2006) Correlating nanoscale titania structure with toxicity: a cytotoxicity and inflammatory response study with human dermal fibroblasts and human lung epithelial cells. *Toxicol Sci* **92**(1):174–185.

Semmler-Behnke M, Kreyling WG, Lipka J, Fertsch S, Wenk A, Takenaka S, Schmid G, Brandau W. (2008) Biodistribution of 1.4- and 18-nm gold particles in rats. *Small* **4**(12):2108–2111.

Warheit DB, Webb TR, ReedKL, Frerichs S, Sayes CM. (2007) Pulmonary toxicity study in rats with three forms of ultrafine-TiO2 particles: differential responses related to surface properties. *Toxicology* **230**(1):90–104.

Zhang W-S. (2003) Nanoscale iron particles for environmental remediation: an overview. *J Nanoparticle Res* **5**:323–332.

Appendix

Appendix

Basic medical concepts

David Baker, Lakshman Karalliedde,
and Virginia Murray

Learning outcomes

At the end of this chapter and any recommended reading the student should be able to:

1. understand the basic structure and function of cells and how they are vulnerable to toxic substances;

2. understand the structure and function of the systems of the human body;

3. understand how body systems are vulnerable to toxic substances;

4. use the knowledge gained to better understand the content of other chapters of this book, and

5. apply acquired knowledge in the analysis and management of hazardous situations.

A1 Introduction

This appendix is designed to provide basic knowledge about the structure and function of the human body for those who have received no formal education in medicine, biological sciences, or human biology. Readers will find this section useful for understanding the terminology used in the main body of the book, as will lecturers on the *Essentials in Toxicology for Health Protection* course. The appendix is also designed to stimulate interested health professionals to learn more of the disease states and disorders of organs and systems in the body that follow exposure to toxic chemicals.

The human body can be divided into a number of systems on the basis of both structure (anatomy) and function (physiology). Each of these systems can be affected by exposure to toxic agents and some play an essential role in combating toxic effects.

The information presented will describe the essentials of normal function of body systems and so provide reference points for the toxic effects described in other chapters.

A2 Cells: the fundamental building blocks of body systems

Humans have evolved from life forms that were originally just single cells in the primordial ocean. The function of the whole body depends on providing each of its 30 trillion cells with a suitable chemical environment, water, and oxygen. The cells of the body require a constant environment which is independent of changes in the outside world. This is ensured by the chemical composition of the extracellular fluid in the body, which bathes each of the cells.

For the amount of a substance in the body to remain constant, the amount gained each day must not exceed the amount required by the cells to function and that is excreted or lost from the body each day.

If intake exceeds the amounts required by cells daily to function normally and that of loss, there will be an imbalance. The amount of this imbalance will determine whether the cells will function abnormally (dysfunction or malfunction).

It will also determine whether cells would multiply abnormally (producing growths—tumours or malignancies) or die. This is the basis of toxicology, where the amount taken by the body is in excess of its needs and/or exceeds the amount that can be lost from the body by normal mechanisms, resulting in malfunction, disease, or death.

The amounts of foreign substances that enter the body depend on ingestion and absorption from the gut, the amounts inhaled (taken in during breathing), and the amounts absorbed through the skin. Foreign substances may cause toxic effects by entering the cells directly or from the fluid that surrounds them.

Toxic substances can also enter by other means, such as when venomous animals bite or sting.

The essential points about the structure and function of body cells are shown in Box A1.

A2.1 Specialized cells

Cells in the body have developed from primary stems cells to perform specific functions (e.g. muscle cells for movement, nerve cells for transmission of impulses or messages, liver cells for metabolism). This process is called cell differentiation. Approximately 200 distinct types of such cells can be identified in the human body. In the body cells migrate to different locations, adhere to each other, and form multicellular structures or tissues (e.g. muscle tissue, nerve tissue, epithelial tissue, and connective tissue). Different types of tissues come together in varying proportions and arrange in differing forms, such as layers or bundles, to form organs, such as the heart and kidney. Most organs possess similar functional sub-units, each contributing to the functions of an organ. Organs with similar functions are often grouped together as systems. There are 10 organ systems in the human body classified on the basis of both structure (anatomy) and function (physiology). Each of these systems can be affected by environmental toxic agents whilst some play an essential role in protecting the human body or minimizing harm following toxic environmental exposures.

A2.2 Body systems

Specialized cells give rise to the systems that make up the body, which are:

1. the nervous system, comprising the central nervous system and peripheral nervous system, including the autonomic nervous system (sympathetic and parasympathetic nervous systems), neurotransmitters, and the neuromuscular junction

Box A1 Structure and overall function of cells

Cell structure and function determine life, disease, and death. Almost all cells have fundamental activities that are necessary for maintaining cell integrity and function, i.e. for a cell to be alive. The thousands of chemical reactions taking place within the human body all the time are collectively referred to as metabolism. Fundamentally, there is a balance between synthesis of substances (anabolism) and breakdown of excess waste products (catabolism). Many of these processes require enzymes (catalysts). Essential products are often the result of enzyme-mediated reactions, which are called metabolic pathways.

Cells: the fundamental building blocks of body systems. Each cell of the body consists of a closed membrane (double layer of lipid (fat) molecules with embedded proteins) which contains functional units within the cell. The membrane itself contains key cell organelles acting as a selective barrier to the passage of molecules, detecting chemical messengers and linking adjacent cells together to form tissues and organs. A space of at least 20 nm exists between the opposing membranes. The membrane is a vital component of the overall structure of the cell.

The cell membrane encloses the main constituents of the cell, the nucleus and cytoplasm.

Nucleus: This comprises the nucleolus, which is composed of DNA and coiled threads of protein-chromatin. These condense to form chromosomes, which store genetic information that is transferred during cell division via RNA. Not all cells have the same nuclear structure, for example skeletal muscle cells have multiple nuclei and red cells none.

Cytoplasm: This is the cell material outside the nucleus and contains:

- endoplasmic reticulum involved in packaging of proteins to be secreted by the cell and for lipid synthesis;
- ribosomes: a large number of proteins and several RNA molecules, which synthesize proteins from amino acids using genetic information.
- mitochondria (spherical or elongated rod-like structures) with iron-containing proteins (cytochromes) which require oxygen to generate adenosine triphosphate (ATP) as a fuel supply for the cell. Carbon dioxide is a waste product of these metabolic processes. Lack of sufficient oxygen, e.g. from decreased oxygen concentration in inhaled air or toxicity to cytochromes from cyanide, will cause cell dysfunction/death due to lack of energy.
- liposomes: these break down bacteria and dead cells within the cell and are an important intracellular digestive system in the specialized cells that make up the defence system of the body.

2. the respiratory system, comprising the lungs and breathing (including transport of oxygen and carbon dioxide)

3. the heart and circulation (the cardiovascular system), including blood and blood components, blood pressure, and the blood vessels

4. the gastrointestinal system, including the stomach and intestines
5. the liver, including normal functions and the important feature of the metabolism of foreign substances (xenobiotics)
6. the kidney and reproductive system
7. the endocrine system, i.e. the production and role of hormones in the body
8. the immune system and body defence mechanisms.

In addition to these systems the body comprises cartilage, bone, ligaments, tendons, and skeletal muscles, which support and protect and allow movement of body.

Finally, all these systems are enclosed inside the skin, which can be regarded as an organ in itself. It is constantly being renewed and provides protection against injury and dehydration, defence against entrance of foreign substances, and regulation of body temperature.

A3 The nervous system

The main functions of the nervous system are to monitor, integrate (process), and respond to information from inside and outside the body. The nervous system controls or regulates many body functions essential to life such as breathing (respiratory centre), circulation (vasomotor centre), hormonal secretions, temperature, and indirectly the activity of the lungs, blood vessels, heart, kidneys, and several other organs. Fundamentally, the role of the nervous system is to maintain normal body function by making the necessary adjustments or responses to changes that may eventually cause harm or ill-health.

The nervous system controls body functions and receives information from the outside world by means of transmission of electrical impulses passing along nerve cells (neurons). In various parts of the system these signals are passed from cell to cell by special relay stations called synapses, where the signal is passed by a chemical messenger. These chemical messengers are called neurotransmitters. Special synapses are found at the end of nerves which pass a signal directly onto an organ, also through a neurotransmitter. Synapses can be regarded as being amplifiers of the electrical signals transmitted through the nervous system.

Overall, the nervous system consists of the central nervous system (CNS), comprising the brain and spinal cord, and the peripheral nervous system (PNS), which is composed of nerves extending to and from the CNS. The major constituent systems of the central and peripheral nervous systems, shown in Box A2, are described in the following sections.

A3.1 The central nervous system

The brain and spinal cord are made up of dense accumulations of nerve cells and their associated fibres. The cell bodies give rise to grey matter and the fibres, with a special coating called myelin, make up the white matter. The whole central nervous system is carefully protected. Three connective tissue membranes called meninges enclose the brain and the spinal cord. These meninges cover the nerves entering and leaving the brain and the spinal cord to varying lengths. The meninges also enclose blood vessels and venous sinuses (large veins into which blood drains from the nerve cells). Meninges retain

Box A2 The major parts of the nervous system

Central nervous system

Peripheral nervous system	→ autonomic	→ sympathetic
		→ parasympathetic
	→ somatic	

cerebrospinal fluid (CSF), which is a watery liquid similar, but not identical, in composition to blood plasma, which supports, cushions, and nourishes the brain. The meninges form artitions within the skull and brain. Inflammation of these lining membranes gives rise to the serious condition called meningitis whilst inflammation of the brain tissue itself (nerve cells) is referred to as encephalitis.

The major regions of the brain are the cerebrum, the midbrain, pons, the medulla oblongata, and the cerebellum, which are shown in Figure A1.

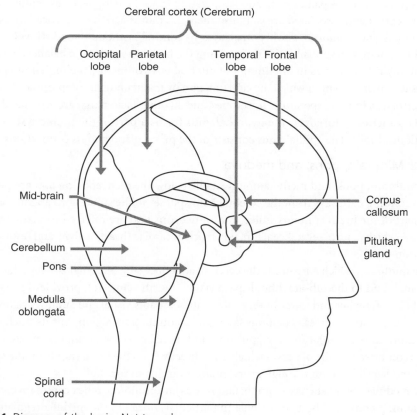

Fig. A1 Diagram of the brain. Not to scale.

A3.1.1 The cerebral hemispheres (cerebrum)

The cerebral hemispheres are the uppermost part of the brain and are separated by the longitudinal fissure formed by the meninges. They make up approximately 83% of total brain mass and are collectively referred to as the cerebrum.

The cerebral cortex (cerebrum) constitutes a 2–4 mm thick grey matter surface layer. Because of its many convolutions, the grey matter accounts for about 40% of total brain mass. It is responsible for conscious behaviour and contains three different functional areas: the motor areas, sensory areas, and association areas. Also located internally in the cerebral cortex are the white matter, responsible for communication between cerebral areas and between the cerebral cortex and lower regions of the CNS, as well as the basal nuclei (or basal ganglia), involved in controlling muscular movement and several bodily functions. CSF is contained in the lateral ventricles located in the cerebral hemispheres.

The diencephalon is located centrally within the forebrain (the anterior or front part of the brain). It consists of the thalamus, hypothalamus, and epithalamus, which together enclose the third ventricle (a sac containing cerebrospinal fluid found within the brain which is connected to the lateral ventricles in the cerebral hemispheres and to the fourth ventricle in the brain stem). The thalamus acts as a grouping and relay station for sensory inputs (inputs such as pain, touch, and temperature from the periphery), ascending to the sensory cortex and associated areas. It also mediates motor activities, cortical arousal or wakefulness, and memories. The hypothalamus, by controlling the autonomic (involuntary) nervous system, is responsible for maintaining the body's homeostatic balance, which is commonly referred to as maintaining the internal environment ('the milieu interior'). This is the environment in which the cells function by maintaining the appropriate balance of electrolytes, ions, temperature, hormones, and all other factors that are associated with normal function. Moreover, the hypothalamus forms a part of the limbic system, the 'emotional' brain. The epithalamus consists of the pineal gland and its connections.

A3.1.2 Midbrain, pons, and medulla

The midbrain, pons, and medulla oblongata lie below the diencephalon and are part of the continuing pathways from the cerebral hemispheres to the spinal cord and its nerves. This part of the brain contains collections of neurons that are referred to as 'nuclei' or 'centres', which control several vital functions such as cardiac (heart) activity and respiration (breathing).

The midbrain, which surrounds the cerebral aqueduct (the duct that conveys the cerebrospinal fluid to the sub-arachnoid space via the fourth ventricle), provides fibre pathways between higher and lower brain centres, and contains visual and auditory reflex and subcortical motor centres. The pons is mainly a conduction region, but its nuclei also contribute to the regulation of respiration and nuclei of some cranial nerves. Cranial nerves comprise 12 pairs of nerves which arise directly from the brain (not from the spinal cord) and leave the brain through apertures or foramina in the skull.

The medulla oblongata has an important role as an autonomic reflex centre involved in maintaining body vital body functions. In particular, nuclei in the medulla regulate respiratory rhythm (the respiratory centre), heart rate (cardiac centre), and blood pressure (vasomotor centre), and contain the nuclei of several cranial nerves. Moreover, the medulla oblongata provides important conduction pathways between the spinal cord and higher brain centres.

A3.1.3 Cerebellum

The cerebellum, which is located behind the pons and medulla, accounts for about 11% of total brain mass. Like the cerebrum, it has a thin outer cortex of grey matter, internal white matter, and small, deeply situated paired masses (nuclei) of grey matter. The cerebellum processes impulses received from the cerebral motor cortex, various brain stem nuclei, and sensory receptors in order to 'fine-tune' skeletal muscle contraction (the muscles that control movement, walking, running etc), thus giving smooth, co-ordinated movements.

A3.1.4 Spinal cord

The spinal cord is the direct continuation of the brain from the brainstem into the verte-bral column. It contains the nerve pathways through which messages are sent from the brain (efferent pathways) and to the brain (afferent pathways). Like the brain itself, the spinal cord is composed of central grey matter containing nerve cells and white matter which comprises nerve fibres. Not all messages controlling the body have to go up to the brain and return. The nerves of the grey matter in the cord can act on their own in response to a sensory stimulus. This action is known as a 'spinal reflex' and the knee jerk is perhaps the best-known example.

The structure of the spinal cord and its connections are shown in Figures A2, A3, and A4.

A3.2 The peripheral nervous system

This contains motor nerves that control voluntary movement together with sensory nerves that carry information concerning touch, pain, temperature, and position to the brain.

Nerves arise from nerve cells and the basic structure of a nerve cell is shown in Figure A5.

Nerve cells have a cell body, dendrites and an axon. The nerve cell and its processes are called neurons. The nerve cell and its processes behave like a small electrical battery: the resting voltage inside the nerve cell is −70 mV, one millivolt being one thousandth of a volt. The fluid inside the nerve cell, like that of other cells in the body, contains a high concentration of potassium ions (K^+). In contrast, the nerve cell is surrounded by tissue fluid which contains mainly sodium chloride, which gives rise to sodium ions (Na^+). In the resting state, the sodium ions are removed from the interior of the cell by the sodium pump. The pump effectively exchanges sodium ions for potassium ions. Both sodium ions and potassium ions diffuse across the cell membrane. Potassium diffuses much more rapidly than sodium, thus generating the resting membrane potential of about −70 mV (interior negative to exterior).

A nerve impulse is a transient event which for a very short period of time alters the permeability of the cell membrane and allows sodium ions to enter the cell. These positively charged sodium ions change the potential inside the cell from −70 mV to +40 mV—a process called depolarization. The sudden change from negative to positive voltage inside the cell is

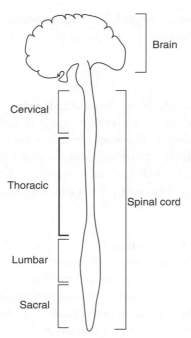

Fig. A2 Diagram of the spinal cord. Not to scale. The spinal cord is an extension of the brain itself and is divided into cervical, thoracic, lumbar, and sacral sections according to the vertebrae which surround and protect it.

termed an action potential, and is propagated along the cell membrane. Each action potential corresponds to a nerve impulse or message which is conveyed to its destination by the membrane, changing its 'behaviour' along the whole nerve, causing a propagation of the nerve impulse.

A nerve impulse lasts about 1 ms and each nerve impulse in both motor and sensory nerves (i.e. nerves that carry messages or impulses to the spinal cord and brain from the peripheral tissues as regards pain, temperature, and touch) is associated with sodium entering and potassium leaving the cell momentarily. Following the action potential, i.e. during the resting phase, there is gradual expulsion of the sodium that entered the nerve cell. The maximum rate of discharge from an anterior horn cell is considered to be approximately 200 impulses a second.

The rate of propagation of an impulse along a nerve or nerve conduction varies with the size of the nerve fibre, the large nerve fibres, with a diameter of 20 μm, have a velocity of conduction of 120 m/s. These large fibres have a sheath made up mainly of fatty material called a myelin (i.e. the nerves are myelinated), and the gaps in this sheath, called nodes of Ranvier, enable a nerve impulse to 'leap-frog' down the nerve as the exchange of sodium and potassium ions only occurs at these interruptions in the myelin sheath.

The smaller fibres, such as those that convey pain impulses to the brain, are about 1 μm in diameter and are not individually myelinated. They therefore conduct impulses slower, at about 5 m/s.

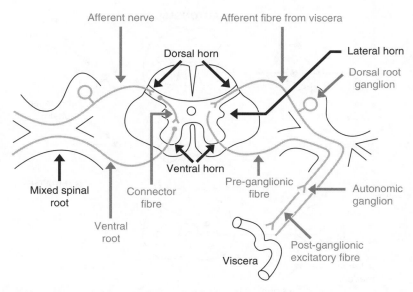

Afferent nerve

Afferent fibre from viscera

Dorsal horn

Lateral horn

Dorsal root
ganglion

Ventral horn

Mixed spinal
root

Connector
fibre

Pre-ganglionic
fibre

Autonomic
ganglion

Ventral
root

Viscera

Post-ganglionic
excitatory fibre

Fig. A3 Diagram of the somatic nervous system and visceral nervous system. Not to scale. Impulses are received via afferent nerves—the cells of the afferent nerves are in the dorsal horn. Transmission of impulses from the dorsal horn to cells in the ventral horn takes place via connecting neurons. The cell in the dorsal horn which sends the nerve fibre or axon is called the internuncial cell. The ventral horn cell and its nerve fibre (axon) send impulses (efferent) to skeletal muscle cells to help us move. Impulses from viscera (e.g. intestines) are sent to the spinal cord via afferent nerves with the cell in the dorsal root (dorsal root ganglion)—the central process enters the spinal cord (grey matter). Connecter cells are in the grey matter. The connector fibres or pre-ganglionic fibres pass to a peripheral ganglion. From these peripheral ganglia (which may receive more than one pre-ganglionic fibre), nerves arise to supply the viscera. These are therefore post-ganglionic fibres.

A3.2.1 Autonomic nervous system

The part of the peripheral nervous system that supplies smooth muscles (in contrast to the striated or skeletal muscles found in our limbs etc.) is termed the autonomic nervous system. The autonomic nervous system also controls the heart, the digestive and urinary systems, and the secreting glands such as sweat and salivary glands. In general, the autonomic nervous system is concerned with involuntary nerve impulses. The part of the peripheral nervous system that controls voluntary actions, such as movement, is known as the somatic or motor nervous system.

The autonomic nervous system itself is subdivided into:

1. the sympathetic nervous system

2. the parasympathetic nervous system.

These systems differ in the chemical transmitter involved in the transmission of impulses at synapses. In the sympathetic nervous system the chemical transmitter is predominantly noradrenaline, whereas in the parasympathetic nervous system the chemical messenger is

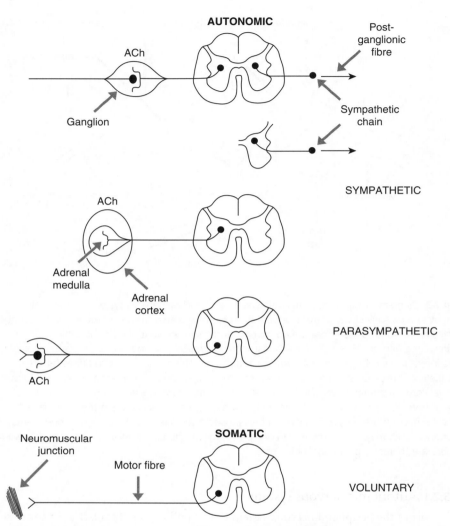

Fig. A4 Diagram of efferent pathways from the spinal cord. Not to scale. These are either autonomic (sympathetic and parasympathetic) or somatic (the nerves controlling muscles). The autonomic system goes through a series of relay stations called ganglia, some of which lie alongside the spinal cord itself, e.g. the sympathetic chain.

acetyl choline. The actions of these two sections of the autonomic nervous system are shown in Table A1 and Figure A6.

The sympathetic nervous system The sympathetic nervous system is active in states of emotional excitement and stress. The system gives rise to what has been called the 'flight or fight' reaction.

Increased sympathetic nerve activity causes the heart to beat faster and also increases the force of contraction of the ventricles of the heart (the force with which the heart muscle contracts). These effects cause an increase in the output from the heart (cardiac output)

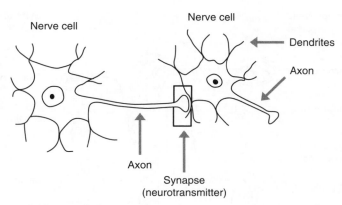

Nerve cell

Nerve cell

Dendrites

Axon

Axon

Synapse
(neurotransmitter)

Fig. A5 Diagram of a nerve cell. Not to scale.

and therefore the blood pressure increases. In addition, the pupils of the eye dilate, the air passages increase in diameter, allowing an individual to breath in more air, and the muscles associated with sweat glands and skin contract, causing the hair to 'stand on end' and goose pimples to form. The rate at which breathing occurs also increases because of the excitement of the respiratory centres in the brain. In addition, sympathetic stimulation slows down the contractions of the digestive tract.

Structure of the sympathetic nervous system The nerve cell (the neuron) in the spinal cord sends a fibre (axon), referred to as the pre-ganglionic fibre, to the ganglion (a collection of nerve cells and their fibres), which is called the sympathetic ganglion. A second fibre starts from the synapse within the ganglion and terminates in the organ (e.g. smooth muscle) it supplies. The preganglionic fibre is covered by a white fatty sheath made of myelin. For this

Table A1 Actions of the autonomic nervous system

Organ supplied	Sympathetic activity	Parasympathetic activity
Pupil of the eye	Dilates	Constricts
Air passages, bronchi, and bronchioles	Dilates	Constricts
Salivary glands	–	Increased salivary secretion and dilatation of blood vessels
Heart	Speeds up, increases force of ventricular contraction	Slows heart rate
Digestive tract	Reduces motility	Increases motility
Sphincters of the digestive tract	Constricts	Relaxes
Rectum	Allows filling	Empties and relaxes internal anal a sphincter
Bladder	Allows filling	Empties and relaxes internal sphincter
Blood vessels	Vasoconstriction	Nil (except salivary gland and external genitalia-vasodilatation)
Sweat glands	Sweating	Nil

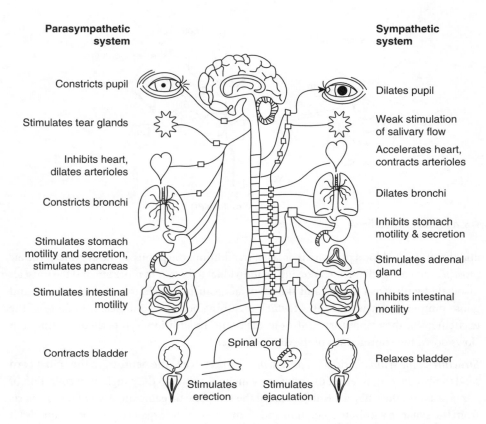

Parasympathetic system

Constricts pupil

Stimulates tear glands

Inhibits heart, dilates arterioles

Constricts bronchi

Stimulates stomach motility and secretion, stimulates pancreas

Stimulates intestinal motility

Contracts bladder

Spinal cord

Stimulates erection

Stimulates ejaculation

Sympathetic system

Dilates pupil

Weak stimulation of salivary flow

Accelerates heart, contracts arterioles

Dilates bronchi

Inhibits stomach motility & secretion

Stimulates adrenal gland

Inhibits intestinal motility

Relaxes bladder

Fig. A6 Diagram of the autonomic nervous system and the organs it controls. Not to scale.

reason, the bundle of pre-ganglionic fibres is called the white ramus. The fibre after the ganglion is termed the post-ganglionic fibre and does not have a myelin sheath, therefore it is grey in colour and is referred to as the grey ramus.

In the spinal cord, the pre-ganglionic outflow takes place between the first thoracic segment and the second lumbar segment. The cells of origin are in the lateral horn of the spinal grey matter in these segments and the fibres leave the spinal cord with the nerves to the voluntary or skeletal or striated muscles. All the fibres from these cells in the lateral horns run to a chain of neurons called the sympathetic chain, which lies very close to the spinal cord. The sympathetic trunk extends upwards towards the neck to the angle of the jaw (superior cervical ganglion of the sympathetic chain) and extends downwards across the back of the thoracic and abdominal cavities to the pelvis.

The chemical transmitters found in the sympathetic nervous system are adrenaline (epinephrine) and noradrenaline (norepinephrine). Chemically, noradrenaline and adrenaline are amines of the benzene derivative catechol and are referred to collectively as catecholamines. Noradrenaline is rapidly removed after release, mainly by re-uptake into the nerve, so that the target organ is capable of responding to further nerve impulses.

Effects of sympathetic nervous activity Over-activity of the sympathetic nervous system leads to narrowing of blood vessels (vasoconstriction) and consequently a reduction of the blood supply to the organ or tissue. If it is widespread, the narrowing of the blood vessels will lead to an increase in blood pressure (hypertension), profuse sweating, and dilatation of the pupils.

Sympathetic nerve fibres can cause either contraction or relaxation of the smooth muscle of the innervated structure. When noradrenaline causes contraction, the receptor responding to the neurotransmitter is referred to as an alpha receptor. If the action of the sympathetic nerve system is to cause relaxation, the receptor concerned is called a beta receptor. The alpha and beta receptors found in the sympathetic system are called Ahlquist receptors. These can be blocked selectively by either alpha or beta blockers. Blockade of beta receptors in the heart is used to reduce blood pressure. Stimulation of beta receptors in the airways is used in the treatment of asthma to dilate or increase the lumen through which air can move in the small airways or bronchioles of the lung.

In addition there are ganglion-blocking drugs that block transmission at the sympathetic ganglia, thereby preventing the transmission of the nerve impulse from the pre-ganglionic fibre to the post-ganglionic fibre. These ganglion blockers are used to treat very high blood pressure in cases of emergency.

A3.2.2 Parasympathetic nervous system

The parasympathetic fibres originate in the cranial nerves and the lower end of the spinal cord (the sacral region). The 12 cranial nerves have their cells of origin in the brainstem. The third, seventh, ninth, and tenth cranial nerves all contain parasympathetic fibres. The tenth cranial nerve or the vagus nerve is the principal parasympathetic nerve and its stimulation causes a slowing of the heart amongst many other effects, such as those on the stomach and stomach secretions, oesophagus, and the small airways of the lungs.

As in the sympathetic system, the parasympathetic nervous system has two neurons which give rise to the pre-ganglionic and post-ganglionic nerves. However, the post-ganglionic nerve is usually very short. In the heart, the ganglion and the post-ganglionic nerves lie within the organ of innervation, the cardiac muscle.

The neurotransmitter at ganglions (synapses), which are junctions between the pre-ganglionic fibres and the post-ganglionic fibres, in both the parasympathetic nervous system and the sympathetic nervous system is acetylcholine (see Figure A4 of the peripheral nervous system). Acetylcholine is also the neurotransmitter at the post-ganglionic nerve endings of the parasympathetic nervous system, and acts as the neurotransmitter at some post-ganglionic nerve endings of the sympathetic nervous system.

Acetylcholine (ACh) has two distinct actions within the autonomic nervous system and at the neuromuscular junction, which are described as nicotinic or muscarinic. These terms were used since early experimenters applied the two chemicals nicotine or muscarine (found in toadstools) directly to autonomic nerves. Acetylcholine activity in the ganglia of the parasympathetic systems and the neuromuscular junction is called nicotinic, while the activity at the junction between the end of the nerve and the organ supplied, other than skeletal muscle, is termed muscarinic.

Like noradrenaline, the effects of acetylcholine are terminated very quickly after its release. However, for acetylcholine this is due to the activity of the enzyme acetylcholine esterase (AChE) which breaks down acetyl choline. Inhibition of this enzyme is the basis of poisoning by organophosphate pesticides and nerve gases (see Chapter 17).

In most parts of the body, the action of the parasympathetic nervous system is the opposite of that of the sympathetic nervous system (Table A1). Thus it slows the heart rate, lowers blood pressure, constricts the pupils, and constricts or narrows the airways. In addition, the parasympathetic nervous system speeds up digestion and plays an important role in defaecation and emptying of the bladder, and increases secretions from several glands such as the salivary glands and tear glands.

A3.3 Neurotransmitters

In 1921, the Austrian scientist Otto Loewi discovered the first neurotransmitter. In his experiment (which came to him in a dream), he used two frog hearts. One heart (heart 1) was still connected to the vagus nerve. Heart 1 was placed in a chamber that was filled with saline. This chamber was connected to a second chamber that contained heart 2. Fluid from chamber 1 was allowed to flow into chamber 2. Electrical stimulation of the vagus nerve caused heart 1 to slow down. Loewi also observed that after a delay, heart 2 also slowed down. From this experiment, Loewi hypothesized that electrical stimulation of the vagus nerve released a chemical into the fluid of chamber 1 that flowed into chamber 2. He called this chemical 'Vagusstoff'. We now know this chemical as the neurotransmitter called acetylcholine.

Neuroscientists (scientists who study the nervous system) consider the following criteria necessary for a chemical to be termed a neurotransmitter:

- the chemical must be produced within a nerve cell;
- the chemical must be found within a nerve cell;
- when a nerve cell is stimulated, the nerve cell must release the chemical;
- when the chemical is released it must act on a specialized area, usually in the adjacent or neighbouring nerve cell (the post-synaptic nerve cell) and cause a biological effect where usually there is a change that alters the movement of ions across a cell membrane;
- after the chemical is released it must be inactivated—this may occur due to re-uptake of the chemical by the nerve cell that released it or by an enzyme which alters its chemical structure and therefore prevents further action at the receptor or specialized nerve ending; and
- if this chemical is applied on the post-synaptic membrane (i.e. the membrane of the adjacent nerve cell), it should produce the same effect as when the chemical is released by a nerve cell.

There are many types of chemical that act as neurotransmitters. The more common neurotransmitters and those of particular interest in toxicology are:

- acetylcholine
- norepinephrine (originally called noradrenaline)

- epinephrine (originally called adrenaline)
- dopamine
- serotonin
- histamine
- gamma-amino butyric acid (GABA)
- glycine, and
- glutamate aspartate.

Acetylcholine is found in both the central and peripheral nervous systems. Choline is taken up by the neuron. When the enzyme choline acetyltransferase is present, choline combines with acetyl coenzyme A (CoA) to produce acetylcholine.

Dopamine, norepinephrine, and epinephrine are a group of neurotransmitters called 'catecholamines'. Each of these neurotransmitters is produced in a step-by-step fashion by different enzymes.

Neurotransmitters are made in the cell body of the neuron and then transported down the axon to the axon terminal. Molecules of neurotransmitters are stored in small packages called vesicles. Neurotransmitters are released from the axon terminal when their vesicles 'fuse' with the membrane of the axon terminal, spilling the neurotransmitter into the synaptic cleft.

Neurotransmitters will bind only to specific areas (receptors) on the post-synaptic membrane that recognize them.

A3.3.1 Some neurotransmitters and their effects

Norepinepherine (noradrenaline) Norepinepherine functions in:

- arousal, energy, drive
- stimulation
- stimulation
- fight or flight.

Norepinepherine deficiencies result in:

- lack of energy
- lack of motivation
- depression.

Dopamine Dopamine functions in:

- feelings of pleasure
- feelings of attachment/love
- sense of altruism
- integration of thoughts and feelings.

Dopamine deficiencies result in:

◆ anhedonia: the loss of the capacity to experience pleasure, which is a core clinical feature of depression, schizophrenia, and some other mental illnesses
◆ lack of ability to feel love, sense attachment to another
◆ lack of remorse about actions
◆ distractibility.

Serotonin Serotonin functions in:

◆ emotional stability
◆ reducing aggression
◆ sensory input
◆ sleep cycle
◆ appetite control.

Serotonin deficiencies result in:

◆ irritability
◆ irrational emotions
◆ sudden unexplained tears
◆ obsessive-compulsive disorder
◆ sleep disturbances.

Gamma-aminobutyric acid GABA functions in:

◆ control of anxiety
◆ control of arousal
◆ control of convulsions
◆ keeping brain activity 'balanced'.

GABA deficiencies result in:

◆ 'free-floating' anxiety
◆ racing thoughts
◆ rapid heart
◆ inability to fall asleep
◆ constant 'fight or flight' state
◆ panic.

A3.4 The neuromuscular junction

The junction between the motor nerve and the skeletal muscle fibre which it supplies is the neuromuscular junction. This is very important both in health and disease for several reasons. Firstly, there is a gap between the nerve fibre endings and the muscle fibres, and the messages across this gap are carried by the neurotransmitter acetylcholine.

The acetylcholine is synthesized in the nerve fibre and is discharged when an impulse reaches the end of the nerve fibre. This chemical messenger reaches specialized parts of the muscle fibre called end plates, which contain specific receptors through which sodium ions pass into muscle fibre and produce a change in membrane potential called the end plate potential. This movement of ions—depolarization—spreads to the whole muscle fibre (propagated action potential), causing calcium ion release, and muscle contraction follows.

Acetylcholine stays only for a very brief period at the neuromuscular junction as it is quickly hydrolysed or inactivated by the enzyme acetylcholinesterase. This enables the next impulse to release acetylcholine again and cause another muscle contraction.

The neuromuscular junction functional activity is vulnerable to many toxic substances. Firstly, toxic substances can interfere with the production and release of the chemical messenger acetylcholine. The specialized parts of the muscle fibres may be damaged or altered in disease states such as myasthenia gravis. The enzyme cholinesterase, which restricts acetylcholine in time and space, can be inactivated by several toxic substances, of which the best known are the pesticides belonging to the class of compounds called organophosphates. Some chemical warfare agents (nerve agents), such as sarin, tabun, and soman, also are organophosphates and produce the same effect.

Importantly in medical practice, particularly in the speciality of anaesthesia, drugs are used to prevent transmission at the neuromuscular junction and thus produce muscle relaxation (the drugs used are called muscle relaxants) to facilitate surgery. Historically the Indians of South America used an arrow poison to paralyse their prey during hunting and this arrow poison was refined to become one of the best known muscle relaxants: curare or tubocurarine.

Every muscle in the body consists of muscle fibres, which are the units that cause muscles to contract and enable all forms of motor activity such as walking, running, and talking. Every muscle fibre needs a nerve supply in order to contract. Nerves controlling muscle fibres have their origins in the spinal cord (anterior horn cells) and as there are more muscle fibres than nerve cells, each nerve cell or anterior horn cell innervates more than one muscle fibre. For example in the leg as many as 200 muscle fibres may share a single anterior horn cell. Where eye muscles are concerned, only about five muscle fibres share one anterior horn cell.

These nerves leaving the anterior horn cell are called axons or motor nerves, and branch to supply a group of muscle fibres on reaching the muscle. The anterior horn cell and the muscle fibres supplied by this neuron are called the motor unit. The motor unit forms the basis for voluntary movement (movements which are intentional). If the motor nerve or axon is cut or damaged, paralysis of muscles occurs.

Nerves from the anterior horn cells carry nerve impulses or messages that enable the muscle fibres to contract. If an anterior horn cell discharges slowly or at a very low frequency, the muscles tend to be relaxed or flaccid. When the rate of discharge from the neurons increases, one may see co-ordinated contractions. However, these motor neurons are capable of discharging at very fast rates, usually in disease states, leading to either tremulous contractions (clonus) or sustained contractions (tetanus). Tetanus is also the name given to an infection (lock-jaw) caused by the tetanus bacillus *(Clostridium tetani)*, which occurs when wounds become contaminated with soil/faeces that contain the bacteria. Tetanus was a serious consequence of accidents and war injuries before immunization against the disease became available.

A4 The heart and circulatory system—the cardiovascular system

The heart and the cardiovascular system are involved in the transport of blood. Blood is transported through the body via a continuous system of blood vessels. Blood is pumped away from the heart in arteries and returned to the heart through veins. Arteries usually carry oxygenated blood away from the heart into capillaries supplying tissue cells. The exception is the pulmonary artery, which carries venous blood from the right side of the heart to the lungs. Veins collect the blood from the capillary bed and carry it back to the heart, and carry deoxygenated blood, except for the pulmonary vein, which brings oxygenated blood from the lungs to the left side of the heart (Figure A7).

The circulatory system is divided into:

- the pulmonary circulation, which takes unoxygenated blood from the right side of the heart to the lungs and returns to the left side of the heart with oxygenated blood;
- the systemic circulation, which takes oxygenated blood from the left side of the heart to all cells in the body and returns unoxygenated blood (i.e. blood from which oxygen has been extracted and which carries carbon dioxide generated in the cells) to the right side of the heart.

The circulation or the cardiovascular system also:

- carries food from the digestive tract to the cells to provide nutrition for growth and energy;
- carries waste products from cells in the body to the kidneys to enable the body to get rid of (excrete) these unwanted products in the urine;
- carries hormones from the glands that produce them (endocrine glands) to other organs of the body, and
- carries heat from parts of the body where heat is produced to the skin so that surplus heat can be given off.

A4.1 The heart

The heart is an organ consisting essentially of two pumps, right and left, which circulate blood round the body. Each pump has two chambers: the atrium and the ventricle. The atrium collects blood from either the lungs (the left atrium) or the tissues (right atrium) and passes it through valves to the major pumping chambers, the ventricles. The left ventricle pumps oxygenated blood which has entered the chamber from the left atrium, whilst the right ventricle pumps the blood that has returned from the cells or tissues after extraction of oxygen and nutrients. This blood is pumped through the lungs where carbon dioxide is removed and oxygen combines with the haemoglobin in the red cells. A small amount of oxygen also dissolves in the blood.

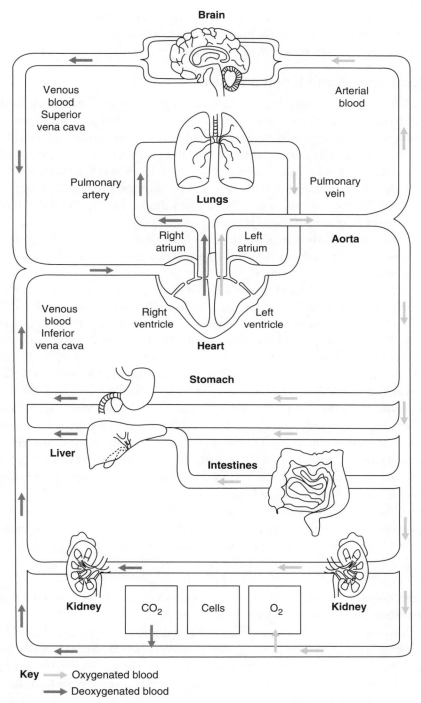

Brain

Venous
blood
Superior
vena cava

Arterial
blood

Pulmonary
artery

Pulmonary
vein

Lungs

Right
atrium

Left
atrium

Aorta

Venous
blood
Inferior
vena cava

Right
ventricle

Left
ventricle

Heart

Stomach

Liver

Intestines

Kidney

CO_2

Cells

O_2

Kidney

Key ⟶ Oxygenated blood
⟶ Deoxygenated blood

Fig. A7 Diagrammatic representation of the circulatory system. Not to scale.

Each time the heart beats, each ventricle pumps out about 70 ml of blood, and this volume is termed the stroke volume. The heart beats about 70 times a minute, which is termed the heart rate. This is usually measured in patients by counting the pulse rate at the wrist.

A4.2 Blood vessels and blood pressure

From the left side of the heart, oxygenated blood is pumped by the left ventricle to the aorta, which carries blood to the whole body. From the aorta arise the large arteries and their branches, which carry the oxygenated blood to the various parts of the body. For example, the carotid arteries arising from the aorta supply the brain, and the renal arteries arising from the aorta supply the kidneys. From the arteries blood is transported to smaller vessels called arterioles as it nears the organs or cells for which the blood supply is intended. From arterioles the blood goes into the very thin-walled capillaries that travel between cells providing oxygen and taking up carbon dioxide. Now the blood, which has provided oxygen and nutrition to the cells, passes from the end of the capillaries to the venules, veins, and then to the larger veins (the superior and inferior vena cava) and finally back to the right side of the heart.

The capacity of the venous side of the circulation is much greater than that of the arterial side and often accommodates 75% of the blood volume. This is because the walls of the vessels on the venous side are not as thick and contain less muscle than the vessels on the arterial side. The left ventricle contracts each time the blood is pushed into the aorta and this flow of blood causes a wave of flow commonly referred to as a pulse. This pulse can be felt only in arteries, which are often not visible. Some veins run just beneath the surface of the skin and are visible. The blood flow in them is non-pulsatile.

Blood pressure is the force applied to the wall of the arteries as the heart pumps blood to the cells in the body through the arterioles and capillaries. The measurement of blood pressure is dependent on the amount of blood pumped, which in turn is dependent on the volume of blood in the body (blood volume), the force with which the heart pumps the blood, and the diameter and elasticity of the arteries. This pressure from behind (driven by the left ventricle) is termed in Latin *vis a tergo*.

In order to have a blood pressure there has to be a flow from the heart (**cardiac output**) and a resistance to flow on the arterial or systemic side of the circulation. This resistance (the peripheral resistance) determines the blood pressure according to the equation:

$$\text{blood pressure} = \text{cardiac output} \times \text{peripheral resistance}$$

The resistance to blood flow is mainly in the small arterioles as it is the smaller diameter vessels that offer the greatest resistance to flow through them.

There are two components to a measurement of blood pressure. The first is the systolic pressure, which is the maximum pressure exerted when the left ventricle is contracting. The second component, the diastolic pressure, represents the pressure in the arteries when the left ventricle is refilling. In 'normal' people these components are recorded as 120/70 mm Hg (mm of mercury).

The arterioles have smooth muscle in their walls, which is arranged circularly. When the muscle contracts it makes the blood vessels smaller. The sympathetic nervous system provides a nerve supply to these vessels and stimulation of this system causes contraction of the smooth muscle in the walls and thus vasoconstriction and an increase in peripheral resistance and hence of blood pressure. When the arterioles are relaxed or when the sympathetic nerve stimulation is not present, the vessels are vasodilated or there is vasodilation. The diameter of these vessels is directly under control of the sympathetic nerve outflow regulated by the vasomotor centre in the medulla oblongata of the brain.

There are many nerve cell groupings that influence the activity of the vasomotor centre. The best known are the baroreceptors, which are found in a special area, the carotid sinus, of each carotid artery (arteries supplying blood to the brain). The higher centres in the brain (regions of the brain where conscious thoughts occur) also influence the activity of the vasomotor centre. Emotional stress and excitement cause stimulation of the vasomotor centre and an increase in blood pressure. Carbon dioxide content in the blood also influences vasomotor centre activity. When the carbon dioxide content and tension are low, as in patients who are breathing rapidly, the activity of the vasomotor centre is reduced. A shortage of oxygen, in contrast, would increase the activity of the vasomotor centre.

There are several factors affecting blood pressure. These include disease of arteries such as thickening or loss of muscle fibres (arteriosclerosis, which usually occurs with ageing), psychological factors such as stress, anger, and fear, kidney disease, and pain. Certain hormonal disorders are also associated with high blood pressure. An increase in blood pressure may occur during pregnancy in some individuals.

A4.3 The blood (haematopoietic system)

An adult has approximately 5 litres of blood in the body. A new born baby has only 300 ml (80 ml per kg body weight). Blood is composed of cells (45%) and plasma (55%). Blood cells are formed in the bone marrow, which is found in cavities of bones. Blood cells can be broadly divided into red and white blood cells and platelets.

Red blood cells

There are approximately 5 million red blood cells per cubic mm of blood. These contain the pigment haemoglobin, which is bright red in colour when combined with oxygen and purple-blue in colour when deoxygenated. Every 100 ml of blood has about 15 g of haemoglobin and this haemoglobin plays an important role in the carriage of not only oxygen but also of carbon dioxide. The life span of the red cell is about 100 days. For the formation of red blood cells (and also of proteins), iron is required, and deficiency of iron leads to iron deficiency anaemia. Other requirements for the formation of red blood cells are vitamin B12 and folic acid. Lack of vitamin B12 and folic acid leads to the formation of abnormally large red blood cells and a state called megalobalstic anaemia.

The hormone erythropoietin, which is formed in the kidney, also plays a role in the production of red blood cells as this hormone is produced in increased amounts when the body is lacking in oxygen, often for long periods of time. This hormone stimulates the bone marrow to produce more red blood cells.

White blood cells

The classification and function of white blood cells is considered in the immunology section (section A11 below).

Platelets and blood clotting

Platelets have two main functions in the human body. They are able to clump together and block small holes in the blood vessels by forming platelet plugs. This is a very important step in preventing loss of blood or bleeding from blood vessels, particularly after injuries.

Blood clotting is a process by which the body prevents loss of blood from blood vessels. It is initiated by a platelet plug and also by the breakdown of platelets, which causes the release of a factor called thromboplastin and converts a component of the blood called prothrombin to thrombin in the presence of calcium ions. Thrombin acts on another component in the blood called fibrinogen, and changes the fibrinogen to fibrin, which forms the blood clot.

There are a few inherited diseases where the clotting of blood is affected due to lack of specific substances in the person's blood. These diseases include haemophilia and Christmas disease.

Plasma

Plasma is the straw-coloured fluid in which the blood cells are suspended. It consists of a watery solution of plasma proteins and plasma electrolytes, and all the substances transported in the blood. It also contains the factors or ingredients necessary for blood clotting. If the factors necessary for blood clotting are removed from plasma, the remaining fluid is called serum.

A4.4 Common medical terms used to describe symptoms and signs of heart and blood vessel disorders

Hypotension: an abnormally low blood pressure that can occur following blood loss, failure of the heart to pump efficiently (heart failure), or as a result of toxic effects on the arterioles causing a decrease in peripheral resistance. Abnormally low blood pressure is seen in the clinical state referred to as shock.

Hypertension: defined as a sustained normally high blood pressure. Transient high blood pressures are part of a normal circulation. Hypertension causes a strain on the left ventricle, which has to pump the blood against a higher pressure. Initially the heart muscle increases in size (left ventricular hypertrophy). This can lead to failure of the heart to maintain normal function, i.e. heart failure. High blood pressure may also cause blood vessels to burst. This may occur in the blood vessels in the brain and cause a stroke. If this occurs, it may result in paralysis on the side opposite to the site where the blood vessel burst, due to the anatomy of the nervous system and brain circulation.

Ischaemic heart disease: a disease of the blood vessels resulting in an insufficient supply of the heart muscles with oxygen that is severe enough to cause temporary strain, or even permanent damage to the muscle with death of muscle fibres.

Myocardial infarction: a term used to describe irreversible injury to heart muscle, which results in loss of function or inability of the muscle to pump blood. Common symptoms include crushing central chest pain that may radiate to the jaw or arms. Chest pain may be associated with nausea, sweating, and shortness of breath.

Angina pectoris: a chest pain that occurs secondary to the inadequate delivery of oxygen to the heart muscle. It is often described as a tight, constricting, or crushing pain in the midsternal area of the chest, which may also be felt on the inside of the arms or in the neck. It arises when the blood supply to the heart muscle is reduced, due usually to a partial or complete obstruction of the blood flow in the arteries supplying the heart muscle (the coronary arteries).

Dyspnoea: difficult or laboured breathing; shortness of breath. Dyspnoea is a sign of serious disease of the airways, lungs, or heart.

Oedema: the presence of abnormally large amounts of fluid in the intercellular tissue spaces of the body and usually means demonstrable accumulation of excessive fluid in the subcutaneous tissues. Oedema may be localized, due to venous or lymphatic obstruction or to increased vascular permeability (which may follow stings from insects), or it may be more widespread due to heart failure or renal disease. Collections of oedema fluid are designated according to the site, for example ascites (peritoneal cavity), hydrothorax (pleural cavity), and hydropericardium (pericardial sac). Oedema due to heart failure is usually first detected as a swelling around the ankles (ankle oedema). Oedema may also occur in the back in front of the end of the spinal cord (sacral area), where it is referred to as sacral oedema.

A5 The respiratory system

Respiration or breathing has three main functions:

1. to deliver oxygen to the cells;

2. to eliminate carbon dioxide, and

3. to regulate the pH of the blood.

The oxidation of carbon and hydrogen from food in order to produce energy and heat requires oxygen from the air, obtained through breathing. In the cells, oxygen is delivered to the mitochondria, intracellular structures that are the 'powerhouses' of the cells. Mitochondria have cytochromes which combine oxygen, hydrogen, and carbon atoms to generate energy in the form of adenosine triphosphate (ATP), and produce carbon dioxide as a waste product.

At rest, 250 ml of oxygen are absorbed per minute during breathing to satisfy the metabolic requirements of the body. The energy requirements depend on the level of activity of the individual. For example, during heavy exercise, the oxygen requirement may be as high as 5000 ml of oxygen per minute.

The lungs fill the thoracic cavity. During breathing, the thoracic cavity expands and creates a negative pressure. This causes the lungs to expand and sucks air in through the structures shown in Figure A8. This is referred to as inspiration. When the thoracic cavity returns to its normal (resting) size, the lungs also decrease in size and air is forced out through the respiratory tract. This is called expiration.

Physiologically, four phases of respiration are recognized:

1. ventilation: the movement of air to and from the lungs;

2. distribution: air entering the lungs is distributed to all parts, including the small air sacs (alveoli) where gas transfer to and from the blood takes place;

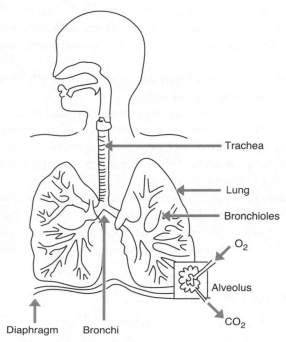

Fig. A8 Diagram of the respiratory system. Not to scale.

3. diffusion: the oxygen from the air diffuses through the walls of the alveoli to the adjacent blood vessels and carbon dioxide from the blood vessels diffuses back in to the alveoli;

4. internal respiration: blood rich in carbon dioxide and low in oxygen is pumped to the lungs via the pulmonary arteries, by the right ventricle of the heart. Blood low in carbon dioxide but loaded with oxygen is returned to the heart via the pulmonary veins. Matching of ventilation and perfusion (the blood supply to the alveoli—air sacs) within the lung ensures normal gas exchange.

The alternating increase and decrease in the size of the chest during normal breathing is under the control of collections of nerve cells in the medulla oblongata (the respiratory centre). Nerves from the anterior horn cells in the cervical and thoracic regions of the spinal cord supply the muscles of respiration. The main muscles involved are the diaphragm and the intercostal muscles (the muscles between the ribs). These muscles are all striated (skeletal) muscles, which are muscles that are usually under voluntary control (by the somatic nervous system). For this reason, the normal reflex action of breathing can be overridden by voluntary activity, such as taking a deep breath.

The respiratory system can be affected by a wide range of agents, including drugs such as morphine, one of the group of opiates that are compounds derived from or containing the active principles of the poppy (including morphine, heroin, methadone, and codeine), and by many toxic substances such as pesticides (particularly the herbicide paraquat) and nerve gases.

The lungs are elastic structures and outside the thoracic cavity they collapse like deflated balloons. In the thoracic cavity they are fully expanded and fill the cavity. Should air enter the space between the outside of the lungs and the inside of the thoracic cavity, the lungs will collapse and this is referred to as a pneumothorax, which severely interferes with respiration.

A5.1 Definitions of lung volumes and capacities

A number of terms are used to describe the movement of gas during breathing:

- Tidal volume (TV): The volume of air breathed in and out in one breath during normal breathing. This is usually around 400–500 ml.
- Minute volume (MV): The volume of air breathed in and out during a minute, which is tidal volume multiplied by respiratory rate (rate of breathing per minute). In exercise, the minute volume may increase from the average 6000–8000 ml to 50,000 ml per minute.
- Dead space: The region of the lung where there is no exchange of gases.
- Alveolar ventilation (AV): This is the volume available for exchange of gases, approximately (tidal volume – dead space) × respiratory rate.
- Inspiratory reserve volume (IRV): The volume of air that can be taken in after a normal breath (inspiration) has already been taken, i.e. the volume of air that can be inspired in addition to the tidal volume (approximately 3500 ml in a 70-kg adult).
- Expiratory reserve volume (ERV): The volume of air that can be breathed out after a normal expiration, i.e. the additional amount that can be breathed out after the end of a normal breath (approximately 1200 ml in a 70-kg adult).
- Residual volume (RV): The volume of air left in the lung after a maximal exhalation, i.e. the amount of air that is always in the lungs after breathing out as far as possible (approximately 1200 ml in a 70-kg adult).
- Inspiratory capacity (IC): The volume of air that can be inhaled after breathing out normally, i.e. after exhaling the tidal volume.
- Functional residual capacity (FRC): The volume of air left in the lung during normal breathing (approximately 2500 ml in a 70-kg adult).
- Vital capacity (VC): The maximum volume of air that can be forced out of the lungs after a maximal inspiration, i.e. the largest tidal volume that the individual is able to make (approximately 4600 ml in a 70-kg adult). This is IRV + TV + ERV.
- Total lung capacity (TLC): Volume of air after a maximal inspiration. This is IRV + TV + ERV + RV (approximately 6000 ml in a 70-kg adult).

Lung capacities are defined as sums of volumes, thus:

- inspiratory capacity = IRV + TV
- vital capacity = IRV + TV + ERV
- functional residual capacity = ERV + RV.

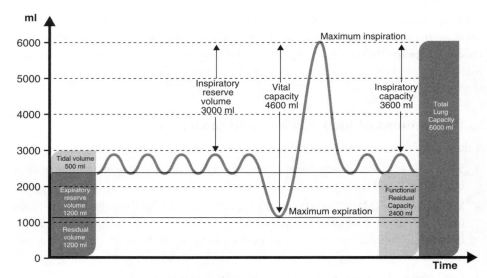

Fig. A9 Lung volumes and capacities. Courtesy of Pneupac Ventilation, Smiths Medical International, Luton, UK.

Spirometry is the direct measurement of lung volumes from a subject breathing spontaneously. Lung volumes as determined by spirometry are illustrated in Figure A9.

A5.2 The carriage of oxygen and carbon dioxide

The alveoli of the lungs contain oxygen, carbon dioxide, nitrogen, and water vapour. These four together make up a pressure equal to the total barometric pressure of 760 mm Hg. The water vapour when it is fully saturated exerts a partial pressure of 47 mm Hg. The other three gases (oxygen, carbon dioxide, and nitrogen) also exert partial pressures depending on the proportion of each in the mixture. In the alveoli of the lung, the pressure of these gases is measured as the total barometric pressure (760 mm Hg) minus the pressure of the water vapour (47 mm Hg), resulting in a pressure of 713 mm Hg. Oxygen contributes 14% and carbon dioxide contributes 6% to this pressure, therefore the pressure due to the oxygen is 14% of 713, i.e. 100 mm Hg.

Oxygen carriage

Gases diffuse across membranes in amounts that are determined by the difference in the partial pressures of that gas between the two compartments. With a partial pressure of 100 mm Hg in the alveoli, oxygen diffuses into the blood with a lower oxygen tension, which is brought by the pulmonary artery, and this continues until the partial pressure in the blood reaches equilibrium with the alveolar gas. The blood leaves the lungs with a tension of 100 mm Hg and usually arrives at the capillaries with a similar tension of oxygen. As the blood flows through the tissue capillary it comes into contact with the tissue fluid with a much lower oxygen tension (e.g. 40 mm Hg). The tension of oxygen in the tissue fluid is low because oxygen is being continually taken up by cells for metabolism.

As the blood flows through the capillary, the oxygen tension falls to 40 mm Hg (the pressure of the surrounding tissue fluid) and returns to the right side of the heart (to the right atrium and ventricle) with an oxygen tension of 40 mm Hg. Then it comes into contact with alveolar air with an oxygen tension of 100 mm Hg and equilibrium occurs when the tension of oxygen in the blood reaches 100 mm Hg and thus becomes referred to as arterial or oxygenated blood.

Gases carried in the blood are now measured routinely. This process is referred to as blood gas analysis and indicates the partial pressure of oxygen and carbon dioxide in the blood and also measures the pH of the blood. These measurements provide valuable information about disease processes and the effects of treatment.

The quantity of oxygen carried in the blood depends on the affinity of oxygen to haemoglobin, found in red blood cells. Haemoglobin allows far more oxygen to be carried than would be possible than in solution alone. One gram of haemoglobin has the ability to combine with 1.34 ml of oxygen. Thus a person who has 15 g of haemoglobin in every 100 ml of blood would theoretically be able to carry approximately 20 ml of oxygen in every 100 ml of blood. This is termed the oxygen capacity of the blood. In venous blood that is returning from the tissues via the veins to the right side of the heart, only 14 ml of oxygen are present in every 100 ml of blood. As noted above, the tension has fallen to 40 mm Hg. Thus, as blood passes through the tissues 5–6 ml of oxygen is taken up by the tissues; during exercise this amount is much more.

Carbon dioxide carriage

The tension of carbon dioxide in the lungs is 40 mm Hg whilst in the tissues it is 46 mm Hg. Therefore as the blood passes through the capillaries in the lung, carbon dioxide diffuses into the alveoli due to the difference of tension of the carbon dioxide in the venous blood and that in the alveoli. Therefore carbon dioxide moves in a direction opposite to that of oxygen in the alveoli of the lungs. The carbon dioxide content of the blood leaving the lungs is 48 ml carbon dioxide per 100 ml blood. As it passes through the cells and tissues, the carbon dioxide content increases to 52 ml of carbon dioxide per 100 ml of blood.

What emerges from the above is that the changes in oxygen content are greater than the changes in carbon dioxide content. This is because carbon dioxide is not only a waste product. An adequate level of carbon dioxide has to be maintained in the blood in order to maintain an acceptable blood pH (a measure of the acidity) to enable cells to function normally (normal range 7.36–7.42).

Carbon dioxide is carried in the blood in three ways, firstly in simple solution as carbonic acid and secondly as sodium bicarbonate in the plasma and potassium bicarbonate in the red blood cells. Thirdly, it is carried as neutral carbamino protein, mainly with haemoglobin in the red cells.

The transport of the acid-gas carbon dioxide in the blood is closely associated with the maintenance of the normal blood pH. Carbon dioxide dissolves in water, or plasma, and forms carbonic acid. This weak acid is in equilibrium with its salt, the bicarbonate ion. The ratio of bicarbonate ions to molecules of carbonic acid defines the acidity of the blood. Under normal circumstances, this ratio is 20:1. Bicarbonate ions are produced in red blood cells in systemic capillaries as carbon dioxide diffuses into these cells and forms carbonic acid. The formation of carbonic acid is catalysed by the enzyme carbonic anhydrase. Bicarbonate ions diffuse from the red cells to the plasma, being replaced by chloride ions moving into the red cells. Hydrogen ions produced during the formation of bicarbonate ions are buffered by haemoglobin in its deoxygenated state. This process is precisely reversed in the capillaries of the lung; bicarbonate ions enter red cells, chloride ions leave red cells, and hydrogen ions released from oxygenated haemoglobin combine with bicarbonate ions to produce carbonic acid, carbonic anhydrase catalyses the formation of carbon dioxide, and water from carbonic acid and the carbon dioxide diffuses out of the cell into the plasma. Note that carbonic anhydrase catalyses both the formation and breakdown of carbonic acid; the direction of the reaction is defined by the law of mass action and the rate of the reaction is controlled by the catalyst, i.e. carbonic anhydrase.

A5.3 Common signs, symptoms, and terms used for disorders of lung or respiratory function

A5.3.1 Asphyxia

This is a state in which there is excess of carbon dioxide and lack of oxygen in the body. This occurs when respiratory function or activity is insufficient to meet the demands of the body or when there is obstruction to respiration, e.g. during strangulation, or when an individual is breathing in a confined space when the expired air has to be inhaled. Asphyxial states stimulate respiration or breathing, as carbon dioxide is a potent stimulus of the respiratory centre, as is a lack of oxygen.

A5.3.2 Hypoxia

This is defined as a shortage of oxygen without a concurrent shortage of carbon dioxide. This is very often encountered when there is insufficient oxygen in the inspired air or when for some reason the tissues are deprived of the normal amount of oxygen, possibly because of poor circulation or a blood clot. In this case, tissue hypoxia results and if this occurs in the heart muscle it results in heart attacks or ischaemic heart disease. Hypoxia also depresses brain function as the brain is dependent on sufficient oxygen supplies for the proper functioning of nerve cells. When hypoxia of the brain occurs, a person becomes disorientated, loses all sense of danger, loses consciousness, and coma sets in. For example, this happens when carbon monoxide displaces oxygen from haemoglobin and deprives the tissues of oxygen.

Hypoxia may be due to a decreased amount of oxygen in the air breathed in (inspired oxygen), as at high altitude, or to lung disease when the oxygen cannot enter the red blood cells in the blood that flows through the lungs.

In contrast to asphyxia, where an individual will struggle to breathe with all the available resources in the body, in hypoxia the individual will soon lose control and become unconscious.

If the supply of oxygen to the brain cells is interrupted for more than 4 minutes (as seen when the heart ceases to pump blood effectively, commonly referred to as cardiac arrest), the nerve cells in the brain may be irreversibly damaged and 'brain death' may result. If there is a deficiency of haemoglobin to transport the oxygen, as is seen an anaemic patients due to either poor nutrition or prolonged blood loss, the term used is anaemic hypoxia. The hypoxia associated with carbon monoxide poisoning is an anaemic hypoxia as there is insufficient haemoglobin to transport the oxygen due to its preferential binding with carbon monoxide, which has an affinity about 250 times greater for haemoglobin than oxygen.

If blood flow through the body tissues is slow, there is insufficient oxygen for the cells to function. This is referred to as stagnant hypoxia.

Finally the cells may be unable to utilize the oxygen brought to them by the blood due to the enzymes within the cells being inactive or destroyed. This occurs in cyanide poisoning, where vital enzymes such as the cytochromes are destroyed by the cyanide and the cells cannot extract the oxygen in the blood.

A5.3.3 Pulmonary oedema

In the lungs, the pulmonary arterial systolic pressure is usually 25 mm Hg compared to about 130 mm Hg in arteries arising from the aorta from the left ventricle. When the pressure in the left atrium or pulmonary veins is elevated (for example when the atrium cannot empty its contents to the left ventricle either because the atrium muscle is not contracting in the normal manner or when there is an obstruction to the flow of blood from the atrium to the ventricle such as narrowing ostenosis of the valve between the two chambers, commonly referred to as mitral stenosis), the pressure in the pulmonary capillaries could be exceeded to such an extent that fluid passes from the capillaries into the alveoli. This fluid would interfere with diffusion of gases. The presence of fluid in the alveoli or in the lung created in this way is referred to as cardiac pulmonary oedema. Pulmonary oedema leads to difficulty in breathing (as there is insufficient oxygen and accumulation of carbon dioxide, which are both stimuli for the respiratory centre) and the patient will become dyspnoeic, that is conscious of breathing and difficulty in breathing, and breathless. Pulmonary oedema may also occur due to the action of poisonous gases such as chlorine or phosgene, where the structure of the alveolar walls and capillaries are damaged, leading a leakage of fluid into the alveoli. If the left side of the heart fails, the heart muscle on the left side of the heart does not function or contract adequately and there is a build up of pressure in the pulmonary veins bringing blood from the lungs. This type of fluid accumulation in the lung is called toxic pulmonary oedema.

A5.3.4 Cyanosis

Cyanosis is a bluish discolouration, especially of the skin and mucous membranes, caused by an excessive concentration of deoxygenated haemoglobin (haemoglobin not bound to oxygen) in the blood. A point of interest to those in countries where anaemia is very common, is that the haemoglobin levels may be so low that the amount of haemoglobin without oxygen (deoxygenated haemoglobin) is insufficient to cause cyanosis.

A6 The gastrointestinal system

Food or water entering the body through the mouth passes down the oesophagus and enters the stomach. From the stomach, partially digested food passes on to the duodenum, jejunum, and ileum (small intestine). That which has not been absorbed proceeds to the caecum and then to the ascending, transverse, descending, and sigmoid colon (large intestine), the rectum and finally the anal canal (Figure A10).

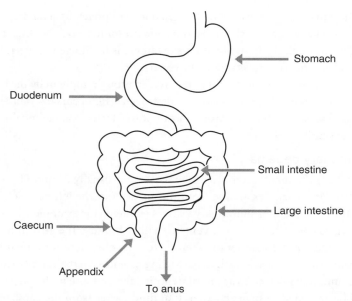

Fig. A10 Diagram of the gastrointestinal system. Not to scale.

In the mouth, saliva is produced by three paired salivary glands: parotid, submandibular, and sublingual. Saliva is secreted by these glands, usually in response to the thought, site, taste, or smell of food. Secretion of saliva is under the control of the parasympathetic nervous system. Thus when there is over-activity of the parasympathetic nervous system and there is more secretion of the neurotransmitter of that system (acetylcholine), there will be excessive secretions, for example as in organophosphorus insecticide poisoning. If the action of acetylcholine on the receptors is blocked by drugs such as atropine, dryness of the mouth results.

The food formed into a bolus in the mouth passes down the oesophagus due to propulsive contractions of the muscle of the oesophagus, which are controlled by another parasympathetic cranial nerve, the vagus. Then the food enters the stomach where digestion begins aided by secretions (pepsin and hydrochloric acid for digestion of proteins) from the cells lining the stomach wall. The secretions of the stomach are also under the control of the vagus nerve and a hormone called gastrin.

At regular intervals of minutes, small quantities of food pass through an opening at the distal end of the stomach, called the pyloric sphincter, to the duodenum. The contents of a stomach usually empty in about 4 hours. However, with a very fatty meal, the emptying of the stomach becomes much slower due to the release of a hormone called enterogastrone.

Stomach ulcers and duodenal ulcers, commonly referred to as peptic ulcers, occur because pepsin, which aids in digesting proteins, acts on the cells of the stomach wall. Digestion of stomach wall cells is aided by the presence of hydrochloric acid, which is also secreted by the cells lining the stomach.

The stomach also has a role in vitamin B12 metabolism. Loss of the stomach or a large part of it can lead to a condition known as pernicious anaemia, which is due to lack of vitamin B12.

A6.1 The pancreas

The pancreas is a gland which sends its secretions into the bloodstream and also into the duodenum. The secretion of insulin and glucagon, which are necessary for the control of blood sugar in the human body, is from the pancreas. The secretions from the pancreas which enter the duodenum are known as the pancreatic juices and contain the enzymes trypsinogen and chymotrypsinogen, which are precursors of the protein-splitting enzymes trypsin and chymotrypsin.

Pancreatic secretion is also under the control of the vagus nerve. Insulin secretion is from specialized cells called the Islets of Langerhans. Failure to produce sufficient insulin results in diabetes mellitus.

Secretions from the liver also enter the duodenum via the bile duct. The bile is stored and concentrated in the gall bladder, which also contracts due to the action of the vagus nerve, and can also contract due to the action of some hormones. The bile constituents may concentrate and give rise to gall stones. Inflammation of the gall bladder is referred to as cholecystitis.

A6.2 The small intestine

The small intestine is concerned primarily with the absorption of sugars or carbohydrates and produces the related enzymes maltase, sucrase, and lactase. Although the nerve supply to the small intestine is both from the parasympathetic and sympathetic nervous systems, these nerves regulate motility or contractions of the small intestine (peristalsis) and have no role in the production of the digestive enzymes. The absorption of food takes place mainly in the small intestine. Amino acids and fats are also absorbed here.

A6.3 The large intestine

The main function of the large intestine is the absorption of water, sodium and other minerals. 90% of the fluid coming from the small intestine is removed here to form semi-solid faeces which may contain important biomarkers following toxic exposure. The large intestine is not essential to life.

A6.4 Common medical signs, symptoms, and terms used for gastrointestinal disorders

Dyspepsia: the impairment of the function of digestion, usually applied to epigastric discomfort following meals.

Peptic ulcer: an ulcer in the wall of the stomach or duodenum resulting from the digestive action of the gastric juice on the mucous membrane, when the latter is rendered susceptible to its action.

Cholecystitis: acute or chronic inflammation of the gallbladder.

Gall stones: stones within the gall bladder, usually of cholesterol (non-opaque) or of calcium bilirubinate (bilirubin), opaque and commonly associated with haemolytic anaemia (sickle cell disease, spherocytosis, thalassaemia). Gall stones are considered to have an increased incidence in individuals commonly referred to as having the five Fs: fat, female, fertile, flatulent, and over 40.

Pancreatitis: an acute or chronic inflammation of the pancreas, which may be asymptomatic or symptomatic, and which is due to autodigestion of a pancreatic tissue by its own enzymes. It is caused most often by alcoholism or biliary tract disease. Less commonly it may be associated with hyperlipaemia (increased fat content in blood), hyperparathyroidism (increased activity of the parathyroid glands), abdominal trauma (accidental or operative injury), vasculitis, or uraemia (increased content of urea in blood usually due to kidney disease).

Ileus: distension of the intestines, usually due to an obstruction such as a tumour. When a lesion causes a cessation of peristalitic movements in the intestines, the term paralytic ileus is used.

A7 **The liver**

The liver is the chemical factory of the body, both producing essential molecules and modifying and detoxifying ingested toxic substances (Figure A11).

The main functions of the liver are given below.

- Production of essential proteins such as albumin.

- Synthesis of factors that are involved in the clotting of blood.

- Maintaining the level of sugar in the blood. The excess carbohydrate absorbed by the blood from food is converted to glycogen, which is also formed from excess fat and protein. The liver glycogen maintains the normal blood glucose level in the blood when glucose is used up by the cells.

- Formation of urea from the ammonia which collects after amino acids have been used up (deaminated). The urea is eliminated through the kidney.

- The bile salts produced by the liver along with products from an anatomically closely related organ, the pancreas, play a vital role in digestion and absorption of fat. The liver also stores fat-soluble vitamins (A and D).

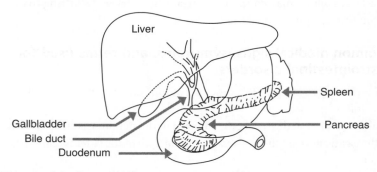

Fig. A11 Diagram of the liver and biliary system. Not to scale.

◆ The destruction of used red blood cells and removal of the breakdown product of haemoglobin (bilirubin) in the bile via the bile duct to the intestine (duodenum). The liver stores vitamin B12, which is necessary for the maturation of blood cells.

◆ In relation to toxicology, the liver plays a vital role by modifying the toxicity of foreign substances (toxins, drugs) that gain entry into the body by any route. Some drugs used in medical treatment are administered as pro-drugs, which depend on the liver to produce the active drug through the action of liver enzymes. The liver also has the ability to bind toxic substances to other compounds to make them more water soluble and thus enable to kidney to excrete them from the body.

A7.1 Jaundice

One of the important roles of the liver, as noted above, is the formation of bilirubin from the red cells that die. Approximately 200 mg of bilirubin, which is insoluble in water, are made each day. It is bound to albumin and brought to the liver, where the albumin is replaced by glucuronic acid (an acid made from glucose), which makes the bilirubin water soluble. The water-soluble complex passes down the bile duct, which is the channel through which the liver eliminates its waste products, into the intestine (duodenum). Water-soluble bilirubin is responsible for the characteristic colouration of the faeces.

The failure to excrete bilirubin gives rise to yellowish discolouration of the whites of the eyes, the skin and nails, and mucosal membranes, which is called jaundice. Jaundice is essentially a sign of liver failure. Several toxic compounds, such as some pesticides, solvents such as carbon tetrachloride, and dry-cleaning fluids, damage the liver cells and prevent them from functioning normally to bind the bilirubin to the glucuronide. There are many drugs used in the treatment of disease which also damage the liver cells and are termed hepatotoxic. For example, high levels of the common drug paracetamol can cause liver damage, liver failure, and jaundice. Another common and important cause of damage to liver cells which often results in liver failure is excessive alcohol (ethanol) consumption.

In liver failure, jaundice occurs, the blood urea falls (as urea is no longer formed from ammonia), there is insufficient production of proteins, of which albumin is the most important, which may lead to swelling of ankles or oedema (as proteins are essential to maintain plasma osmotic pressure, which keeps fluid within capillaries), and blood clotting will be impaired. The most important effect is that the blood will not have sufficient glucose for cells to function normally.

In addition, when liver cells fail to function properly, their ability to make foreign substances less toxic by metabolic enzymes fails and the toxicity of some drugs used in medicine, such as morphine, is increased.

A7.2 Role of the liver in metabolism of xenobiotics

Humans are constantly and unavoidably exposed to foreign chemicals or xenobiotics, which include both synthetic and natural chemicals such as medical drugs, industrial chemicals, pesticides, pollutants, plant alkaloids and plant metabolites, and toxins produced by moulds, plants, and animals.

The physical property that enables many xenobiotics to be absorbed through the skin, lungs, or gastrointestinal tract is their fat solubility or lipophilicity. Lipophilicity is also an obstacle to their elimination as they can be readily reabsorbed. Another important consideration is that lipophilicity facilitates the entry of toxic substances into cells. Therefore, the elimination of xenobiotics often depends on their conversion to water-soluble compounds by a process called biotransformation, which is catalysed by enzymes in the liver and other tissues. An important result of biotransformation is the conversion of a lipophilic substance to one that is more water soluble (hydrophilic) (see phase 1 and phase 2 reactions below).

This transformation is probably one of the most important defence mechanisms of the body. Xenobiotics such as drugs exert beneficial effects and others may cause deleterious effects, as in the case of poisons. The effect a xenobiotic produces in the human body is dependent on its physicochemical properties and thus the results of xenobiotic exposure would be altered by this process of biotransformation.

Some drugs must undergo biotransformation to be effective because the metabolite of the drug and not the drug itself produces a therapeutic or beneficial effect. Similarly, some xenobiotics undergo biotransformation to produce their harmful or toxic effects. However, in the vast majority of situations, biotransformation terminates the effectiveness of the xenobiotic in the human body, be it beneficial or harmful. In the context of toxicology, this means that many potentially toxic substances are made relatively innocuous by biotransformation by liver enzymes. These are predominantly the cytochrome P450 group of isoenzymes, which are responsible for the majority of oxidation reactions that xenobiotics undergo.

The enzymes catalysing biotransformation reactions often determine the intensity and duration of the action of drugs and play a key role in chemical toxicity. The xenobiotic biotransforming enzymes catalyse two types of reactions. These are:

Phase I reactions: addition of a functional group (e.g. –OH, –NH$_2$, –SH, or –COOH) to produce a slight increase in water solubility or hydrophilicity.

Phase II reactions: include glucuronidation, sulfation, acetylation, methylation, conjugation with glutathione and conjugation with aminoacids (e.g. glycine, taurine, glutamic acid). These reactions cause a large increase in water solubility and thus increase the excretion of the xenobiotic, for example:

> Morphine, heroin, and codeine are all converted to morphine-3-glucuronide. In the case of morphine, this is a result of direct conjugation with glucuronide. In the instance of heroin and codeine, conjugation with glucuronic acid is preceded by phase I biotransformation—hydrolysis or deacetylation—with heroin and demethylation involving oxidation by cytochrome P450 isoenzymes with codeine.

A7.3 The cytochrome P450 enzyme system

The liver is the organ with the highest concentration of enzymes catalysing biotransformation reactions. These enzymes are also located in the skin, lungs, nasal mucosa (mucosa of the nose), eyes, and gastrointestinal tract. In the liver and in most other organs, they are located in the cells, primarily in the endoplasmic reticulum (microsomes) or in the soluble fraction of the cytoplasm, with a smaller concentration in the mitochondria, nuclei, and lysosomes.

Amongst the phase I biotransformation enzymes, the cytochrome P450 system is responsible for most oxidation reactions and is probably the most versatile, detoxifying more xenobiotics than any other enzyme system.

In humans, about 40 different microsomal and mitochondrial P450 enzymes play a key role in catalysing reactions in the following areas:

- the metabolism of drugs, environmental pollutants and other xenobiotics;
- the biosynthesis of steroid hormones;
- the oxidation of unsaturated fatty acids to intracellular messengers, and
- metabolism of fat-soluble vitamins.

The liver microsomal P450 enzymes involved in xenobiotic biotransformation belong to three main P450 gene families: CYP1, CYP2, and CYP3. The level and activity of each P450 enzyme varies from individual to individual due to genetic and environmental factors.

It is important to remember that the activity of the CYP isoenzymes can be altered by several agents. For example, there are many drugs that increase the activity of the isoenzymes and these are called enzyme inducers. Similarly some xenobiotics can inhibit the activity of CYP450 isoenzymes and these are called enzyme inhibitors. The induction of CYP450 isoenzymes by drugs such as phenobarbital (a barbiturate used primarily in the treatment of epilepsy) or rifampicin (an antibiotic used in the treatment of tuberculosis) can prevent the effectiveness of the oral contraceptive drug ethinyl oestradiol.

A7.4 Common medical signs, symptoms, and terms associated with liver dysfunction

Jaundice: a yellowing of the skin (and whites of eyes) by bilirubin, a bile pigment, frequently caused by a liver problem.

Ascites: an accumulation of serous fluid within the inner lining of the abdominal cavity (the peritoneal cavity), which causes a 'bulging' abdomen.

Hepatic encephalopathy: a term used to describe the deleterious effects of liver failure on the central nervous system. Features include confusion, dementia, and often unresponsiveness (coma). A common cause is alcoholic cirrhosis.

A8 The kidney

The kidneys are two bean-shaped organs about the size of a fist lying below the rib cage. Although they are small in size (about 0.5% of the body weight), the kidneys receive approximately 20% of the blood that is pumped out from the heart via the renal arteries. The main parts of the kidney are an outer lightly coloured cortex and an inner darker medulla (Figure A12). The renal (kidney) pelvis is the funnel which collects the urine from nephrons (the basic functional unit of the kidney) and enables the urine to flow to the ureters. The ureters are the tubes that carry the urine from the kidneys to the urinary bladder.

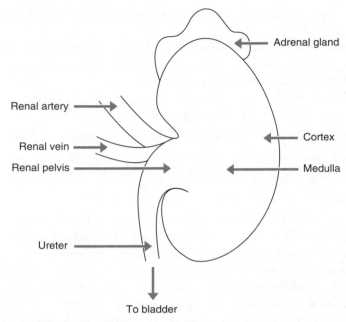

Fig. A12 Diagram of the kidney. Not to scale.

The blood brought to the kidneys by the arteries is filtered under pressure by a part of the nephrons (Figure A13). There are approximately one million nephrons and each nephron is a thin long convoluted tube, surrounded by capillaries, which is closed at one end, where the filtering takes place. The filtered fluid is then absorbed from within the nephron, according to the needs of the body. The cells of the tubules also have the ability to secrete waste substances into the lumen of the tubule of the nephron into the urine. These waste substances include many toxins and drugs.

The kidney plays a key role in the elimination of waste products and unwanted substances from the blood. The blood supply and blood vessels and the structure of the kidney enable the entire blood volume of an individual to be filtered 20–25 times a day. The 'cleaned' blood is returned to the circulation by the renal veins.

Essentially, three basic processes take place in the nephron: filtration, absorption or reabsorption, and secretion or excretion.

The principal function of the kidney is to produce urine, which is excreted from the body and ensures the maintenance of the correct chemical environment (milieu interior) for body cells: water balance, electrolyte balance, and the pH of the blood. It has other functions such as producing substances necessary for the formation of red blood cells (erythropoietin), converting vitamin D to an active form which promotes the absorption of calcium from the intestine, and also producing some hormones associated with the regulation of blood pressure.

Urine normally contains surplus water and electrolytes, waste products such as urea, which is formed from the amino acids, uric acid, which is produced from nucleic acids

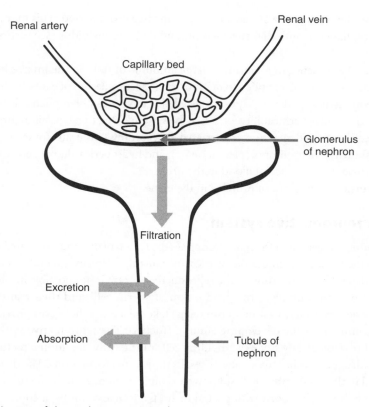

Fig. A13 Diagram of the nephron. Not to scale.

and purines, and creatinine from muscle. Urine also gets rid of excess amounts of acids or alkalis that have either been ingested or are formed following metabolic processes.

It is important to note that most toxic substances and even beneficial substances such as drugs that are used in treatment are eliminated in the urine and the measurement of the relevant constituents can confirm either the use of drug(s) or the exposure to toxic compounds. Thus examination and analysis of the urine is an important investigation in toxicology and acts as a biomarker of exposure. The amounts excreted in the urine may also be an indicator of the severity of exposure to a toxic substance.

A8.1 Common symptoms associated with disease of the kidneys

Anuria: the complete suppression of urinary secretion by the kidneys.

Uraemia: in current usage, this is the entire constellation of signs and symptoms of chronic renal failure leading to increased urea in the blood. These include nausea, vomiting, anorexia, a metallic taste in the mouth, a uraemic odour of the breath, pruritus, uraemic 'frost' on the skin, neuromuscular disorders, pain and twitching in the muscles, hypertension, oedema, mental confusion, and acid base and electrolyte imbalances.

Dysuria: painful or difficult urination.

Polyuria: the passage of a large volume of urine in a given period. This may be a characteristic of diabetes, both diabetes mellitus and diabetes insipidus (see section A10 on hormones).

Oedema: the presence of abnormally large amounts of fluid in the intercellular tissue spaces of the body, usually applied to demonstrable accumulation of excessive fluid in the subcutaneous tissues. Oedema may be localized, due to venous or lymphatic obstruction or to increased vascular permeability, or it may be systemic due to heart failure or renal disease. Collections of oedema fluid are designated according to the site, for example ascites (peritoneal cavity), hydrothorax (pleural cavity), and hydropericardium (pericardial sac).

Haematuria: the presence of blood in the urine.

Proteinuria: the presence of proteins in the urine.

A9 The reproductive system

The reproductive system in the male comprises the testes, penis, and associated ducts and glands. In the female it includes the ovaries, uterine tubes, uterus, vagina, and mammary glands. A detailed consideration of the reproductive system is not possible in a text of this length but overall it involves the production of sperm cells and their transfer to the female. In the female, fertilization of ova (eggs) takes place and the uterus provides a suitable environment for the developing embryo (foetus). The reproductive system is very important toxicologically since the dividing cells of the early developing foetus are vulnerable to drugs and other toxic substances, leading to malformations. The drug thalidomide, used in the 1960s, was the first known example of damage to the foetus in this way, leading to babies being born with partial or total absence of limbs, a condition called phocemelia.

A10 The endocrine system and the production of hormones

The activities of the organs of the body are primarily controlled by nerve impulses. The other important mode of control of activity is by hormones. These are chemical messengers produced by endocrine glands. They enter the bloodstream directly following secretions by the glands and are brought to all parts of the body by the cardiovascular system. Most organs are under the influence of both nerve impulses and hormones.

The word 'hormone' is derived from the Greek word *hormao*, which means to excite. A hormone is a naturally occurring substance secreted by specialized cells that affects the metabolism or behaviour of other cells possessing functional receptors for the hormone. Hormones may be hydrophilic, like insulin (from the pancreas), in which case the receptors are on the cell surface, or lipophilic, like steroids (from the adrenal cortex), where the receptor can be intracellular. Thus hormones are substances which circulate in the blood and bring about an effect on distant organs.

The main endocrine glands are:

- pituitary
- thyroid
- parathyroid glands

- adrenal glands
- ovaries in the female
- testes in the male
- placenta during pregnancy
- pancreas, which is both exocrine and endocrine (secretions of exocrine glands reach the bloodstream through ducts whilst those of endocrine glands reach the bloodstream directly).

A10.1 Pituitary gland

The pituitary gland lies in a bony cavity in the skull called the pituitary fossa. The posterior part of the pituitary is suspended by a structure called the pituitary stalk from a part of the brain called the hypothalamus. The gland has two parts: the anterior pituitary or adenohypophysis, and the posterior pituitary or neurohypophysis (Figure A14). Whilst the posterior pituitary has neural or nerve connections with the brain, the anterior pituitary has vascular connections with the brain.

A10.1.1 The posterior pituitary

The **posterior pituitary** is composed mainly of nervous tissue descending from the hypothalamus and produces two hormones:

- antidiuretic hormone (vasopressin), and
- oxytocic hormone (oxytocin).

Antidiuretic hormone

Antidiuretic hormone (ADH) is involved intimately with water balance as it controls or regulates the amount of water that is reabsorbed in the kidney. Large doses of ADH cause high blood pressure or hypertension as it causes vasoconstriction or contraction (narrowing) of blood vessels. The amount of ADH secreted is controlled by the amount of water in the blood. If the body is short of water, more ADH will be secreted and more water will be reabsorbed by the kidney tubules and less urine will be formed.

The posterior pituitary may fail to produce ADH, in which case the condition is called diabetes insipidus. In this condition excessive amounts of urine are formed and lost from the body and patients are always very thirsty.

The oxytocic hormone

The oxytocic hormone is only important during pregnancy. It causes contraction of the pregnant uterus and facilitates the ejection of milk during lactation.

A10.1.2 The anterior pituitary

The hormones released by the anterior pituitary gland are:

- growth hormone;
- thyrotrophic hormone;
- adrenocorticotrophic hormone, and
- gonadotrophic hormones.

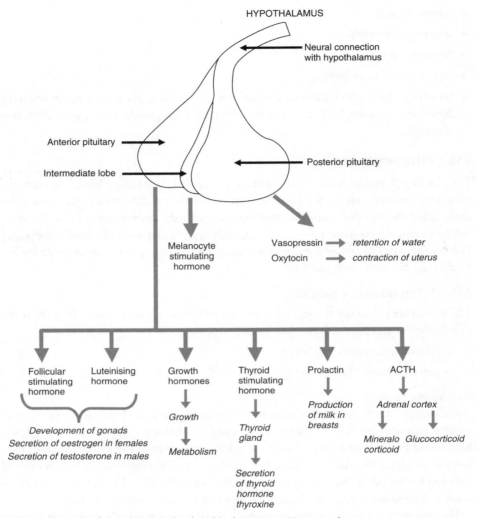

Fig. A14 Diagram of the pituitary gland and its hormones. Not to scale.

Growth hormone

This hormone stimulates the growth of bone and muscle tissue during childhood. If there is excessive production of this hormone before puberty (when the long bones fuse with the growing ends or epiphyses and no further increase in growth can occur), gigantism results. Insufficient production causes dwarfism. Increased production after puberty leads to an increase in the size of facial bones and the bones of the hands and feet—a condition called acromegaly.

A10.2 Thyroid-stimulating hormone and the thyroid gland

The thyroid-stimulating hormone acts on the thyroid gland in the neck and stimulates the release of the thyroid hormones thyroxine and tri-iodothyronine. The thyroid hormone stimulates metabolism by acting on the cells to speed up the rate at which food is used up and converted to heat and energy. The thyroid gland is unique in that it stores its hormones as a colloid in small vesicles in the gland. The other glands store their secretions in the cells themselves. The formation of the thyroid hormone requires iodine ingested in the diet. In regions where populations may encounter a deficiency of iodine in their diets, the addition of iodine to salt (iodized salt) has helped in the prevention of thyroid disease, particularly the enlargement of the thyroid gland known as goitre. Deficiency of the thyroid hormone (also called hypothyroidism) in a child causes cretinism, where the development of the nervous system is affected and the child is mentally retarded. In an adult, deficiency of thyroid hormone causes myxoedema, where the body temperature is low, the heart rate is slow, brain activity is sluggish, and there is deposition of fluid-like material under the skin. The face and eyelids become puffy.

If there is increased production of thyroid hormone (hyperthyroidism), metabolism is stimulated and more heat is produced, the heart beats faster, and the heart excitability is increased, which may give rise to disorders of heart rhythm (cardiac arrhythmias). In this situation, which is called thyrotoxicosis, the person is irritable, anxious, and nervous. They lose weight although the appetite is good. They often have protrusion of the eye balls (exophthalmos).

In addition, the thyroid gland produces calcitonin, which is important in the regulation of calcium balance.

A10.3 Parathyroid

Parathyroid glands are adjacent to the thyroid gland but are not controlled by the secretions of the anterior pituitary gland. There are four parathyroid glands, two on either side of the thyroid. The hormones from the parathyroid gland control the calcium levels in the blood. Another factor affecting the blood calcium level is calcitonin, which as stated above is a secretion of the thyroid gland. Calcitonin acts by trapping calcium in the bones. Another important factor determining the level of blood calcium is vitamin D.

With increased activity of the parathyroids (hyperparathyroidism), the plasma level of calcium increases to about 20 mg calcium per 100 ml of blood from a normal of 5.5 mg of calcium per 100 ml of blood. This calcium comes from the bone and the kidney gets rid of it from the body. Thus the bones become thin and fragile, and are likely to fracture more easily than normal bones with sufficient calcium.

With decreased production of parathyroid hormone (hypoparathyroidism), the blood calcium level falls, which causes increased excitability of the nerves and of the neuromuscular junctions, leading to a condition called tetany (this has to be distinguished from the disease tetanus, which follows infection with a bacillus *Clostridium tetani*). In tetany, there is spasm of the hands and feet (carpo-pedal spasm). Increased excitability of the nerve cells in the brain may lead to convulsions.

A10.4 Adrenocorticotrophic hormone and the adrenal gland

The adrenal glands are located on the top of each kidney (see Figure A12). Each adrenal gland consists of a central medulla and an outer cortex.

The adrenal medulla releases the hormones adrenaline and noradrenaline (epinephrine and nor-epinephrine) in response to nerve stimuli that enter the medulla from the sympathetic nervous system. Thus the adrenal medulla is an integral part of the sympathetic nervous system and is intimately involved in the fight or flight responses to stress, where increased sympathetic activity is life saving. It is common to state that a person should have sufficient adrenaline to perform well. The secretions of the hormones from the adrenal medulla are not under the control of the anterior pituitary adrenocorticotrophic hormone (ACTH).

The adrenal cortex has three layers and each layer produces a different hormone and at least two of the layers are controlled by ACTH from the anterior pituitary gland.

The outer layer—the zona glomerulosa—produces aldosterone, which is necessary for reabsorption of sodium in the kidney. An excess of aldosterone causes salt and water retention. The secretion of aldosterone is considered to be regulated by a hormone secreted by the kidney, renin.

The inner two layers of the adrenal cortex—the zona fasciculalta and the zona reticularis—produce hormones collectively known as cortcosteroids. The main corticosteroid secreted is cortisol (hydrocortisone). The corticosteroids have several actions:

◆ they favour the utilization of proteins for the production of heat and energy in preference to the use of carbohydrates;

◆ anti-allergy;

◆ anti-inflammatory, and

◆ aldosterone-like effects causing retention of sodium and of water and loss of potassium. The salt and water retention may lead to oedema and/or high blood pressure (hypertension).

Cortisol reduces the utilization of carbohydrates for energy, thus the blood sugar level often increases (a diabetogenic effect). When body proteins are broken down, wound healing is impaired and the effect on suppression of immune or inflammatory response can lead to 'masking' of infections (which may cause delays in diagnosis) and also an increased susceptibility to infections.

Over-production of the adrenal cortex hormone leads to Cushing's syndrome, which is characterized by a 'moon face' that is caused by redistribution of fat and swelling of the face. Redistribution of body fat leads to 'an egg on match sticks' appearance with an expanded abdomen and chest with 'skinny' limbs, particularly lower limbs, diabetes, and increased blood pressure. The skin tends to bruise easily and purple striae appear on the skin; females develop hirsutism. There may also be psychological changes.

Changes similar to Cushing's syndrome follow treatment with corticosteroids over a period of time for several common disease states. An excessive production of aldosterone leads to Conn's disease, which is associated with muscular weakness, increased loss of potassium, and water in the urine.

Decreased activity of the adrenal gland leads to Addison's disease. This was common following tuberculosis affecting the adrenal gland when both the medulla and cortex were affected. In Addison's disease, sodium and water are lost from the body and this causes a lowering of blood pressure, muscle weakness, nausea, and vomiting. The production of catecholamines (e.g. adrenaline and noradrenaline) is affected and there is increased production of melanin instead. This leads to increased pigmentation, particularly of exposed parts. Episodes of low blood sugar may occur as adrenaline plays an important role in mobilizing glucose, particularly in times of stress.

A11 The immune system

Immunology is the study of the physiological responses by which the body destroys or neutralizes foreign matter or xenobiotics, living and non-living, as well as its own cells that have become altered in certain ways. The ability of the immune response to protect us against bacteria, fungi, viruses and other parasites, and other foreign matter is one of the most important defence mechanisms of the human body.

This immune response—the process by which xenobiotics are destroyed or neutralized—is therefore essential for a healthy disease-free life. The immune response can also destroy cancer cells that arise in the body and also worn out or damaged cells such as old red blood cells or erythrocytes.

Immune responses can be broadly classified into:

1. non-specific immune responses, which recognize in a non-selective manner all foreign substances;

2. specific immune responses against substances that are specifically identified and then attacked.

Bacteria have the ability to cause damage at their sites of invasion or can release into the body fluids (extracellular fluids, of which blood is the most important) toxins that are carried to other parts of the body to cause damage to cells.

The body also needs protection against viruses, which are essentially nucleic acids surrounded by a protein coat. Unlike bacteria, which have their own metabolic processes and can multiply independent of other cells, viruses lack the enzyme processes and other cell constituents such as ribosomes for their own metabolism and energy production. Therefore viruses can only multiply whilst living inside other cells whose biochemical apparatus they make use of. The nucleic acids in the viruses cause the production/manufacture of proteins required for the viruses to multiply and also the energy to multiply.

The cells and associated components that carry out immune responses are collectively called the immune system. Although called a system, it has no anatomical continuity but consists of diverse collections of cells found in both the blood and tissues (cells) throughout the body.

Cells mediating the immune response are the following:

1. White blood cells or leucocytes, including neutrophils, basophils, eosinophils, monocytes, and lymphocytes. The lymphocytes are grouped into B cells and T cells (cytotoxic T cells, helper T cells, and suppressor T cells). White blood cells can leave the circulation or blood (unlike the red blood cells) and enter tissues and function in the tissues.

2. Plasma cells found in peripheral lymph organs. Plasma cells differentiate from lymphocytes in the tissue and are not found in the blood as the name suggests.

3. Macrophages present in almost all tissues and organs are large cells but their structure may vary from tissue to tissue. They are derived from monocytes (white blood cells) that leave the blood vessels to enter the tissues. As their main function is to engulf foreign material, they are strategically located at sites where entry of foreign substances or organisms is likely to take place.

4. Mast cells are also found in all tissues and organs. Mast cells differentiate from basophils that have left the blood vessels and a characteristic feature is that they usually contain large numbers of secretory vesicles and they secrete mainly locally acting chemical messengers such as histamine. These cells are involved in allergic responses such as hypersensitivity reactions.

A11.1 Inflammation

This is the local reaction of the body to injury or infection which essentially destroys or inactivates the foreign invaders and prepares the body to repair the injury caused. The main role is played by phagocytes, which engulf the foreign material by a process called phagocytosis. Once inside the phagocyte, the foreign substance is destroyed. The important phagocytes are the neutrophils, monocytes, and macrophages.

The usual clinical manifestations of inflammation are redness, swelling, heat, and pain, which are produced by a variety of chemical messengers or mediators. The better known of these mediators are the kinins, histamine, complement, and eicosanoids. The kinins are produced from the plasma protein kininogen whilst histamine is released from mast cells.

Two important mediators, interleukin 1 (IL1) and tumour necrosis factor, are protein in nature and are released by monocytes and macrophages during an inflammatory response.

Complement kills microbes without prior phagocytosis. Complement is always present in the blood albeit in an inactive form most of the time. Activation of complement in response to an infection or tissue injury generates active molecules from inactive precursors and the complement system comprises at least 20 distinct proteins. Complement also stimulates the secretion of histamine from mast cells and effectively increases the blood flow to the injured area and facilitates the movement of phagocytes such as the neutrophils to the injured area from within the blood vessels.

Lymphocytes also circulate in the blood but tend to gather in large numbers in group of organs and tissues called lymphoid organs such as bone marrow, the thymus gland (a gland found in the chest which tends to shrink in size after puberty), lymph nodes, spleen, and tonsils. These cells also concentrate in the lining of the intestine and in the respiratory, genital, and urinary tracts.

The lymphatic system is a network of lymphatic vessels and lymph nodes found along these vessels through which lymph, a fluid derived from interstitial fluid, flows. It constitutes a route by which interstitial fluid can reach the blood vessels or the cardiovascular system. This movement of interstitial fluid as lymph to the cardiovascular system is very important because the amount of fluid filtered out of all the blood vessel capillaries (except those of the kidney) exceed that which is reabsorbed by approximately 4 litres each day. These 4 litres are returned to the venous blood via the thoracic duct in the chest. In the process, the small amount of protein that usually leaks out of the capillaries is also brought back into the circulation by the lymphatic system.

Also important is that the lymph node cells encounter the materials that start off their response, that is the immune response via the lymph flowing through them. Each lymph node is a honeycomb of sinuses (enlargements or sac-like dilations containing lymph) lined by macrophages with large clusters of lymphocytes between the sinuses. The spleen is the largest of the organs containing lymphoid tissue and lies on the left side of the abdominal cavity between the stomach and the diaphragm (the large muscle that is essential for breathing and separates the thoracic cavity from the abdominal cavity).

The other structures with large collections of lymphoid tissue are the tonsils, which are small rounded structures in the throat that often get inflamed in children, resulting in the common condition called tonsillitis.

There are multiple populations and sub-populations of lymphocytes termed B lymphocytes, T lymphocytes, cytotoxic, helper, and suppressor T cells. There are two broad categories of specific immune responses. Firstly, a lymphocyte is programmed to recognize a specific antigen. An antigen is a foreign substance that triggers a specific immune response and is not an anatomical description but is a functional description. The ability of lymphocytes to distinguish one antigen from another is the basis of specific immune responses. Recognition of an antigen implies that antigen becomes bound to the lymphocyte which has receptors for that antigen.

Once the lymphocyte has attached itself to the antigen, it divides into different types of cells, and this takes place at the site where the antigen has attached itself to the lymphocyte. Some of the divided cells will attack the antigens, whilst others may influence both the activation and function of these 'attack cells'.

The activated cells attack all the antigens that initiated the immune response. Lymphocytes attack the 'invaders' in one of two ways: antibody mediated or humoral and cell mediated.

Antibodies are proteins that are both present in the plasma membranes of B cells and are also secreted by them. These antibodies travel along the bloodstream to all parts of the body, combine with the antigens, and direct an attack by phagocytes and complement that eliminates the antigen or the cells bearing them. Antibodies belong to a group of proteins called immunoglobulins.

In cell-mediated immunity, the T lymphocytes and natural killer cells travel to the location of cells bearing on their surface antigens that initiated the immune response and directly kill them.

Two broad generalizations can be made. Antibody-mediated responses carried out by B lymphocytes have a large range of targets and are the major defence against bacteria, viruses, and other microbes and against toxic molecules. Cell-mediated killing by T lymphocytes and natural killer cells is against a more limited number of targets, specifically the body's own cells that have become cancerous or infected with viruses. The helper cells activate both humoral and cell-mediated immune responses. The helper cells are essential for the production of antibodies except in the case of a small number of antigens. Suppressor T cells inhibit the function of both B cells and cytotoxic T cells.

A12 **Further reading**

Barrett KE, Ganong WF. (2009) Ganong's Review of Medical Physiology, 23rd edn. McGraw Hill, New York.

Boon NA, Davidson S. (2006) Davidson's Principles and Practice of Medicine. 19th edn. Elsevier Health Sciences, London.

Green JH. (1978) An Introduction to Human Physiology, 5th edn. Oxford University Press, London.

Porth CM, Matfin G. (2010) Handbook of Pathophysiology. 3rd edn. Churchill Livingstone, London.

Glossary and abbreviations

absorption (1) The entry of a substance into the human body usually via skin, lungs, or gastrointestinal tract (2) Take up of a gas by a solid or liquid, or the take up of a liquid by a solid. It differs from adsorption in that the absorbed substance permeates the bulk of the absorbing substance.

acidosis Pathological condition in which the hydrogen ion concentration of body fluids is above normal and hence the pH of blood falls below the normal range (7.4).

acrocyanosis Bluish discolouration of the extremities—hands and feet—due to poor oxygen supply.

acrodynia Form of mercury poisoning, usually seen in children. Symptoms include pain, pink discolouration of extremities (hands and feet), itching, and peeling of the skin (desquamation), and may be accompanied by irritation.

ACTS Advisory Committee on Toxic Substances, Health and Safety Executive.

acute Occurring over a short time.

acute effect Effect of short duration (hours or a few days) immediately following exposure.

acute exposure Contact with a substance that occurs only once (or for a short period usually under 24 hours).

additive effect A biological response to the exposure to multiple substances that equals the sum of responses to all the individual substances under the same conditions.

ADI Acceptable daily intake. Estimate of the amount of a substance in food or drinking water, expressed on a body mass basis (usually mg/kg body weight), that can be ingested daily over a lifetime by humans without appreciable health risk. ADI is normally used for food additives (tolerable daily intake is used for contaminants).

ADI 'not specified' No acceptable daily intake allocated. Terminology used by JECFA in situations where an ADI is not established for a substance under consideration because (a) insufficient safety information is available, (b) no information is available on its food use, (c) specifications for identity and purity have not been developed.

ADMS Atmospheric dispersion modelling system. Commercially available short-range dispersion model developed in the UK.

adsorption The physical or chemical binding of gases or liquids onto the surface of solid particles. See also *absorption*.

adverse health effect A change in the morphology, physiology, growth, development, or lifespan of an organism which results in impairment of functional capacity or impairment of capacity to compensate for additional stress or increase in susceptibility to the harmful effects of other environmental influences.

aerobic Requiring oxygen to survive. Usually applied to bacteria which cannot survive or multiply without oxygen.

agonist (1) A substance that tends to increase the action of another (2) A drug or other substance having a specific cellular affinity that produces a predictable biological reaction.

agonistic effect A positive biological response following the action of a substance at a specific site.

ALARP As low as reasonably practicable.

alkalosis Pathological condition in which the hydrogen ion concentration of body fluids is below normal and hence the pH of blood rises above the normal range (usually a pH above 7.4).

allergen A substance capable of producing a specific immunological response (restricted mainly to immediate hypersensitivity or anaphylactic reactions).

alopecia A general term for loss of hair.

ambient Surrounding (for example ambient air, water, sediment, or soil). Refers to the environment around an individual.

amnesia Loss of memory.

anaemia A reduction in haemoglobin concentration in the blood.

anaerobic Metabolism requiring minimal amounts of oxygen.

analgesia The relief of pain.

anaphylaxis Immediate, often life-threatening, hypersensitivity (allergic) reaction to an antigen (a substance that induces a specific immunological response).

aneugenic Inducing aneuploidy. See *aneuploidy*.

aneuploid A normal human cell has 23 pairs of chromosomes: a cell or organism with missing or extra chromosomes is known as an aneuploid.

aneuploidy The circumstances in which the total number of chromosomes within a cell is not an exact multiple of the normal haploid (see polyploidy) number. Chromosomes may be lost or gained during cell division.

anhydrous A chemical substance without water.

anorexia Loss of appetite. (Anorexia nervosa is the term used to describe a psychological eating disorder.)

anosmia Loss of sense of smell.

anoxia Strictly this is the total absence of oxygen but anoxia is sometimes used to mean decreased oxygen supply in tissues, i.e. hypoxia.

antagonist effect A negative biological response following the blocking of the action of a substance at a specific site.

antidote A general term for a substance used to counteract the toxic effects of a poison.

Antigen A substance that induces an immune response.

anuria No output of urine over a 24-hour period.

aplastic anaemia Type of anaemia where the bone marrow fails to produce an adequate number of all blood cells and platelets.

apnoea Cessation of breathing.

aqueous Water based.

ARDS Acute respiratory distress syndrome.

areflexia Absence of reflexes, usually reflexes assessed by examination of the nervous system.

ARF (1) Acute renal failure (2) Acute respiratory failure.

arrhythmia Any variation from the normal rhythm of the heartbeat.

asbestosis Chronic fibrotic lung disease caused by inhaling airborne asbestos fibres.

aspiration When a liquid or object is inhaled into the lungs. A common cause is inhaling acid in vomit from the stomach.

AST Aspartate aminotransferase. An enzyme normally present in the liver; its level in blood provides a test of liver function (formerly known as glutamic oxaloacetic transaminase).

asymptomatic A subject without any complaints (symptoms).

asystole Absence of contraction of the heart muscle to produce a heartbeat.

ataxia Loss of co-ordination of parts of the body. It affects the parts of the nervous system that control movement and balance, leading to unstable posture or gait.

atrial fibrillation A condition in which the atria (the two upper chambers of the heart) contract at a very high rate and in an irregular way.

atrophy Decrease in size or wasting away of a body part or tissue.

ATSDR Agency for Toxic Substances and Disease Registry, US Department of Health and Human Services.

BaP Benzo[a]pyrene.

bioavailability A term referring to the proportion of a substance which reaches the systemic circulation unchanged after a particular route of administration.

biologic indicators A species or other biological endpoint used as a quantifiable proxy to measure a condition of interest.

biological monitoring/biomonitoring Scientific technique used to assess human exposure to chemicals using biological samples.

biological sample A tissue or fluid sample taken from a person (or animal), e.g. urine, blood, hair etc.

biological uptake The transfer of substances from the environment to plants, animals, and humans.

biomarker Observable change (not necessarily pathological) in an organism related to a specific exposure or effect.

biota All living organisms as a totality.

biotransformation Chemical alteration of a substance within the body, as by the action of enzymes. This process usually leads to less harmful products or those that can be eliminated from the body more easily than the parent substance. Sometimes, it may result in a more active or harmful product.

BMGV Biological monitoring guidance values.

body Total amount of substance of a chemical present in a biological sample at a given time.

bradycardia Slow heart rate.

bronchospasm Narrowing of the small bronchi (bronchioles) by muscular contraction.

bundle branch block Interruption of the conduction of cardiac impulses from the upper chambers of the heart, the atria, to the lower chambers of the heart, the ventricles, which usually results in a slow heart rate.

cancer A synonym for a malignant neoplasm, that is a tumour that grows progressively, invades local tissue, and spreads to distant sites. See also *tumour*.

cancer risk Probability that cancer will be produced by exposure, for example to a hazardous chemical.

carboxyhaemoglobin (COHb) Complex formed between carbon monoxide and haemoglobin in the blood. Haemoglobin has a much higher affinity for carbon monoxide than oxygen, hence the amount of oxygen in the blood is greatly reduced. See *haemoglobin*.

carcinogen The causal agents which induce tumours.

carcinogenic Liable to cause cancer.

cardiac Referring to the heart.

CAS number Number assigned by the Chemical Abstract Service (CAS, a division of the American Chemical Society) to a specific chemical. CAS numbers are assigned sequentially and serve as a concise, unique means of identification. The numbers have no chemical significance.

case (in toxicology) A medical or epidemiologic evaluation of one person or a small group of people (case study) to gather information about specific health conditions and past exposures.

case-control study An epidemiological study where a comparison is made between the proportion of cases (individuals with disease) that have been exposed to a particular hazard (e.g. a chemical) and the proportion of controls (individuals without disease) that have been exposed to the hazard.

catecholamine Group of compounds, including epinephrine (adrenaline) and norepinephrine (noradrenaline), released from the adrenal glands in response to stress. Typical effects produced are an increase in heart rate, blood pressure, and breathing rate.

CBR Chemical, biological, and radiological.

CBRN Chemical, biological, radiological, and nuclear.

CCA Civil Contingencies Act 2004. The legislation that defines UK emergency planning and response, and sets expectations for civil protection.

CCDC Consultant in communicable disease control—a specialist doctor working in public health in the UK.

central nervous system (CNS) The part of the nervous system that consists of the brain and the spinal cord.

CfI Centre for Infections, Health Protection Agency.

CHaPD Chemical Hazards and Poisons Division, UK Health Protection Agency.

CHEMDATA Emergency response computer database available from the National Chemicals Emergency Centre (part of the AEA Group) used by the fire service and other emergency services in the UK and worldwide for chemical information.

CHEMET A service from the Meteorological Office that provides information on weather conditions as they affect an incident involving hazardous chemicals (e.g. the anticipated behaviour of any plume). CHEMETs are available on request by the emergency services.

CHEMSAFE Chemical Industry Scheme for Assistance in Freight Emergencies.

CHIP The Health and Safety Executive's Chemicals (Hazard Information and Packaging) Regulations.

chromatid One of the paired and parallel strands of a duplicated chromosome joined by a central centromere.

chromosomal aberrations Collective term for particular types of chromosome damage induced after exposure to exogenous chemicals or physical agents that damage the DNA. See *clastogen*.

chromosome In simple organisms such as bacteria and some viruses, the chromosome consists of a single circular molecule of DNA containing the entire genetic material of the cell. In the cells of more complex organisms, such as animals and plants, the chromosomes are thread-like structures, composed mainly of DNA, which are present in the nuclei of every cell. They occur in pairs, the numbers varying from one to more than 100 per nucleus in different species. Normal somatic cells in humans have 23 pairs of chromosomes, each consisting of linear sequences of DNA which are known as genes.

chronic effect A prolonged health effect that occurs due to an exposure and tends to persist for a long time even after cessation of exposure.

chronic exposure Continued exposure occurring over an extended period of time or a significant fraction of the lifetime of a human or test animal.

CIMAH Control of Industrial Major Accident Hazards Regulations 1984 (now replaced by the Control of Major Accident Hazards Regulations).

CIMAH/COMAH sites Industrial sites that are subject to the Control of Industrial Major Accident Hazards Regulations 1984. From February 1999, these were replaced by the Control of Major Accident Hazards Regulations.

clastogen An agent that produces chromosome breaks and/or consequent gain, loss, or rearrangement of pieces of chromosomes. Clastogens may be viruses or physical agents as well as chemicals.

clastogenicity Inducing chromosome breaks and other structural aberrations.

CLAW Control of Lead at Work Act 1998.

CLEA Contaminated land exposure assessment model.

cluster investigation A method of sampling where there is review of an unusual number, real or perceived, of health events (e.g. reports of cancer) grouped together in time and location. Cluster investigations may be designed to confirm case reports, determine whether they represent an unusual disease occurrence, and suggest hypotheses regarding possible causes and contributing environmental factors for potential further investigation.

CMO Chief Medical Officer.

CNS depression Decrease in function of the central nervous system resulting in a state that can range from drowsiness to coma.

CO Carbon monoxide.

COC Committee on Carcinogenicity of Chemicals in Food, Consumer Products and the Environment.

COM Committee on Mutagenicity of Chemicals in Food, Consumer Products and the Environment.

COMAH Control of Major Accident Hazards Regulations. See also *CIMAH/COMAH* sites.

COMEAP Committee on Medical Effects of Air Pollution.

concentration The amount of a substance present in a certain amount of soil, water, air, food, blood, hair, urine, breath, or any other media.

congener Substance which by structure, function, or origin is similar to another.

conjunctivitis Inflammation of the conjunctiva, the mucous membrane covering the white of the eye and the inner lining of the eyelids.

contaminant A substance that is either present in an environment where it does not belong or is present at levels that might cause harmful (adverse) health effects.

convulsions Violent involuntary contraction of muscles.

co-ordination The harmonious integration of the expertise of all the agencies involved, with the object of effectively and efficiently bringing the incident to a successful conclusion.

COSHH Control of Substances Hazardous to Health Regulations.

COT Committee on Toxicity of Chemicals in Food, Consumer Products and the Environment (non-food).

cyanosis Bluish discolouration of skin, mucous membranes (lips), fingernails, and other tissues due to deoxygenated haemoglobin (i.e. haemoglobin without oxygen bound to it).

cytochrome C oxidase An enzyme necessary for cells to utilize oxygen. It is the terminal enzyme in the electron transport chain in mitochondria.

delayed health effect A disease or an injury that happens as a result of exposures that have occurred in the past.

dermal Referring to the skin. For example, dermal absorption means passing through the skin.

dermal contact Contact with the skin.

dermatitis Inflammatory disorder of the skin.

descriptive epidemiology The study of the amount and distribution of a disease in a specified population by person, place, and time.

detection limit The lowest concentration of a chemical that can reliably be detected/measured from a zero concentration.

dilated pupils (mydriasis) Large pupils.

dioxin Dioxins are members of a large group of substances with similar structure (chemically they are as polychlorinated dibenzo-p-dioxins). They are not produced intentionally but very small amounts are produced in combustion processes and as a by-product in certain industrial processes. They have similar types of toxicity but vary markedly in their potency. The most potent is the 2,3,7,8-tetrachloro derivative, often referred to as TCDD. This is extremely toxic. The toxicity of other dioxins is expressed relative to TCDD. In some cases this is several orders of magnitude less than TCDD.

diplopia Double vision.

disease prevention Measures used to prevent a disease or reduce its severity.

disease registry A system of ongoing registration of all cases of a particular disease or health condition in a defined population.

diuresis Increased formation and passage of urine.

DNA Deoxyribonucleic acid. The carrier for genetic information for all living organisms except the group of RNA viruses. Each of the 46 chromosomes in normal human cells consists of two strands of DNA containing up to 100,000 nucleotides, specific sequences of which make up genes. DNA itself is composed of two interwound chains of linked nucleotides.

dose (for chemicals that are not radioactive) Total amount of a substance administered to, taken, or absorbed by an organism (latter may be referred to as absorbed dose).

dose-response relationship The relationship between the dose of a substance and the resulting changes in body function or health (response), usually plotted as a graph, with the dose on the x-axis and the response on the y-axis.

dys- Prefix meaning difficult, painful, abnormal.

dysarthria Difficulty in speaking caused by a disturbance of either the speech centre in the brain or the muscles involved in speech.

dyskinesia Difficulty in performing voluntary movement.

dysphagia Difficulty in swallowing.

dysphonia General term covering disorders of voice, including hoarseness.

dyspnoea Difficulty in breathing or shortness of breath.

dystonic movements Neurological movement disorder caused by prolonged, repetitive muscle contractions that may cause twisting, jerking, or repetitive movements.

dysuria Painful urination.

EA Environment Agency.

EC European Commission.

EC Directive Directive to member states of the European Union to draw up national legislation to implement the content of the Directive.

ECG Electrocardiogram. An instrument that measures and records the electrical activity of the heart.

ECG changes Changes in cardiac rhythm, rate, or electrical activity shown on an electro-cardiograph.

eczema General term for a range of inflammatory skin conditions whose characteristic signs may include dryness, redness, itching, oozing blisters, crusts, and scabs.

EEG Electroencephalogram. A record of the electrical activity of the brain.

embolism Sudden blocking of a blood vessel or vein by a clot or foreign body from a site distant to the site of the blockage.

emesis Vomiting.

encephalitis Inflammation of the brain.

encephalopathy Disease states which manifest as altered functions of the brain. May be seen with liver failure (hepatic encephalopathy in alcoholics) and kidney failure.

endarteritis obliterans A disease of arteries, usually of the legs, which causes a marked decrease of blood supply to the muscles in the leg and causes pain during walking; referred to as claudication.

environmental health officer (EHO) A professional officer responsible for assisting people to attain environmental conditions that are conducive to good health. Most EHOs work for local authorities and are concerned with administration, inspection, education, and law enforcement.

environmental media Soil, water, air, biota (plants and animals), or any other parts of the environment that can contain contaminants.

EPA Environmental Protection Act (UK).

epidemiology The study of the distribution and determinants of disease or health status in a population.

epistaxis Bleeding from the nose.

erythema Reddening of the skin due to congestion of blood or increased blood flow to the skin.

erythrocyte superoxidase dismutase An enzyme present in red blood cells involved in the reduction of superoxide radicals to hydrogen peroxide. It acts as an antioxidant protecting against the harmful effects of the active oxygen species.

euphoria Exaggerated feeling of well-being.

exposure The process by which a substance becomes available for absorption by a population by any route, e.g. swallowing, breathing, or contact with the skin or eyes. Exposure may be short-term (acute exposure), of intermediate duration, or long-term (chronic exposure).

exposure assessment The process of finding out how people come into contact with a hazardous substance, how often and for how long they are in contact with the substance, and the amount with which they are in contact.

exposure investigation The collection and analysis of site-specific information and biologic tests (when appropriate) to determine whether people have been exposed to hazardous substances.

exposure pathway The route a substance takes from its source (where it began) to its end point (where it ends), and how people can come into contact with (or be exposed to) it. An exposure pathway has five parts: a source of contamination (such as an abandoned business), an environmental media and transport mechanism (such as movement through groundwater), a point of exposure (such as a private well), a route of exposure (eating, drinking, breathing, or touching), and a receptor population (people potentially or actually exposed). When all five parts are present, the exposure pathway is termed a completed exposure pathway.

exposure registry A system of ongoing follow-up of people who have had documented environmental exposures.

exposure-dose reconstruction A method of estimating the amount of people's past exposure to hazardous substances. Computer and approximation methods are used when past information is limited, not available, or missing.

extrapyramidal symptoms (EPS) Excess involuntary movements.

fasciculations Visible twitching of muscles—distinct from muscle spasms.

furans Dioxins and furans are chlorinated aromatic hydrocarbon species.

G6PD Glucose 6-phosphate dehydrogenase. An enzyme present in red blood cells.

gene The functional unit of inheritance; a specific sequence of nucleotides along the DNA molecule forming part of a chromosome.

good agricultural practice The recommended usage of a pesticide which is necessary and essential for the control of a pest under all practical conditions, bearing in mind any toxicological hazards involved.

haem- Prefix referring to blood.

haematemesis Vomiting of blood.

haematoma Localized accumulation of blood, usually clotted, in an organ, space, or tissue due to a failure of the wall of a blood vessel.

haematuria Presence of blood in the urine.

haemoglobin Oxygen-carrying substance in red blood cells.

haemolysis Breakdown of red blood cells usually due to disruption of the red blood cell membrane which releases haemoglobin into the plasma.

haemoptysis Coughing up of blood.

haemorrhage Bleeding.

hazard Set of inherent properties of a substance, mixture of substances, or a process involving substances that make it capable of causing adverse effects to organisms or the environment, depending on the extent of exposure.

hazard identification A process by which potential hazards are identified.

Hazardous Substance Release and Health Effects Database (HazDat) The scientific and administrative database system developed by ATSDR (see *ATSDR*) to manage data collection, retrieval, and analysis of site-specific information on hazardous substances, community health concerns, and public health activities.

HAZCHEM Hazardous chemical label.

HAZMAT Incidents involving hazardous materials.

head space analysis Chemical analysis of vapour given off by a liquid mixture.

health investigation The collection and evaluation of information about the health of community residents. This information is used to describe or count the occurrence of a disease, symptom, or clinical measure, and to assist in investigating the possible association between the occurrence and exposure to hazardous substances.

heart block Interruption of conduction of cardiac impulses, which usually causes the slowing of the heart.

hepatic Referring to the liver.

hepatitis Inflammation of the liver cells.

HMEI Hypothetic maximally exposed individual.

HPA The United Kingdom Health Protection Agency.

HSE The Health and Safety Executive. Government body in the UK with responsibility for enforcing health and safety legislation and investigation of accidents.

hyper- Prefix meaning above, more than normal, excessive.

hyperactivity Increased activity in an individual or a biological system.

hyperacussis Heightened sense of hearing.

hyperaesthesia Increased sensitivity to touch and other sensory stimuli.

hypercalcaemia Abnormally increased concentration of calcium in the blood.

hypercapnia Excess of carbon dioxide in the blood.

hyperglycaemia Abnormally increased concentration of glucose (sugar) in the blood.

hyperkalaemia Abnormally increased concentration of potassium ions in the blood.

hyperkeratosis Thickening of the outer layer (epidermis) of the skin.

hypernatraemia Abnormally increased concentration of sodium ions in the blood.

hyperpigmentation Increased pigmentation.

hyperpyrexia High body temperature, commonly called fever.

hyperreflexia Increased reflexes.

hypersalivation Increased salivation/drooling.

hypertension High blood pressure. Usually refers to the systemic circulation, i.e. arteries and arterioles from the aorta. May be used to refer to a particular circulation, e.g. pulmonary hypertension (increased blood pressure in the pulmonary circulation) or portal hypertension (increased pressure in portal circulation to liver).

hypertonia Increased muscle tone.

hyperventilation Increased breathing rate.

hypo- Prefix meaning below, less than normal.

hypocalcaemia Abnormally decreased concentration of calcium ions in the blood.

hypoglycaemia Abnormally decreased concentration of glucose in the blood.

hypokalaemia Abnormally decreased concentration of potassium ions in the blood.

hyponatraemia Abnormally decreased concentration of sodium ions in the blood.

hyporeflexia Decreased muscle reflexes.

hypotension Low blood pressure.

hypothermia Low body temperature.

hypotonia Decreased muscle tone.

hypoventilation Reduced rate or depth of breathing.

hypoxia Decreased oxygen content in the body tissues.

IARC International Agency for Research on Cancer.

ICSC International Chemical Safety Card.

ICU Intensive care unit.

IDLH Immediately dangerous to life and health.

incidence The number of new cases of disease in a defined population over a specific time period.

ingestion The act of swallowing something through eating, drinking, or mouthing objects. A hazardous substance can enter the body this way.

inhalation The act of breathing in. A hazardous substance can enter the body this way.

insomnia Inability to sleep.

in vitro A Latin term used to describe effects in biological material outside the living animal. Literally 'in glass'. Used to refer to studies in a laboratory involving isolated organs, tissues, or cells.

in vivo A Latin term used to describe effects in living animals. Literally 'in life'. Refers to studies carried out on a living organism.

IPCS International Programme on Chemical Safety.

irritable Abnormally sensitive to stimuli.

ischaemia Local deficiency of blood supply and hence oxygen to an organ or tissues, usually due to constriction of the blood vessels or to obstruction.

ISO 14001 International (ISO) Standard for Environmental Management Systems.

ISO 9001 International (ISO) Standard for Quality Management Systems.

I-TEQ International Toxic Equivalent Quotient (used for dioxins and furans).

jaundice Pathological condition characterized by deposition of bile pigment in the skin and mucous membranes, including the conjunctivae, resulting in yellow appearance of the patient.

JECFA Joint FAO/WHO Expert Committee on Food Additives.

lacrimator Substance that irritates the eyes and causes tearing.

L_{den} Day–evening–night level in decibels as an indicator for 'annoyance'.

LD_{50} The dose of a toxic compound that causes death in 50% of a group of experimental animals to which it is exposed. It can be used in the assessment of the acute toxicity of a compound but is being superseded by more refined methods.

LDL:HDL cholesterol Ratio of low density lipoprotein cholesterol to high density lipoprotein cholesterol.

lead time The period of time from exposure to the development of adverse health effects.

leucocytosis Increased number of white blood cells in the blood.

leucopaenia Decreased number of white blood cells in the blood.

LFT Liver function test.

limit of detection The lowest concentration that can be measured.

lindane gamma Gamma-hexachlorocyclohexane, a pesticide.

lipophilic Having affinity for lipids (fatty compounds). Dissolves much more readily in lipids than water.

LOAEL Lowest observed adverse effects level.

LTEL Long-term exposure limit.

malaise Vague feeling of lethargy and fatigue.

meiosis Process of 'reductive' cell division, occurring in the production of gametes, by means of which each daughter nucleus receives half the number of chromosomes characteristic of the somatic cells of the species.

MEK Methylethylketone.

MEL Maximum exposure limit. This is an obsolete term that has been superceded by WEL(qv).

melaena Black stools due to altered blood from bleeding into the bowel.

metabolism The conversion or breakdown of a substance from one form to another by a living organism which usually results in the production of a less toxic substance or a substance that could be eliminated from the body more easily. The products of a metabolic process are metabolites.

metabolite Any product of metabolism.

methaemoglobinaemia Presence of methaemoglobin (altered haemoglobin) in the blood.

MetHb Methaemoglobin.

mg/cm² Milligram per square centimetre (of a surface).

mg/kg Milligram per kilogram.

mg/m³ Milligram per cubic metre. A measure of the concentration of a chemical in a known volume (a cubic metre) of air, soil, or water.

MIC Methyl isocyanate.

micronuclei Isolated or broken chromosome fragments which are not expelled when the nucleus is lost during cell division, but remain in the body of the cell, forming micronuclei. Centromere positive micronuclei contain DNA and/or protein material derived from the centromere. The presence of centromere positive micronuclei following exposure to chemicals can be used to evaluate the aneugenic potential of chemicals.

miosis Constricted pupils (the size of the pupil is less than 2 mm).

mitochondria Rod-shaped constituents of a cell involved in cell respiration producing energy for the organism. Referred to as the 'power house' of cells.

mitotic index A measure of the rate of proliferation of cells and the ratio of number of cells dividing (mitotic cells) to cells that are not dividing.

ml Millilitre.

mm Millimetre.

mmol Millimole.

morbidity State of being ill or diseased. Morbidity is the occurrence of a disease or condition that alters health and quality of life.

MRL Maximum residue level. The maximum concentration of residue (expressed as milligrams of residue per kilogram of food/animal feeding stuff) resulting from, for example, the use of a pesticide, likely to occur in or on food and feeding stuffs after the use of pesticides according to good agricultural practice. See *good agricultural practice*.

MSDS Material safety data sheet.

mucosa Surface membrane lining the nose, respiratory tract, and other cavities of the body.

mutagen A substance that causes mutations (alterations or loss of genes or chromosomes).

mutagenic The ability of a substance to increase the occurrence of mutations.

mutation A permanent change in the amount or structure of the genetic material in an organism or cell which can result in a change in phenotypic characteristics. The alteration may involve a single gene, a block of genes, or a whole chromosome. Mutations involving single genes may be a consequence of effects on single DNA bases (point mutations) or of large changes, including deletions, within the gene. Changes in whole chromosomes may be numerical or structural. A mutation in germ cells of sexually reproducing organisms may be transmitted to the offspring, whereas a mutation that occurs in somatic cells may be transferred only to the descendant daughter cells.

mydriasis Dilated pupils.

myo- Prefix referring to muscle.

myocardial infarction Area of necrosis (death of heart muscle cells) resulting from inadequate blood supply to the heart muscle (i.e. heart attack).

myocarditis Inflammation of the heart muscle.

myocardium Heart muscle.

NAMAS National Accreditation of Measurement and Sampling. Accreditation given to laboratories from the UK Accreditation Service (UKAS).

NAME Nuclear accident model. Long-range dispersion model run by the UK Meteorological Service.

ND Not detected.

necrosis Localized death of tissues or cells.

neoplasm See *tumour*.

neoplastic Pertaining to or like a neoplasm.

neuroleptic Describing the effect on cognition and behaviour of antipsychotic drugs.

neuropathy Any disease of the central or peripheral nervous system.

NFAR No further action required.

ng Nanogram (1 billionth of a gram).

NIOSH National Institute for Occupational Safety and Health.

NO_x Oxides of nitrogen, NO and NO_2 are commonly referred to as NO_x.

NOAEL No observed adverse effect level. The highest administered dose at which no adverse effects are observed.

NPIS National Poisons Information Service.

nucleotide The 'building block' of nucleic acids such as the DNA molecule. A nucleotide consists of one of four bases—adenine, guanine, cytosine, or thymine—attached to a phosphate–sugar group. In DNA the sugar group is deoxyribose, while in RNA (a DNA-related molecule that helps to translate genetic information into proteins) the sugar group is ribose and the base uracil substitutes for thymidine. Each group of three nucleotides in a gene is known as a codon. A nucleic acid is a long chain of nucleotides joined together and therefore is sometimes referred to as a 'polynucleotide'.

nystagmus Involuntary, repetitive lateral movement of the eyes.

occupational exposure limit (OEL) The concentration in air of a chemical in the workplace that is thought to be safe. This means that most workers can be exposed at the given concentration or lower without harmful effects for specified periods.

oedema Presence of abnormally large amounts of fluid in intercellular spaces of body tissues, causing swelling.

oedema, cerebral Swelling due to excessive fluid in the brain.

oedema, pulmonary Accumulation of fluid in the lungs. Occurs in the small air sacs or alveoli.

OES Occupational exposure standard.

oliguria Excretion of a reduced amount of urine (less than 400 ml per day in adults).

organoleptic properties Properties relating to taste and odour.

OSHA Occupational Safety and Health Administration (USA).

PAH Polycyclic aromatic hydrocarbon.

palpitation(s) Sensation of rapid or irregular heartbeat felt by a subject. Also refers to undue awareness of the heart beat.

papilloedema Oedema of the optic disc. Usually indicates raised pressure within the skull, for example with a brain tumour.

paraesthesia Number of abnormal sensations anywhere in the body but usually in limbs, e.g. tingling, pricking, burning, pins and needles, partial numbness.

patient group directions (PGDs) Documents that make it legal for medicines to be given to groups of patients, e.g. in a mass casualty situation, without individual prescriptions having to be written for each patient. They can also be used to empower staff other than doctors legally to give the medicines in question.

PBB Polybrominated biphenyls.

PCB Polychlorinated biphenyl.

peripheral neuropathy Any disease of the peripheral nerves.

pH Acidity/alkalinity scale.

photophobia Abnormal intolerance to light of the eyes.

pica A craving to eat non-food items, such as dirt, paint chips, and clay. Some children exhibit pica-related behaviour.

plumbosolvency Solvency of lead in water.

PM Particulate matter.

PM10 Particulate matter between 2.5 and 10 μm in diameter.

PM2.5 Particulate matter less than 2.5 μm in diameter.

pneum- Referring to the lungs.

pneumonitis Inflammation of the lungs.

point of exposure The place where someone can come into contact with a substance present in the environment.

point source emission Single emission source in a defined location.

polydypsia Excessive intake of water (increased thirst), a common symptom of diabetes.

polyneuropathy Any disease which involves several nerves.

polyploidy Having three or more times the haploid (single set of unpaired chromosomes as found in germ cells) number of chromosomes. Somatic cells from animals generally contain a diploid set of chromosomes, with pairs of equivalent chromosomes, so that twice the haploid number is present.

polyuria Passage of a large volume of urine.

population A group or number of people living within a specified area or sharing similar characteristics (such as occupation or age).

portal vein A vein in the liver that receives many tributaries, including the splenic vein from the spleen and pancreas, the gastric vein from the stomach, the mesenteric vein from the small and large intestines, and the rectal vein from the rectum and anus.

ppb Parts per billion.

PPE Personal protective equipment.

ppm Parts per million.

ppt Parts per trillion.

prevalence The number of people with a condition (e.g. disease or symptom) at any one time related to the size of the population.

prevalence survey The measure of the current level of disease(s), symptoms, or exposures. This is often carried out using a questionnaire that collects self-reported information from a defined population.

proteinuria Excretion of excessive amounts of protein (derived from blood plasma or kidney tubules) in the urine.

prothrombin time A laboratory measurement of the time taken for blood to clot.

proximal Nearest to the head.

psychosis Any major mental disorder characterized by derangement of the personality and loss of contact with reality.

PTSD Post traumatic stress disorder.

pupils constricted Small pupils.

pupils fixed Condition when pupils do not react to light, i.e. constrict when a light is directed to the pupil.

PVC Poly vinyl chloride.

pyrexia Fever, high temperature.

QRA Quantitative risk assessment.

REACH Registration, evaluation, authorization and restriction of chemical substance.

reference dose (RfD) A US Environmental Protection Agency term used for an estimate (with uncertainty spanning perhaps an order of magnitude) of a daily exposure to the human population (including sensitive subgroups) that is likely to be without appreciable risk of deleterious effects during a lifetime.

renal Referring to the kidneys.

rhabdomyolysis Breakdown of muscle tissue resulting in release of myoglobin into the bloodstream.

rhinorrhoea Discharge from the nose.

risk Possibility that a harmful event (death, injury, or loss) may arise from exposure to a chemical or physical agent that may occur under specific conditions.

risk assessment Identification and quantification of the risk resulting from a specific use or occurrence of a chemical or physical agent, taking into account possible harmful effects on individual people or societies of using the chemical or physical agent in the amount and manner proposed, and all the possible routes of exposure. Quantification ideally requires the establishment of dose–effect and dose–response relationships in likely target individuals and populations.

risk communication Interpretation and communication of risk assessments in terms that are comprehensible to the general public or to others without specialist knowledge.

risk reduction Actions that can decrease the likelihood that individuals, groups, or communities will experience disease or other adverse health conditions.

route of exposure The way people come into contact with a hazardous substance. Three common routes of exposure are breathing (inhalation), eating or drinking (ingestion), or contact with the skin (dermal contact).

safety factor See *uncertainty factor*.

sample (1) In statistics, a group of individuals often taken at random from a population for research purposes (2) One or more items taken from a population or a process and intended to provide information on the population or process (3) Portion of material selected from a larger quantity in some manner chosen so that the portion is representative of the whole.

sample size The number of units chosen from a population or an environment.

SGOT Serum glutamic oxaloacetic transaminase (also known as aspartate aminotransferase, AST).

sinus tachycardia Increased but regular heart rate.

sister chromosome exchange (SCE) Exchange of genetic material between two subunits of a replicated chromosome.

'SLUDGE' Acronym used to describe the clinical effects of acute organophosphorous intoxication: salivation, lacrimation, urination, defaecation and gastric emesis.

SNARL Suggested no adverse effect level. Maximum dose or concentration that on current understanding is likely to be tolerated by an exposed organism without producing any harm.

SO_x Oxides of sulphur, SO and SO_2, are commonly referred to as SO_x.

solvent A liquid capable of dissolving or dispersing another substance (for example acetone or mineral spirits).

somatic (1) Pertaining to the body as opposed to the mind (2) Pertaining to non-reproductive cells or tissues (3) Pertaining to the framework of the body as opposed to the viscera.

stakeholders Those with a personal or professional interest in a particular issue.

statistics A branch of mathematics that deals with collecting, reviewing, summarizing, and interpreting data or information. Statistics are used to determine whether differences between study groups are meaningful.

STEL Short-term exposure limit.

synergism Pharmacological or toxicological interaction in which the combined biological effect of two or more substances is greater than expected on the basis of the simple summation of the pharmacological toxic effects of each of the individual substances.

synergistic effect Biological effect following exposure simultaneously to two or more substances that is greater than the simple sum of the effects that occur following exposure to the substances separately.

tachy- A prefix meaning rapid.

tachypnoea Increased frequency of respiration (breathing).

TDI Tolerable daily intake. An estimate of the amount of contaminant, expressed on a body weight basis (e.g. mg/kg bodyweight), that can be ingested daily over a lifetime without appreciable health risk.

temporary ADI Used by JECFA when data are sufficient to conclude that use of the substance is safe over the relatively short period of time required to generate and evaluate further safety data, but are insufficient to conclude that use of the substance is safe over a lifetime. A higher-than-normal safety factor is used when establishing a temporary ADI and an expiration date is established by which time appropriate data to resolve the safety issue should be submitted to JECFA. The temporary ADI is listed in units of mg/kg body weight.

temporary MRL Temporary maximum residue limit. Used by JECFA when a temporary ADI has been established and/or when it has been found necessary to provide time to generate and evaluate further data on the nature and quantification of residues. Temporary MRLs are expressed in terms of milligrams of residue per kilogram of food.

TEQ Toxic equivalent quotient. See also *I-TEQ*.

teratogen A substance which, when administered to a pregnant woman or animal, can cause congenital malformations (structural defects) in the baby or offspring.

THOR The Health and Occupational Reporting Activity, Centre of Occupational and Environmental Health, University of Manchester.

time-weighted average Concentration of a hazardous substance, usually in air, averaged over a specified period of time. For example, for occupational exposures it is usually averaged over 8 hours.

Tinnitus Ringing in the ears.

TOXBASE Online information resource developed by the UK National Poisons Information Service (NPIS).

toxic agent Chemical or physical (for example, radiation) agents that, under certain circumstances of exposure, can cause harmful effects to living organisms.

toxicant Synonym for toxic agent/substance.

toxicity Ability of a substance to cause damage to living tissue.

toxicology The study of the harmful effects of substances on humans or animals.

toxin Toxic substance produced by a biological organism such as a microbe, animal, or plant.

TOXNET US National Library of Medicine toxicology data service.

TREM CARD Transport emergency cards.

triage Process of assessment and allocation of priorities by the medical or ambulance staff at the site or casualty clearing station prior to evacuation. Triage may be repeated at intervals and on arrival at a receiving hospital.

tumour A mass of abnormal, disorganized cells arising from pre-existing tissue which are characterized by excessive and unco-ordinated proliferation and by abnormal differentiation. Benign tumours show a close morphological resemblance to their tissue of origin, grow in a slow expansile fashion and form circumscribed and (usually) encapsulated masses. They may stop growing and they may regress. Benign tumours do not infiltrate through local tissue and they do not metastasize. They are rarely fatal. Malignant tumours resemble their parent tissues less closely and are composed of increasingly abnormal cells in terms of their form and function. Well-differentiated examples still retain recognizable features of their tissue of origin but these characteristics are progressively lost in moderately and poorly differentiated malignancies; undifferentiated or anaplastic tumours are composed of cells which resemble no known normal tissues. Most malignant tumours grow rapidly, spread progressively through adjacent tissues, and metastasize to distant sites.

TWA Time-weighted average.

uncertainty factor Value used in extrapolation from experimental animals to humans (assuming that humans may be more sensitive) or from selected individuals to the general population, for example a value applied to the NOAEL to derive an ADI or a TDI. The value depends on the size and type of population to be protected and the quality of the toxicological information available. (In the past the term 'safety factor' was used rather than 'uncertainty factor'.)

-uria Suffix referring to urine.

urinary incontinence Inability to control urination.

urinary retention Inability to pass urine despite a full bladder.

urticaria Vascular reaction of the skin marked by the transient appearance of smooth, slightly elevated patches (wheals, hives) that are redder or paler than the surrounding skin and often associated with severe itching.

ventricular fibrillation A life-threatening disturbance of cardiac rhythm which leads to ineffective pumping of blood from the heart and can cause death.

ventricular tachycardia A type of arrhythmia in which the heart beats at an abnormally fast rate and which may lead to potentially lethal ventricular fibrillation if untreated or prolonged.

vertigo Dizziness associated with the sensation of movement or spinning. May be associated with height reached whilst walking or climbing.

VOC Volatile organic compound. An organic compound that evaporates readily into the air. VOCs include substances such as benzene, toluene, methylene chloride, and methyl chloroform.

vulnerable populations People who might be more sensitive or susceptible to exposure to hazardous substances because of factors such as age, occupation, sex, or behaviours (for example cigarette smoking). Children, pregnant women, and older people are often considered vulnerable populations.

WEL Workplace exposure limit.

WHO World Health Organization, United Nations.

Sources: the explanations used in this glossary are derived from many sources, including:

ATSDR Glossary of terms. Agency for Toxic Substances and Disease Registry, US Department of Health and Human Services, www.atsdr.cdc.gov.

IPCS JECFA glossary of terms. International Programme on Chemical Safety, World Health Organization, www.who.int/ipcs.

SIS Glossary for Chemists of Terms Used in Toxicology. Specialized Information Services, United States National Library of Medicine, www.sis.nlm.nih.gov.

Index

Note: page numbers in *italics* refer to boxes, figures, and tables. The suffix 'g', for example 315g, refers to glossary entries.

pneumothorax 293
Pneupac VR1 ventilator *224*
Pocket Guide to Chemical Hazards, NIOSH 63
point of exposure 330g
point source emission 330g
poisoning, difference from chemical
    agent release 212
poisons, history 4–5
polonium 210 28
polychloride 247
polychlorinated biphenyls (PCBs)
  combustion products 242–3
  tissue sampling *53*
polychlorinated dibenzofurans (PCDFs) 242–3, 247
polychlorinated dibenzo-*p*-dioxins (PCDDs) 242–3
polycyclic aromatic hydrocarbon compounds
    (PAHs)
  air pollution 121
  health effects 241–2
  production during combustion 241, 247, 248
polydipsia 330g
polyethylene glycol, whole bowel irrigation 74
polymers, combustion products 234, 235, 239, 240,
    242–3, 244–5, 247
polymorphisms
  glutathione production 117
  influence on susceptibility 49, 90
polyneuropathy 330g
polynucleotides 328g
polyploidy 330g
polyurethane foams, combustion
    products 243–4, 247
polyuria 306, 330g
polyvinyl chloride, combustion products 234
pons *273*, 274
population selection, biomonitoring studies 51
populations 330g
portal vein 330g
potassium dichromate 184
potency of drugs 13, *14*
potentiative interactions 101
pralidoxime, in organophosphate poisoning 79
precipitin reactions 29
prednisolone, presence in herbal medicines 203
pregnancy
  carbon monoxide susceptibility 164, 231
  cautions with herbal medicines 205–6
  dental amalgams 178
  risk from lead 172
  smoke exposure 246
prevalence 330g
prevalence surveys 330g
primary particles 116
private water supplies 137
prolactin *308*
protein binding 12
protein corona, nanomaterials 263
proteinuria 306, 330g
prothrombin time 330g
proximal 330g
psychosis 330g
PTFE, combustion products 244–5

public health protection 5–6
public water supplies 137
pulmonary circulation 286
pulmonary oedema 297, 329g
pulmonary oedemagens 218–19
pulmonary toxins *7*
pupils
  constricted 330g
  effects of toxins 20, 30–1
  fixed 330g
pyrethrins /synthetic pyrethroids 194
pyrexia 330g
pyrolysis 228–9

quantum dots 260

radiological weapons 212
Ramazzini, Bernadino, study of occupational
    disorders 96–7
Ranvier, nodes of 276
Rasa Shastra 170
Raynaud's phenomenon
  and arsenic exposure 179
  and vinyl chloride exposure 99
REACH *see* Registration, Evaluation, Authorisation
    and restriction of Chemicals (REACH)
    regulations (EU)
reactive airways dysfunction syndrome (RADS,
    irritant-induced asthma) 98, 235
reactive oxygen species
  generation by macrophages 262
  generation by ultrafine particles 259
recognition of chemical incidents 69–70
red blood cells 27–8, 289
reference concentrations *see* health criteria
    values (HCVs)
reference nutrient intakes (RNIs)
  copper 184
  zinc 174
Registration, Evaluation, Authorisation and
    restriction of Chemicals (REACH)
    regulations (EU) 102, 105, 331g
relative bioavailability *133*
relative risk 16
renal 331g
renal transplant patients, cautions with herbal
    medicines *204*
repeated dose toxicity studies 35–7
reproductive system 30, 306
  effects of lead 172–3
  effects of mercury 178
reproductive toxicity testing 38–9
reproductive toxins *7*
Research Ethics Committees (RECs) 54
residual volume 293, *294*
respiration 291–2
  external 26–7
  internal 27–8
respiratory centre 274, 292
respiratory control 26
  depression 27
respiratory off-gassing 68, 69, 73